*P*rimary *P*revention *P*ractices

Martin Bloom

Issues in Children's and Families' Lives

Volume 5

SAGE Publications
International Educational and Professional Publisher
Thousand Oaks   London   New Delhi

For information address:

 SAGE Publications, Inc.
2455 Teller Road
Thousand Oaks, California 91320
E-mail: order@sagepub.com

SAGE Publications Ltd.
6 Bonhill Street
London EC2A 4PU
United Kingdom

SAGE Publications India Pvt. Ltd.
M-32 Market
Greater Kailash I
New Delhi 110 048 India

Printed in the United States of America

Library of Congress Cataloging-in-Publication Data

Bloom, Martin, 1934-
    Primary prevention practices / author, Martin Bloom.
        p.   cm.—(Issues in children's and families' lives; v. 5)
    Includes bibliographical references and index.
    ISBN 0-8039-7151-6 (cloth: acid-free paper).—ISBN
    0-8039-7152-4 (pbk.: acid-free paper)
    1. Social service—United States.   2. Family services—United
States.   3. Preventive health services—United States.   I. Title.
II. Series.
HV91.B575   1996
362'.0424—dc20   95-41736

This book is printed on acid-free paper.

96 97 98 99 00 01 10 9 8 7 6 5 4 3 2 1

Sage Production Editor: Diane S. Foster
Sage Typesetter: Andrea D. Swanson

BRIEF CONTENTS

CONTENTS

PREFACE

This book is a celebration. I celebrate the small but growing number of theories used in primary prevention described briefly in this book. I celebrate the larger and rapidly growing number of substantial research studies that are testing primary prevention ideas across the spectrum of personal and social challenges facing us and our world today—and tomorrow.

The major celebration, however, and the purpose of this book is to describe primary prevention practice, the specific and reproducible methods by which practitioners have sought to prevent predictable problems, to protect existing states of healthy functioning, and to promote desired life objectives. I describe 50 specific practice strategies or tactics, as they have been used in particular studies and as they may be generalized for use with other challenges.

I also celebrate people because, locked in common experiences, as in worldwide folklore, is the ideology that it is far better to prevent than to cure. I celebrate you, gentle reader, whose countless preventive, protective, and promotive actions have given life and meaning to this topic with all its tensions. The day I wrote this preface, I took a break for my daily swim. There I had an epiphany, a tiny experience that reflects this universe of primary prevention. A mother was teaching her eager young son to dive—he would soon be enthusiastically leaping into space several meters above the water's surface—while at the same time she was cautioning him not to run at the pool's edge as it was slippery. This delicious result was tension between risk taking to achieve some desired goal combined with a protectiveness to prevent predictable problems. Both are necessary to nurture the body and to feed the mind and the spirit.

I celebrate especially those who have contributed to the rapid developments in this field of study and action: the ABCs of primary prevention—George Albee, Albert Bandura, Bernard Bloom, Gerald Caplan, Emory Cowen, and Edward Zigler. For a complete enumeration of my heroes, please see the author index to this book. My friends and colleagues gave help in various ways: Waldo Klein, Tom Gullotta, Baker Salsbury, Karen Potter, Valeria Sloan, and Frank Reeves. I celebrate the 15th anniversary of the *Journal of Primary Prevention* and its sole and singular editor, Tom Gullotta.

I also celebrate my personal good fortune: our first grandson, Paul Alexander Bloom (and his parents, Sara and Laird). The newest member of the family, Vicki Borah, engaged to our son Bard. And most of all, my wife, Lynn—I celebrate 37 years of a vital and stimulating marriage and other secrets.

1

Frame of Reference for
Primary Prevention Practice

This chapter sets the stage for presenting state-of-the-art methods for the practice of primary prevention. An ecological orientation (termed the *configural equation*) is offered to guide understanding and action regarding any social behavior: What are the pushes and pulls on relevant actors in a situation that determine the resulting flow of events? Subsequent chapters focus on different components of this equation, illustrating how primary prevention practices have been described in the current literature.

A. Introduction to Primary Prevention
B. The Configural Equation: Components of an Interactive Ecology
C. The Preventive Problem-Solving Process
   1. Preproject Responsibilities
   2. The Problem-Solving Process
   3. Postproject Responsibilities
D. Preview of Subsequent Chapters: How Best to Use This Book

A. Introduction to Primary Prevention

This book provides a brief guide to the wide range of strategies or tactics used in primary prevention research and demonstration projects as

1

reported in the major journals and selected books in this field over the past two decades. The specific tactics used in practice are described, with reference to the original studies from which they are derived, but I attempt to generalize these tactics as practice principles when possible so as to encourage their experimental usage in a wider array of circumstances. Users should consult the primary references for full details.

The domain of this discussion is primary prevention, defined as coordinated actions seeking to prevent predictable problems, to protect existing states of health and healthy functioning, and to promote desired potentialities in individuals and groups in their physical and sociocultural settings over time. The term prevention developed its contemporary meaning at least by the 15th century (Oxford English Dictionary, 1971): to anticipate, to take precautions against (a danger or evil), and hence to evade that danger. Its Latin root—to come before—is still the core meaning: to take action before some untoward set of events occurs so as to preclude, delay, or reduce its occurrence in some population or person at risk. There was also a positive sense of the word, however, meaning to excel, which has reappeared in the contemporary promotive sense. Consider this definition in a recent social work dictionary, with its dual prevention and promotion emphases:

> Prevention: Actions taken by social workers and others to minimize and eliminate those social, psychological, or other conditions known to cause or contribute to physical or emotional illness and sometimes socioeconomic problems. This includes establishing those conditions in society that enhance the opportunities for individuals, families, and communities to achieve positive fulfillment. (Barker, 1987, p. 124)

Workers in many professions have contributed to the current definition, including some terms that have complicated as well as clarified common understanding. Leavell and Clark (1953) provided an early public health interpretation; Caplan (1964) expanded those terms for preventive psychiatry. Table 1.1 illustrates these terms and definitions. Klein and Goldston (1977) proposed to simplify the discussion by using the distinctions primary prevention, treatment, and rehabilitation in place of Caplan's primary, secondary, and tertiary prevention. (Although there is some meaning in "preventing an existing problem from getting worse," the term *treatment* fully encompasses this, whereas *secondary prevention*

Table 1.1 Definitions of Primary Prevention

Public Health (Leavell & Clark, 1953)	Preventive Psychiatry (Caplan, 1964)	Configural Approach (Bloom, 1990)
1. Health promotion: Furthering health and well-being through general measures: education, nutrition, social services, and so on aimed at host populations.	1. Primary prevention: Lowering the rate of new cases of mental disorder in a population over a certain period by counteracting harmful circumstances before they have a chance to produce illness.	1. Primary prevention: Promotive activities are actions that support persons achieving high-level potentials or making environmental changes for same ends.
2. Specific protections: Measures applicable to particular diseases to intercept the pathogenic agent before it affects host population.	2. Secondary prevention: Reducing the disability rate due to a disorder by lowering the prevalence of the disorder in the community by	2. Primary prevention: Protective activities are actions that maintain or move people into a zone of adequate functioning or make environmental changes for same ends.
3. Early recognition and prompt treatment: a. Screening and periodic exams of population at risk b. Disease control through standard medical practice c. Surveillance of pathogenic conditions in the environment	a. Lowering the number of new cases b. Shortening the duration of old cases. (Primary prevention focuses on the former, whereas secondary prevention focuses on the latter. Thus secondary prevention includes primary prevention.)	3. Primary prevention: Preventive activities are actions that forestall predictable untoward events, either by eliminating the harmful environmental agent or by strengthening people's resistance to agents or both.
4. Disease limitation: Preventing or delaying the consequences of clinically advanced or incurable diseases in identified hosts.	3. Tertiary prevention: Reducing the rate in a community of defective functioning due to mental disorders; defects may be due to the disability caused by disordered functioning or lowered capacity remaining as a residue	4. Advanced service or treatment: Actions that screen, detect, and treat subclinical problems through use of high technology; clients are unaware of problem.
5. Rehabilitation: Affected persons brought back to useful place in society, as far as possible.		5. Acute treatment: Actions that treat observable problems promptly through standard medical practice; clients are aware of problem.

(continued)

Table 1.1   Definitions of Primary Prevention (Continued)

Public Health (Leavell & Clark, 1953)	Preventive Psychiatry (Caplan, 1964)	Configural Approach (Bloom, 1990)
	after the disorder has terminated. (Tertiary prevention focuses on the latter, whereas primary and secondary prevention address the former. Thus tertiary prevention includes the other two.)	6. Rehabilitation: Actions that assist people in regaining the highest level of functioning possible, including use of personal or environmental prostheses, permanent or temporary. 7. Palliative actions: Activities that recognize the terminal phase of a person's condition and seek to reduce pain and to promote personal contentment and social fulfillment with (and of) family and friends.

clouds the prevention emphasis of acting before a problem exists.) I follow Klein and Goldston's terminology in this book for ease of communication.

There has been an enormous growth in the literature of primary prevention in the past decade, so much so that it is difficult to keep up with the great variety of new theories, methods, and results. Journals have become specialized in focus; anthologies address limited themes. Fortunately, there are accessible sources in which theories, research, practice, and policy statements are presented. Appendix A presents a selection of these sources.

Only few resources, however, bring together the many strategies or tactics used in achieving the objectives of primary prevention. This is the major purpose of this book. In addition to presenting summaries and descriptions of these practice methods, I illustrate an approach to primary prevention that enables one to bring into view the complex array of interacting events. The more one is able to take into account the multiple interacting factors in real-life situations, the more likely one is able to deal effectively with social and personal problems and possibilities (Barnett & Escobar, 1989; Begley & Biddle, 1988; Dew, Bromet, Brent, & Greenhouse, 1987; Schmidt & Tate, 1988).

B. The Configural Equation:
Components of an Interactive Ecology

No one seriously disputes the ecological perspective: that each element in a given situation is ultimately related to every other element, often in an interactive way. But the implications of this systems perspective appear at first to be overwhelming so that it is difficult to grasp the whole perspective, let alone use it in a practice situation. One may take shortcuts in the mistaken belief that such simplifications—*X* causes *Y* in a linear fashion—will provide enough of the story to guide a successful intervention.

I have taken a different tack as a guiding frame of reference for this book. I offer a configural equation that identifies classes of factors to be considered in any thorough analysis of a given situation. (Readers should consider other ecological or systems approaches, such as those of Bronfenbrenner, 1979; Germain & Gitterman, 1995; Harwood & Weissberg, 1992; Killen et al., 1988; Lutzker, Wesch, & Rice, 1984; Maton, 1989b; Shannon, 1989; Srebnik & Elias, 1993.) In some situations, some of the components in the equation will not be as relevant as others and may be temporarily ignored. (They may reemerge as important later.) The point is that one chooses what to do based on an analysis of all potentially relevant and interactive ingredients, the entire array of components in the ecology of the problem or the potential. This checklist function of the equation is helpful for planning purposes to keep the full range of forces acting on events in mind as one decides what, when, and where preventive actions should be applied.

The configural equation also provides a road map for the chapters of this book. Each major component is addressed in a subsequent chapter, where, for the most part, distinctive preventive tactics are employed. As one identifies the nature of the preventive problem or potential in a given situation, one can consider how various methods might be relevant components of that situation. Then the entire group of relevant methods may be reconsidered as to how they may be packaged as one unified

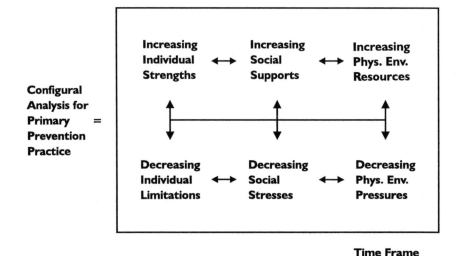

Time Frame

Figure 1.1. The Configural Equation

program, because what one does in one situation may augment or interfere with what one does in another area.

The configural equation owes much to Albee's (1983) equation on factors related to the incidence of mental disorders:

$$\frac{\text{Incidence of}}{\text{Mental Disorder}} = \frac{\text{Organic Factors} + \text{Stress} + \text{Exploitation}}{\text{Coping Skills} + \text{Self-Esteem} + \text{Support Groups}}$$

For variations, see Dusenbury and Botvin (1992, p. 192) and Elias (1987). Generalizing from Albee's equation, I offer a configural analysis (Figure 1.1) of any social behavior that emphasizes the strengths in social situations (top line) reduced by limitations in that situation (bottom line), all viewed within a given time frame (Bell, 1986). Because this is a service-oriented equation, I indicate the direction of each effort—increasing strengths and decreasing limitation across all contexts. The double-headed arrows indicate reciprocal interactions, such as the individual affecting and being affected by sociocultural factors. Each component can be analyzed separately—but only at great risk of misinterpreting the whole situation. Figure 1.2 identifies the conceptual components of the configural analysis.

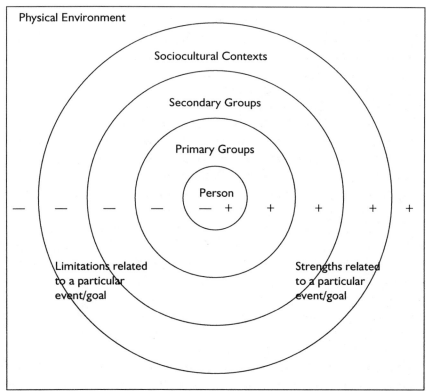

Components of the Configuration:

PERSON—Cognitive, affective, behavioral, physiological-biological aspects

PRIMARY GROUPS—For example, family, peer groups, close associates at work
for which interactions are face-to-face and personal

SECONDARY GROUPS—For example, large-scale organizations in which there
are specialized roles in a division of labor

SOCIOCULTURAL GROUPS—Collectivities sharing systems of symbols that
supply meaning to life, such as laws, social mores, ethnic heritage, language,
subcultural lifestyle, and spirituality

PHYSICAL ENVIRONMENT—Includes both the natural environment (land, water,
air) and the built environment (buildings, roads, planned open spaces,
playgrounds)

TIME FRAME—Life course events occurring to individuals and groups over time,
including historical changes, group evolution, and personal growth and
development

Figure 1.2. Configuration of Factors to Be Considered in the Study of Any Human
Problem or Potential

In addition, each component may be broken down into relevant subheadings—indeed, these terms are the subheadings of subsequent chapters. For example, personal strengths encompass cognitive, affective, behavioral, and physiological components; past work has proven these distinctions useful, and specific tactics have emerged in each of these specialized areas. The next section of this chapter presents an overview of these headings and subheadings as a preview of the rest of this book.

Beyond identifying distinctive tactics, I want to emphasize the integrative or synthesizing aspect of the configural equation. The pieces must be put back together again with some indication of what weight each component has in relation to the whole. How much weight do individual characteristics have in a given situation, relative to the social and environmental forces and structures that push and pull the actors? Particular theories, in effect, supply their suggested weightings. For example, Freud's theory ascribes greatest weight in the actions of an individual to the unconscious affective conflicts he or she experiences. For Freud, the particular nature of the society or culture is of far lesser importance. Not so with a Marxian interpretation of social behavior, where social class is the primary driver of events, so much so that personal characteristics are essentially without weight in Marx's equations.

One example of putting pieces of research and practice together into a general set of policy recommendations is Glynn's (1989) summary of the synthesizing efforts of a National Cancer Institute expert advisory panel on school-based smoking prevention programs. On the basis of the available evidence, the institute recommends that an effective smoking prevention program consider and integrate the following concepts:

- Audience: Dropouts, lower socioeconomic status students, and minority students have been least likely to be reached by existing programs.
- Focus and timing: Either a smoking-only or a multicomponent health focus can be effective, if enough time is devoted to the sessions.
- Content: Information should include social consequences, short-term physiological effects, social influences pushing smoking, and resistance training.
- Program length: A minimum of two 5-session blocks should be delivered in separate school years between Grades 6 and 9; preferred are 10 sessions each year in Grades 6 through 9.
- Age at intervention: Intervene in all grades where possible, but at least starting at Grade 6 or 7—the transition to middle or junior high school.

- Peer involvement: Use a peer leader to assist a trained teacher in implementing specific portions of the program.
- Parental involvement: Active involvement can be very helpful.
- Teacher training: Training is essential and should involve experiential activities, such as role-playing and refusal training.

On the basis of a close reading of the empirical literature, a practitioner would be well advised to combine these elements into a coordinated plan of action. What specific combination a practitioner decides to use in a real situation is, ipso facto, his or her theory of human behavior, a system of ideas about how events interact to produce certain outcomes. The choices of personal, social, or environmental service components represent the weightings ascribed by the practitioner to the particular situation. For example, if a practitioner designs a smoking prevention program that places emphasis on teaching youths to resist peer pressures to smoke rather than providing each individual with factual information about the harmful effects of smoking, this would represent a program based on a theory that conformity to peer pressure is stronger than cognitive information at this stage in the person's development. Few theories instruct users as to how much of one component to use in combination with other components, even though this is a crucial piece of information. This is where the art of program design emerges—in the best guesses as to how much of each possible intervention to use in combination (Albino, 1984; Dumas, 1989).

Program evaluation may reveal, after the fact of intervention, what contribution each component made to the overall outcome. Sophisticated statistical analysis (such as path analysis) attempts to tease out the contribution of each component toward the overall outcome. Such results may help theorists reshape their conceptual models to provide clearer guides to practice.

The configural equation, as a general frame of reference, places a demand on practitioners to be more explicit regarding the components of a service plan and the weightings assigned to each component. How much investment of time, energy, and resources is expended on particular components of the configural equation? The answer to this question is the weighting that practitioners assign to the factors in the situation, reflecting their implicit or explicit use of strategy to guide practice. The primary prevention program is a manifestation of its creators' theory, understanding of the empirical literature, experiences with similar life situations, and values in the context of the reality factors in which they are working. The validity and wisdom of their choices must await evaluation in the individual situation.

C. The Preventive Problem-Solving Process

The use of tactics, such as described in Chapters 2 through 6, requires an orientation to practice. How do these tactics fit together with basic practice methods? I propose to use a general problem-solving process for primary prevention (Bloom, 1981). I will summarize and update that discussion over the next few pages. The general process is represented in Figure 1.3. Let me describe briefly the steps leading up to the tactics and the steps following these actions.

1. Preproject Responsibilities

Before I begin discussing the preventive problem-solving process that is at the heart of the service program, I must provide some orientation: One must understand the negative and positive concerns people face, knowingly or not, in particular contexts and must be sensitive to the ethical issues these concerns raise. (For discussions of ethical issues in prevention, see Conner, 1990; O'Neill, 1989; Pope, 1990; Wallack, 1984; Walters, 1988). One must be aware of how these concerns and sociocultural and political contests will energize would-be friends or potential opponents (Goldston, 1986, 1991; Mason & McGinnis, 1990). "Good ends" never justify the use of "bad means." One must keep one's goals and methods synchronized with the contextual norms and personal values of all relevant parties to the preventive enterprise as far as possible. Yet, as a prevention professional, one must accept the risks of leading public opinion so that people will understand the health potentials and risks of current and proposed programs (Bloom, 1993).

2. The Problem-Solving Process

Identifying the Problems and Potentials

The core problem-solving process for primary prevention consists of at least five discrete phases. I would like to offer some rough practice principles for enacting each of these steps. First, one must identify the

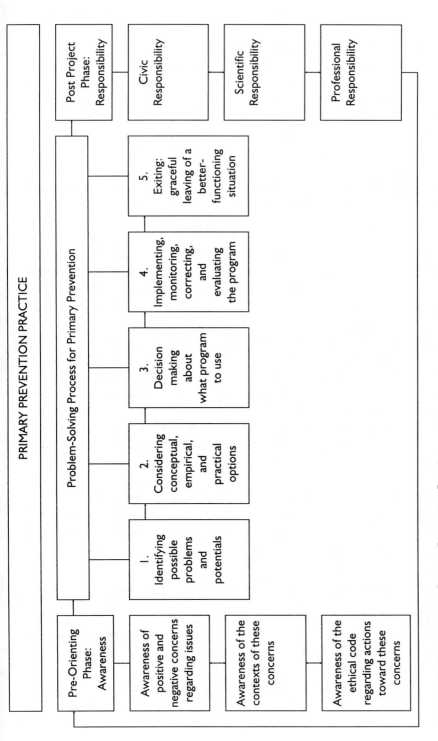

Figure 1.3. Orientation to Primary Prevention Practice

11

specific problems or potentials of the relevant groups of people involved in the situation (knowingly or not). What risks do they face, what goals do they have, and how do the circumstances of one group impinge on the others? One can approach this complex set of questions by being clear about what risks and goals one is discussing, obtaining the best available information about them, and putting the information together as a system of interactive pressures and opportunities (Long, 1992).

Operational Definitions of Key Terms. The following are some guidelines for developing a clear understanding of the preventive problems and goals:

1. Become thoroughly steeped in the real-life context regarding the topic under study. Learn how people involved in the situation view these topics. This commonsense meaning becomes the basis for a conceptual definition, an abstracted and generalized understanding of the topic. If one doesn't fully understand the local context, then unexpected turns of events may occur (Wittman, 1989).

2. Attach an operational definition to this underlying conceptual understanding: What are the specific things one can do (or observe others doing) that would represent a clear example or experience of the conceptual idea? This set of specific directions is a first approximation of an operational definition, a working definition.

3. Check out this working definition to see if it makes sense to relevant parties in the situation, including the original participants and colleagues. Can a new professional follow the specific directions of the working definition and come up with the same or similar identified experience? Modify the working definition until a reasonably common set of operations produces a reasonably consistent set of common experiences. This becomes the operational definition of the key concepts in the project, a tentative yet strong basis for acting.

Gathering Epidemiological and Social-Psychological Information

Now that we have conceptual and operational terms in mind, we can review the literature to see what is known about these events (Ginter, Duncan, & Capper, 1991; Robins & Rutter, 1990).

1. The concepts are likely to be the key terms used in information systems for retrieval of specific articles. Check this out with the psycho-

logical and sociological thesauri, which list the scientific terms currently used as retrieval words (along with nontechnical language synonyms) from which one will be able to choose those most like the search terms.

2. Go to the psychological and sociological abstracts and the hundreds of specialized abstracts, many of which are on computerized databases, to locate specific information about the topic.

3. Epidemiological information refers to the distribution in time and space of specific instances of psychosocial health and illness (MacMahon & Pugh, 1970). The categories of people who get or do not get the illness or condition lead one to speculate on possible underlying causal patterns, which then can be brought into the design of preventive projects for testing. For example, Werner (1989a, 1989b) notes that about one third of her subjects who emerge from highly stressful life circumstances become relatively healthy adults, whereas others in this same situation have significant problems. Werner's epidemiological analysis suggested that the at-risk children who turned out to be resilient had good relationships with teachers or other adults, among other distinguishing factors (Chess & Thomas, 1986). This kind of information leads to the possibility of setting up such supportive relationships for similar children who lack them. Thus one has learned about the epidemiology of resilience and generated some preventive or promotive service hypotheses: One can try to ensure that all children living in stressful circumstances receive those social supports and other services, which may promote the resilience observed in the Werner studies (1989a, 1989b; see Chapter 2, I.E.4 for further details).

4. Social-psychological information emerges from various sources, including laboratory studies, field demonstration projects, and anything in between. This information may present data that are like micro-epidemiological patterns on a specific sample, which may be reformulated into a new practice hypothesis. For example, Okwumabua, Okwumabua, Hayes, and Stovall (1994) describe a study of (Piagetian) cognitive levels as correlated with correct health decision making in school children. They found that children testing at the highest cognitive level were significantly better at making correct health decisions than those at lower cognitive levels. The implication is that any future study attempting to train children to make correct health decisions should take into account their cognitive levels (cf. Gondolf, 1987).

Combining Epidemiological and Social-Psychological Patterns

To optimize available information for guiding preventive projects, one needs to link these data sources in one integrated program. For example, Durkheim's (1951) early studies of anomic suicide—in part showing that people who lacked linkages with a community were more likely to suffer emotional stresses, some of which led to suicide—may be linked with the many studies that show that having social supports reduces chances of emotional stress. Felner and Adan (1988) describe a study in which students entering a new school (an anomic situation for many) were given social supports to reduce the expectable stresses they faced. Thus combining epidemiological and social-psychological information may help optimize the construction of fruitful primary prevention projects. (See Birkel & Reppucci, 1983, and Gensheimer, Roosa, & Ayers, 1990, on recruitment of participants; see Meichenbaum & Turk, 1987, and Shumaker, Schron, & Ockene, 1990, on facilitating adherence to preventive programs.)

Considering Conceptual, Empirical, and Practical Options

The second major step of the preventive problem-solving process involves building on what others have thought, studied, and tried in real-life situations. These options run in the thousands; I present some discussion here and appendixes to help readers sort out possibilities. Appendix A lists some basic information sources with regard to conceptual and empirical studies in primary prevention; the references for this book present sources of practice options. Appendix B describes the major concepts and propositions of theories particularly relevant to primary prevention: the health belief model (Rosenstock, 1990), the theory of reasoned action (Fishbein & Ajzen, 1975; Fishbein & Middlestadt, 1989), a model on social stress (Dohrenwend, 1986; Israel & Schurman, 1990), the social cognitive theory (Bandura, 1986, 1989a, 1989b), the recurrent themes model (Caplan, 1989), and some social models for changing behavior.

The main point of this step in the problem-solving process is that one has much to gain by couching preventive efforts in a conceptual framework that gives meaning to what one does. Theories help describe, explain, predict, and thus potentially control events—vital elements in any prevention project. Theories offer different explanations and predictions and thus guide practice in quite different directions—so one must choose theories wisely.

And how shall one choose theories wisely? Probably the best advice is to see what empirical results have emerged in other studies as a result of using or testing the propositions from a given theory. No theory is ever a perfect guide to reality but, rather, offers probabilities to successful conclusions. Most of the time—but not always—positive reinforcement of some behavior tends to see that behavior repeated. Some of the time—but perhaps not a very large proportion of the time—psychodynamic therapy leads to a successful conclusion. New research keeps changing the picture of what results derive from given theories, so the task of keeping up to date with theories as guides involves keeping up with the literature and one's own experience with given models.

And how shall one incorporate one's own experience with models that guide behavior? Some less empirically supported model may appear to work better than a better-supported model. If so, and if one is using both models as intended, then one must factor this information in the choice of a guiding theory. All things considered, use the best supported models as beginning points—not the models that sound interesting but lack objective evidence of support. If one can learn to use a model with successful results, then this model should be added to the practice repertoire.

Making Decisions About What Program to Use

Eventually, one has to make a decision from among all the options and sources of evidence. As one makes this decision, some important considerations should be added.

Individualizing Abstract Theories. By definition, theories do not fit any specific individual situation, so one has to translate the concepts back into the real world to apply what one has gained from using an abstract model. Schinke, Gilchrist, and Small (1979) describe this personalizing process using a cognitive behavioral model on preventing unwanted teen pregnancy:

1. Provide general information on the topic one wishes to teach participants. For example, on the topic of birth control, one might discuss abstinence along with alternative forms of socializing, or, for the sexually

active, inform students that the use of condoms is an effective method that has other health-promotive features as well.

2. Test whether the overall information presented is understood, stored, and retrievable on demand. Conventional testing methods may be used here.

3. Individualize the general learning to fit the learner's own life situation. With regard to condoms, "Jack" is taught to think about and to say "when Jill and I have sex without using a condom, Jill is in danger of getting pregnant, which neither of us wants at this time." Translating the abstract into one's own life situation increases the likelihood that the specific action will be performed.

4. Reinforce the person's individualized solution with appropriate means, such as peer and teacher approval in role-taking situations, which add to the learner's self-efficacy (see Chapter 2, I.E.1) under realistic practice conditions.

These four steps provide a useful and portable set of modifications of any educational or training program.

Synchronizing Individual Values and Collective Norms. Developing an effective primary prevention project will be optimized if the individual values of the participants are synchronized with the collective norms of relevant groups and the community. One can approximate this synchronization as follows:

1. Identify the nature and strength of personal values of participants relevant to the topic. In general, values, as persistent preferences regarding goals of action and acceptable means for attaining those goals, tend to be consistent. But not always. For example, a person may favor self-determination but oppose abortion.

2. Identify the nature and strength of collective norms relevant to the same topics. Norms are reflected in the patterns of action the group has taken over time, perhaps as influenced by charismatic leaders or traumatic events. Norms are likely to be reflected in laws and social mores, which can be learned from resource persons in a given setting.

3. Value or norm conflicts can appear within an individual or a group or between an individual and a group. Then the degree of centrality becomes important. Central conflicts must be resolved; peripheral con-

flicts may be ignored, because they are not serious enough to cause breakdown in the social system. The general rule to resolve value conflicts is to appeal to a higher value or law, if possible, that mediates or controls the conflict. A variation is to seek amicable separation on this issue and isolate it from other continuing communications between these parties. It is very hard to convince another that his or her central values are "wrong."

Avoiding Stigmatization of Participants. Stigmas are disincentives that make participants less likely or less motivated to take part in voluntary prevention programs. Although preventers think they have the best interests of the participants at heart, the very act of defining people as "at risk" for some devalued status or event is de facto labeling them as tainted or damaged in some way—despite appearances that they are healthy and well functioning regarding the point in question. Although preventers think their programs are wonderful and helpful, in fact, something will be done to participants putting them into a receiving end of an uninvited relationship. Records are to be kept, whose ultimate disposition is not known and is out of the client's control. There is always some degree of intrusiveness in the affairs of people and, to that degree, some loss of their own control. It is a wonder that preventers are ever surprised when would-be participants say "no thanks" to all these problems in the best of prevention programs. Many people have dealt directly with the stigmatization issue (e.g., Hess, 1983; Munoz, 1986; Pilisuk, Parks, Kelly, & Turner, 1982; Shaffer, Garland, Gould, Fisher, & Trautman, 1988; Stilwell & Manley, 1990). The following are some general guidelines for avoiding stigmatizing participants in primary prevention programs:

1. Instead of picking out some people at high risk for an untoward outcome, arrange the preventive or promotive program to be offered to all people in a geographic area where there is a high concentration of the target group. Take in enough clients until there are sufficient numbers in the true target group. Serve all, and use the others as a kind of comparison group.

2. The name of the preventive service should not suggest weakness or limitation. Emphasize the strengths of people—this is always a recommendation in primary prevention. A positive or neutral name, such as Family Life Education or Positive Parenting, can include some specific

skills, such as disciplining, that may be especially useful for people at high risk for child abuse but that is relevant for a wide range of patients.

③ Involve people from the community and the subculture to help define the general goals of the program as ones relevant to their needs. When participants "own" the program, the stress is removed from a potentially threatening topic imposed from outside. Involve local residents in such administrative procedures as is possible, such as intake workers who can make good use of their familiarity with the local situation while maintaining genuine respect for their neighbors. Working together toward a common and positive goal will help the project as well as reduce stigmatization.

Contracting: Who Is to Do What With Whom? Developing an effective prevention program will be optimized if each party understands and agrees to the various roles involved in carrying out the program: Who is to do what, with whom, and under what circumstances—in a word, *contracting* (Reid & Epstein, 1972). The following are guidelines to set up formal or informal contracts:

1. First, have the parties involved select some mutually agreed-on goals and objectives. These should be clearly (operationally) defined so there is little room for error in working together to attain a goal.
2. The tasks involved in achieving these goals and objectives are identified as a sequence of behaviors that each party is to perform.
   a. Who?
   b. Does what? (Make sure each party understands and can actually perform the steps required.)
   c. With whom?
   d. Where? When?
   e. Under what circumstances? (This includes frequency, intensity, and duration of the action.)
   f. How will each party know when the action has been performed appropriately? (This is an evaluation question that may involve monitoring of events. Sometimes, participants join in the evaluation; most of the time independent researchers do it.)

Implementing, Monitoring, Correcting, and Evaluating the Program

Implementation is the heart of any service program, and the monitoring and evaluation components should be concomitant with service. One cannot accurately know about the success or failure of the program unless one keeps objective track of what is achieved, compared with what one sets out to achieve, and take appropriate measures to make use of this ongoing feedback to make corrections in the program activities. Basic research texts present appropriate scientific methods, whereas specialized texts focus specifically on research and evaluation in primary prevention (Bickman, 1983; French, Fisher, & Costa, 1983; French & Kaufman, 1981; Kumpfer, Shur, Ross, Bunelli, Librett, & Millward, 1993; Price & Smith, 1985). Price, Cowen, Lorion, Ramos, and McKay (1988) present 14 exemplar studies in primary prevention. Research studies appear in the major journals in primary prevention (see Appendix A); some are summarized in this book as well. For consideration of cost-benefit analyses, see Schweinhart and Weikart (1988) on preschool education; Schmidt and Tate (1988) on employment assistance programs; Hunter and Chen (1992) on programs related to AIDS; Nuehring, Abrams, Fike, and Ostrowsky (1983) on prevention programs aimed at children; and Bloom (1986) on mental retardation; also see Lee and Moss (1987) on whether cost-benefit analyses are appropriate for AIDS prevention and Russell (1986, 1994), who notes that all preventive measures involve risks and costs and that each topic has to be analyzed in its larger contexts to locate the true costs. Chapters 2 through 6 of this book discuss implementation in detail.

In taking a pragmatic overview of any service program, it is important to note that as one monitors the ongoing status of the services and outcomes, one is bound to discover small or large details that need correcting. This fine-tuning is intrinsic to the nature of every service activity, provided that one monitors the effects the service is having. Monitoring uses the same tools as evaluation, but because it is intended to provide rapid feedback, one ordinarily uses preliminary data rather than a completed study. These preliminary data provide the sense for fine-tuning, and further preliminary data confirm or disconfirm these changes. The more rigorous the preliminary data, the more objective the corrections that can be made. Yet one must be willing to be patient and give time for the service to have its effect. Midcourse corrections are part of the art of evaluated practice.

Exiting: Gracefully Leaving a Better-Functioning Situation

Most prevention programs begin as time-limited experimental projects, which necessarily must come to an end. The task of exiting is not well developed in the professional or prevention literature, but it involves leaving the affected persons and situations functioning better than at the beginning of the study. Exiting refers to disengaging from the various social connections the project formed in the community, formally and informally, and the concomitant replacement of these social bonds with something equivalent or better so that the successful services provided in the project will continue in some form. Exiting must be conducted professionally so that no one is harmed by the closing down of the project. The following ideas are offered to approximate these ideals:

1. Exit leaving a complete set of procedures regarding how the project was conducted so that should others wish to continue one or more aspects of the program, there will be adequate instruction for doing so. Such manuals are helpful but so would be training of indigenous workers who remain in the neighborhood, if not the agency.

2. Exit at time X but prepare for exiting at time 1. This involves having clear definitions of project goals and doing regular assessments to test whether or not these goals have been attained. Progress reports are useful for keeping perspective on the whole project and for being ready with relevant information as termination approaches. The major task is to "give away" the knowledge and skills one has learned in the project to persons who hold institutional roles (at the agency or in the community) so that continuity is possible. Empowering relevant parties to continue to do for themselves what the project staff had done for and with them is a vital element that should be activated from the beginning.

Follow-up studies may be conducted to check on the long-term effects of a time-limited program. (This is also discussed in the section on booster shots, Chapter 3, II.C.5. See also Flay et al., 1989; Murray, Pirie, Luepker, & Pallonen, 1989.)

3. Exiting involves the development of informal professional support groups to maintain the momentum and the esprit de corps that have been generated over the life of the program. Plan and announce reunions of former colleagues after termination as booster shots for the remaining helping professionals. Exit with grace and confidence when those left behind have the ideas, skills, and experience not only to solve ordinary problems but to foresee the solutions to novel challenges because they have learned the underlying problem-solving approach (Comer, 1988).

4. Test one's planned exit by seeing where every client will now be served or where similar clients will be served in the future. If institutional arrangements are in place in the existing community, then the exiting will likely be successful. If one exits when the program is not successful, it is probably best to be straightforward about the lack of overall success while trying to identify whatever components were useful in specific ways.

3. Postproject Responsibilities

After one finishes this preventive problem-solving process, one still has some postproject responsibilities to civic, scientific, and professional colleagues:

1. Civic responsibility is due the founders of the project and those participants who want to know what happened. Reports are written for these different intended audiences, but they should always protect the confidentiality of individual participants. Sometimes, newspapers ask for reports at the beginning and the end of community projects because these are of broad social interest. Contributing to the local media is another responsibility of project staff, but be careful that reporters get the information correctly; it is harder to correct an error than to get the story right the first time.

2. Scientific responsibility involves making scientific reports to colleagues on the use of given conceptual models; the variations, if any, in research designs used; the effects of new instruments developed for this project; and the overall outcome of the study. Connect this work with others from the literature so as to continue the development of lines of thinking and study so that the scientific family may continue to flourish.

3. Professional responsibility involves reporting to colleagues from whom one has borrowed practice methods and approaches. Report what was done, how well it achieved its objectives, and with what side effects. In this way, one extends the common practice wisdom and lead to sharper and more finely tuned methods (Backer, Liberman, & Kuehnel, 1986).

D. Preview of Subsequent Chapters: How Best to Use This Book

The subsequent chapters of this book are linked to the configural equation shown in Figure 1.4. There are several ways to use this book, as

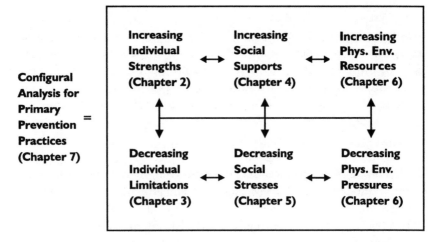

Time Frame

Figure 1.4. The Configural Equation and This Book

I will discuss again in Chapter 7. First, you can use the configural equation itself as a way to orient a project. Take whatever social behaviors you seek to address and consider how each of the six facets of the configuration may play an interactive part. Of these facets, which can you effectively influence? You might want to begin to build the project around these facets and methods.

Second, you can use this volume as a kind of handbook of tactics, each with one or more references to guide you to the primary literature. If your agency includes caseworkers or group workers or community developers, then you might look at the tactics that make use of one-to-one techniques or small group techniques or more systemwide approaches. The main point of the configural equation, however, continues to remind us not to neglect any significant part of clients' life situations.

Third, if you need to do a review of the literature, then one way to begin this effort is to look at the references for specific types of situations. The subject index directs you to the sections of the book where a topic is discussed. From there, you can select the most nearly relevant citations to act as starting points for your own research.

Fourth, if you want to get an overview of the empirical perspective in primary prevention, then reading through the chapters will supply you with a diversity of examples. (The subject index identifies substantive areas throughout the book; in most of them, recent research projects are discussed.) The breadth and depth of current research is exhilarating; it often models good research and practice and should also stimulate ideas more closely linked with your own topic.

Fifth, I hope that you will be motivated by this book to become part of this exciting effort in primary prevention. Whether your current work is in treatment of existing problems or the rehabilitation of victims, it is possible to prevent like problems for others, to protect existing states of health for relatives and friends of the victim, and to promote desired goals for all these people. If you are at a crossroads in occupational or professional choice, then consider some of the extraordinary possibilities that primary prevention practices offer in every substantive field.

2

METHODS OF PRIMARY PREVENTION

Dimension I. Increasing Individual Strengths

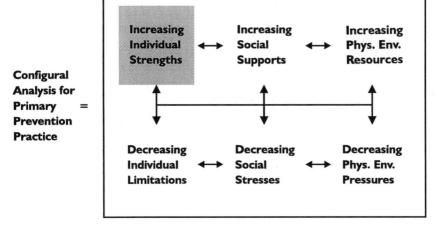

Configural
Analysis for
Primary   =
Prevention
Practice

Time Frame

Figure 2.1. The Configural Equation

This chapter introduces the configural perspective on methods for conducting primary prevention. Like the six faces of a cube, six facets together describe preventive, protective, and promotive actions for increasing individual strengths, social supports, and physical environmental resources while decreasing individual limitations, social stresses, and physical environmental pressures. For each facet, there are a number of distinctive practice methods; this chapter addresses the first dimension—methods related to increasing individual strengths.

Dimension I. Increasing Individual Strengths
    The Configural Equation for Primary Prevention Practice
    A. Cognitive Aspects
        1. General Education Methods
        2. Preventive Problem Solving
        3. Cognitive Stimulation
        4. Anticipatory Instruction
        5. Specific Cognitive Competencies: Coping With Stress
    B. Affective Aspects
        1. Attitude Change
        2. Moral Reasoning, Values Clarification, Character Education
        3. Instigation of Hope, Promotion of Optimism
    C. Behavioral and Skill Aspects
        1. Learning Theories
        2. Social Skills Training
    D. Physiological and Biological Aspects
        1. Nutrition
        2. Lifelong Exercise
        3. Immunization and Vaccination
    E. Holistic or Multifactor Approaches
        1. Perceived Self-Efficacy
        2. Assertiveness and Resistance Training
        3. Affective Education
        4. Resilience

The Configural Equation
for Primary Prevention Practice

The configural equation (see Figure 2.1) (described in Chapter 1 and presented at the beginning of Chapters 2 through 6) presents six general factors that may be active in any social behavior: individual strengths and limitations, social supports and stresses, and physical environmental resources and pressures. To give each factor potentially equal strength in a given situation and to emphasize the continuous transactions among them, it may be useful to conceive of them as facets of a cube that contains any given human event. Each facet is a set of structures and forces interacting with all the others, the result of which is that human event in a particular context. In a real-life situation, one or another facet may have

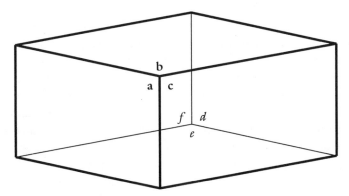

a. Structures and forces acting to increase individual strengths
b. Structures and forces acting to increase social supports
c. Structures and forces acting to increase resources from the physical
   environment
d. Structures and forces acting to decrease individual limitations
e. Structures and forces acting to decrease social stresses
f. Structures and forces acting to decrease pressures from the physical
   environment

Figure 2.2. The Configural Cube

NOTE: This cube represents the six aspects of the primary prevention configural formula, all of which must be considered to understand a situation and used so as to optimize effective preventive interventions.

more influence than the others but any facet might potentially be the predominant one. What is more likely is that the transactions among all six facets make up any given observed event in its context (see Figure 2.2).

As a heuristic device for training practitioners, the cube metaphor is useful because the omission of any facet will break up one's understanding of the whole client and situation. Practitioners need to investigate the realities of each facet in deciding how to plan the primary prevention service. The equation presents constructive and destructive facets, requiring that practitioners attend to both sides—not merely preventing some untoward event but also promoting some positive experience in its place (Bond, 1982; Bond & Wagner, 1988; Harwood & Weissberg, 1992).

Events in the configural equation are constantly changing to some degree, not only because of internal happenings but also because of interactions between and among facets. Moreover, the helping professional influences events and interactions within the cube. This dynamic or moving configuration of events is known only approximately; our language tends to sort things out in linear and paired fashion rather than in the systemic complexity that is more nearly like social reality. Using the cube as a visual reminder of the whole, however, one can begin to make connections among all aspects of the configural equation, even though one does this with a few pieces of a complex situation at any time. The prevention professional operates as if he or she were at the center of the cube, adding to, negotiating among, and coordinating the forces emanating from each of the sides.

This chapter deals with increasing personal strengths, one of the six facets of primary prevention. Personal strengths refer to any aspect of the person that can be used to adapt effectively to inner or outer challenges. I conform to common usage in discussing cognitive, affective, behavioral, and physiological aspects of individual strengths, even though these features tend to blur into one another. I also add holistic or multifactor methods when useful. Hollister's (1967) term *strens* is used to describe any set of forces or structures that increases individual strengths and opportunities.

I use a common organizational structure in this and the following chapters, first offering a definition of terms, then illustrating the method in some research or demonstration study (or common experience), and finally providing some general guidelines (and references) for the use of this method in preventive and promotive practice. These guidelines or general principles for practice are the heart of this book. They are intended to be clear and complete, but readers must retranslate them into terms relevant for their own projects. It may be helpful to read the original sources for nuances that go beyond my summarizing. An overall listing of dimensions and specific practice methods appears at the end of this book, as well as in Figure 7.2.

A. Cognitive Aspects

1. General Education Methods

What people learn in school constitutes a major portion of their core knowledge about themselves and the world, as selected by political and cultural forces in control of public and private education. This includes the formal skills of reading, writing, and arithmetic, as well as a host of other skills that are less clearly labeled, such as critical thinking, historical and futuristic perspectives, and creativity. People also may learn a host of social and interpersonal skills and values at school, as well as prejudices and stereotypes. The existence of schooling does not guarantee either the quality of the lessons or the adequacy of the learning. Many primary prevention projects take place at preschool or school because of the potential scope of access, the overall receptiveness of young minds, and the general cooperativeness of educators and parents in these shared social goals. I discuss specific educational methods throughout the book, but I want to remind readers about some basic aspects of education. The general strategy of formal education involves the following steps, which readers can test against their own experience (Elias, 1989; Elias et al., 1991; Elias & Weisberg, 1990; Kahn, 1984):

1. Introducing a body of knowledge to be learned (previewing to get a sense of the whole; Trad, 1993)
2. Breaking that body of knowledge down into digestible pieces according to the cognitive capacities of the learners (Meade et al., 1994; Plimpton & Root, 1994)
3. Presenting sequences of these learning units over long periods of time, with frequent tests (of memory and comprehension), projects (to test how well the learning is applied to novel situations), or papers (to practice synthesizing the knowledge learned)
4. Arranging the learning experiences and tests so that the students will have frequent experiences of mastering the content—experiences that will increase the students' sense of perceived self-efficacy, the belief that one is able to accomplish some specific task (Bandura, 1986)
5. Providing incentives for mastery, including small rewards for current work and larger rewards for proportionally greater amounts of learning—also including sanctions or alternatives for those who do not perform within acceptable ranges (Glasser, 1969)
6. Forming relationships with teachers and other students and creating a congenial place for learning (the formal objective) and friendship (the informal or integrative objective)—relationships that can be very important in the lives of the individuals involved (Werner, 1989a, 1989b)

It is interesting to note that many forms of preventive service, as well as therapy, make use of portions of the methods used in general and formal education. Cognitive-behavioral theorists have contributed a number of

I. The First Dimension

specific methods that are described on these pages, as in the discussion of individualizing in Chapter 1 (Schinke, Gilchrist, & Small, 1979; see also Anderson & Quast, 1983; Baker & Butler, 1984; Echterling, 1989; Lorion, Hightower, Work, & Shockley, 1987; Meichenbaum, 1977; Meichenbaum & Jaremko, 1983).

Programmed learning also makes use of this sequential learning, testing, and reinforcing process. Similar ideas guide age-paced educational materials addressed to new parents regarding the growth and development of their children during the preschool years (Dickinson & Cudaback, 1992; Laurendeau, Gagnon, Desjardins, Perreault, & Kishchuk, 1991).

2. Preventive Problem Solving

Problem solving is a frequently used method in primary prevention, formally or informally, because it is a general content-free approach applicable to a broad range of concerns. Problem solving involves a planned sequence of cognitive-affective and cognitive-behavioral efforts to enable the person to accomplish a desired end most expeditiously. Problem solving has a long history of generally successful applications (Shure, 1988; Urbain & Kendall, 1980; Weissberg & Allen, 1986).

Problem-solving approaches share the core ideas of identifying a perceived challenge (including predictable problems or desired states to be obtained), surveying possible options to meet that challenge, weighing the probable costs of each option against likely effects, and making a decision as the basis of action. (For variations in problem solving, see Bond & Compas, 1989; Bond & Rosen, 1980; Folkman, 1991; Robin, 1981; Schinke & Gilchrist, 1984.)

The title of this section, "Preventive Problem Solving," connects this general method with primary prevention. A better title would be "Pre-Problem Solving, Protecting, and Potential Achieving," but common usage of the phrase "problem solving" is so strong that this change would create more confusion than enlightenment.

Problem solving is used as the overall framework for this book (see Figure 1.3), but in this section, I want to focus on a specific method used in primary prevention because it illustrates the connection of theory, research, and practice with a significant social concern. The programmatic work of Spivak and Shure and their colleagues is an exemplar of primary prevention, for the continual refinement of its conceptualization, its detailed practice methods, its ongoing evaluation, and the development of materials for dissemination. Let me present some background to their work.

Spivak and Levine (1963) encountered distinct differences in the interpersonal thinking skills used by normal and disturbed adolescents; this discovery led at different times to similar findings for adults and prepuberty-aged children (Spivak, Platt, & Shure, 1976). Spivak theorized that some set of cognitive problem-solving skills was the intervening factor. That is, the way people identified a problem, what they thought was causing it, the number of possible alternatives they saw in trying to solve it, and the consequences that each alternative entailed come together in some way to spell the difference between successful and unsuccessful interpersonal behaviors.

Spivak and Shure (1974) posed the question about how these cognitive skills might be taught and the earliest that they could be successfully absorbed. They assumed that the earlier these skills could be learned, the more life challenges they could be applied to and the greater the cumulative benefit. These investigators also checked to see whether level of intelligence correlated with level of effective problem solving: Do smarter people make better problem solvers? The consistent evidence over at least seven studies reported by Spivak, Platt, and Shure (1976) is that IQ score or general verbal skills are not related to effective problem solving. Another question concerned how overly inhibited children (very shy, passive) or overly impulsive children (quick to act, impatient) would respond to problem-solving training. Both of these extremes share being deficient in the ability to generate solutions to interpersonal problems geared to their age level and foreseeing the consequences of actions, as compared with nonimpulsive and noninhibited peers. Both shy and impulsive children responded well to training in problem solving.

Spivak and Shure (1974) then carried out a series of studies to identify the earliest feasible age for problem-solving training. They first worked with black inner-city nursery school children, randomly dividing them into control and experimental groups. The experimental group received the interpersonal cognitive problem-solving program (ICPS)—the children later nicknamed these initials as "I Can Problem Solve." This program involves one trainer who meets daily with six to eight children in a 20- to 30-minute period for 46 sessions. A carefully constructed script is followed that represents the guiding principles of this problem-solving approach.

I. The First Dimension

1. The children are first taught the necessary cognitive concepts, such as same-different and if-then, that will be used in making comparisons and reaching judgments.
2. Then they learn to identify different emotions in themselves and in other people. By recognizing in him- or herself the unpleasant feelings others may have, a child comes to understand the implications of the effects of his or her actions on others.
3. The basics of problem solving are taught: First a problem is recognized—some felt concern that it is or may become hurtful to some person.
4. Once a problem is recognized, children learn to generate alternative solutions to that problem. They learn to predict the short-term and long-term consequences of a particular proposed solution. (What good feelings or bad feelings will be likely in the various people affected by the action?)
5. A decision is made among the alternative solutions, which involves what Spivak and Shure (1974) call *means-ends thinking*—the ability to plan a series of specific actions to attain a specific objective, along with anticipating possible obstacles.
6. Training in problem solving does not involve instructions on what to think. Rather, the focus is on how to think.

This approach is generic; it is applicable to diverse racial, ethnic, age groups, and social classes; and it is adaptable to different settings, including families in which, for example, mothers can be trained to work with their children on problem solving (Shure, 1988). On balance, the results of various studies using the ICPS have been favorable, but the program is not without its critics (Durlak, 1983; Elias & Clabby, 1992; Shure, 1988; Urbain & Kendall, 1980).

Spivak and Shure (1974) emphasize that the program is not a mechanical process—it has to be sensitively adapted to particular groups. It cannot be delivered in a short time; they suggest at least 4 months for young children.

The ICPS was extended to mothers of inner-city black children after the authors found that mothers' ICPS ability and child-rearing style related to the child's ICPS ability and behaviors—but only in girls (Shure, 1988, p. 176). When both mothers and children (boys and girls) received the ICPS training, the children showed significant gains in alternative solutions skills and in desired behavioral adjustment.

The ICPS approach continues to be developed, extended, and tested. Its detailed training manual offers a primary prevention technology that is available for use and adaptation in a wide variety of circumstances (see Battistich, Elias, & Branden-Muller, 1992; Clabby & Elias, 1986; Elias

& Clabby, 1992; Elias, Gara, Schuyler, Branden-Muller, & Sayette, 1991; Winer, Hilpert, Gesten, Cowen, & Schubin, 1982).

3. Cognitive Stimulation

This section deals with a number of related methods to stimulate the mind, some that augment what parents naturally do, and others that add formal curricula in institutional settings. From a preventive or promotive point of view, one can trace how stimulation applied at the right time and place and in the right manner can have good effects (Olds, 1988; Pierson, 1988; Scarr-Salapetek & Williams, 1973; Wandersman, 1982; Zigler & Styfco, 1993) just as its absence will produce bad effects (Bowlby, 1951, 1969; Parkes, Stevenson-Hinde, & Marris, 1991).

Infants receive all kinds of stimuli from the environment, but some forms of stimuli appear to be more beneficial than others to lead to the kinds of growth and development—perceptual, mental, and physical—that are adaptive to the demands of a middle-class society. Some have termed these enriched experiences the *hidden curriculum* of the middle-class home that seem to be less available in more impoverished environments. On the other hand, life experience in the slums provides training in street survival skills. But if the children of the poor are to make their way into a middle-class world, they need the tools and skills relevant for this. Ojemann (1972) sees in noncausal or punitive styles of communication (such as "shut up and do it because I told you to") the seeds of dysfunctional human relationships and mental illness, whereas a causal orientation (such as "if you don't be quiet, then you'll wake up the baby") could lead to constructive behaviors in this middle-class-dominant society. (See Green, 1995, on the association between parental communication clarity and the academic achievement of children with learning disabilities.)

In a longitudinal study by Levenstein (1988) and her colleagues, low-income mothers and their toddlers received planned sequential stimulation from "toy demonstrators." These demonstrators were people from the community who were trained to demonstrate how mothers could play with their children using age-relevant free toys and books. These toys stimulated verbal interactions between parent and child that were both enjoyable and educational. The successful results led to replications of this program 84 times in 16 states and involved various ethnic groups—including blacks, Hispanics, and Native Americans.

The program consisted of a maximum of 92 visits during the 2-year service period. The toy demonstrators modeled effective verbal and play interactions that appeared to enable the youngsters to develop cognitive skills for dealing with complex intellectual challenges, while at the same time it fostered the mothers' parenting skills and self-esteem. Although national norms showed that more than one third of all urban youth drop out of school, evidence from the Levenstein study and others suggests that if we can reach these young people very early in their lives, we can prevent the academic failures that are so costly to the individuals involved as well as to society (Srebnik & Elias, 1993). Levenstein (1988) summarizes her findings:

> The research results of in-house and outside evaluations indicated that, on the average, the model Program significantly aided low-income children's intellectual growth and later school performance. Their third grade reading, arithmetic, and intelligence scores were at the level of national norms. Their fifth grade reading and intelligence scores also met national norms and significantly surpassed those of Non-Program children of similar background, as had all their previous scores. (p. 205)

Evidence from one follow-up study extending to the eighth grade shows these trends to be maintained (DeVito & Karon, 1984). Indeed, DeVito and Karon noted that Program graduates outperformed comparable Non-Program students (Head Start graduates) in their achievement, and "they met or exceeded national norms."

This finding is in contrast to studies of the "long-term" effects of Head Start, where early initial positive effects tend to be washed out after a few years in school. Levenstein's (1988) follow-up studies also noted this washout of effects, especially in Grades 3, 4, and 5, although dramatic turnarounds appeared evident in Grades 6, 7, and 8. Another important longitudinal study by Schweinhart and Weikart (1988) and Barnett (1993a) shows the cost-benefit ratios of high-quality early childhood education programs. Control group youngsters as compared with the experimental group some 14 years after the beginning of the project cost society more in welfare, special education, or delinquency control. The cost-benefit ratio was at least 3 to 1—$3 returned to society for every $1 it cost to run the program.

The toy demonstrator program was eventually popular with the mothers and children. Indeed, once a mother has been trained in her own home, she may become a toy demonstrator herself, possibly providing her with a first employment experience and spreading the effect of the program (see Chapter 4, III.A.1). Stimulation continues throughout life, sometimes increasing with great zest (see Maccoby & Altman, 1988, and Sprafkin, Swift, & Hess, 1988, on the use of television to stimulate healthy lifestyles) or with violence (see Abbott, 1992; Eron, 1982; Kolbert, 1994, on television violence), and at other times falling into monotonous routine (see Peplau & Goldston, 1984, on disabling loneliness). In some European countries, vacations are legally obligatory, which puts these periods for regenerating physical and mental batteries in a quite different light than our own voluntary vacations. Overall, the value of stimulation as a planned activity related to constructive health concerns is underestimated in American society. The following statements may offer some guidance regarding stimulation:

1. People should be exposed to age-appropriate stimuli in batches that continue to expand their range of experiences, but not so much as to overwhelm them in the process. "Natural" teachers and experiences should be used, as people of all ages learn by doing within a supportive context. It may be necessary to teach natural teachers such as parents how to be more effective in parenting, or sexual partners how to provide enduring forms of comfort and pleasure (especially when practicing safer sex).

2. All people need quiet time that is unscheduled in terms of stimulation. Sleep is a natural quiet time, but people must be able to wind down from stimulation to benefit from this natural rest. A weekly Sabbath provides a much needed day of rest; a yearly vacation provides a more general change of context and renewed energy and direction. Even the humble coffee break offers a change of pace in an often hectic routine that could enable a person to maintain both a reasonable level of efficiency and personal satisfaction at work.

3. The stimulation should permit the receiver to act on the information, in addition to absorbing it cognitively and effectively. I will return to this point in the discussion of lifelong exercise, but in general, active involvement is better than passive reception in learning as in physical activity.

4. Sensory capabilities decline with old age, so there is need for multiple sensory experiences in one situation. Hearing, seeing, and touching together may make a social interchange meaningful when one or another of these sensory modalities may have reduced acuity.

I. The First Dimension

5. Stimulation may be planned. Curricula may be formally developed, even in informal settings, such as the toy demonstrator program. The material aspects of stimulation must not be ignored, such as giving toys to children, books on tapes to people who cannot read, or videos on how to model some complex behavior.

6. Experience in various stimulation projects suggests acquainting participants with the experience slowly without overwhelming them. Ongoing evaluation of the programs provides corrective feedback during the service period as well as assessment of outcomes.

4. Anticipatory Instruction

The strategy I am terming *anticipatory instruction* includes several related approaches such as anticipatory socialization, antecedent systematic desensitization, and anticipatory guidance. This strategy is rare among methods in the preventive armamentarium in being counterintuitive and born from theory. At its core, the strategy suggests that informing consumers of coming stresses will somehow enable them to prepare psychologically for these stresses and be more successful in dealing with them when they actually happen.

I suggest, however, that anticipatory instruction be expanded to include anticipation of the positive outcomes as well as the negative experiences. It is not merely that one is going to undergo a difficult surgery, but also that one may anticipate an improved state of health after the recovery period. Then the details of the pain and suffering to be expected in the surgery make sense. Anticipating a stren (Hollister, 1967), which is a growth-promotive experience, may make the event itself more pleasing and useful. (I will continue this idea in the discussion of instigating hope and optimism, I.B.3.)

Why should knowing about some stressor before experiencing it provide some advantage for the client? How much of that anticipatory experience should be provided under what circumstances? Poser (1970, p. 40) deals with the first question in his concept of antecedent systematic desensitization. From the general desensitization theory, he argues that providing people with increasing amounts of stress at levels they are able to handle at each occasion will eventually enable them to handle large amounts of stress. In antecedent systematic desensitization, he gradually introduces images and actual experiences of potentially stressful situations so that when the real event occurs, the individual will have already had experiences in thinking about the problem and coping with it.

For example, Poser notes that some nursery school children exhibit anxious behaviors after being left at school, whereas others do not. He assumes that the latter group experiences some natural desensitization as parents talk about nursery school, take the child for visits, and in other ways subject the child to small but manageable forms of stress. It might also be the case that these experiences are stimulating and represent growth-promotive strens, rather than growth-inhibiting stresses (Hollister, 1967), by raising the child's curiosity and satisfying it in pleasant ways. For children who do not receive this natural antecedent systematic desensitization, it would be possible to provide an artificial version at every class level, from nursery school (Axtell, 1991, personal communication) to high school (Felner & Adan, 1988) to college. (A concentrated orientation week at college may not be as satisfactory a learning experience as a planned experience at high school distributed over a semester or two, as Felner & Adan, 1988, suggest.)

Felner and Adan (1988) describe a school transitional environment project that involves some anticipatory and concurrent instructions to reduce the untoward affect of moving from elementary to junior high school or from junior high school to high school. Felner and Adan assume this normative transition is stressful and provide social and physical environmental changes to reduce the stresses. All incoming project students are assigned to special homerooms whose teachers serve a new function, to link students (and parents) and school through administrative and counseling functions. Project students attend core subject classes together so as to establish a stable peer support system. This information is supplied to incoming students, which therefore serves as anticipatory instruction.

Results reported by Felner and Adan (1988) support the successful transitions of project students as compared with control group students, both during the school year and longitudinally. Dropout rates for project students are half those of controls, and academic achievements as well as low absenteeism rates favor the project students.

Family life education may also be viewed as a form of anticipatory instruction (see Arcus, Schvaneveldt, & Moss, 1993a, 1993b; Pill, 1981), often dealing in advance of any need with methods of discipline (on the negative side) and with ways to enjoy communications and shared activities (on the positive side; see also Gordon, 1970, 1989). Golann (1986)

I. The First Dimension

discusses important life transition points and how understanding these enables professional helpers to facilitate growth (see also Germain & Gitterman, 1995).

Positive life events may also be stressful, such as a wedding. A known situation is turning into a situation with many unknowns. Although the transition ritual itself is likely to be pleasant, the stresses of going through the ritual may raise tensions and emotions. Planning the package of rituals can supply some structure for one's expectations through a series of manageable objectives. These plans address both the tangible issues—the wedding dress, the license, the reception—and the intangible—the various hopes and fears one experiences in making such a major life decision. The anticipatory instructions in such a complex social event involve many persons, so one doesn't always know what to expect from others at these delicate times. Rehearsal dinners and the like are anticipatory devices to coordinate the behaviors of the many involved persons, whose prompted performance is intended to reduce the stress of the actual affair. Nonetheless, tension is relieved when the ritual is over; a constructive memory smooths over the glitches, and in retrospect, a happy time was had by all.

I will give one last example of a form of anticipatory instruction designed to take place in the context of a serious crisis. Caplan (1989) presents the anticipatory guidance and emotional inoculation component of his Recurring Themes Model of primary prevention (discussed in Appendix B). He employs this approach when a crisis can be predicted, such as when a child is admitted to a hospital for a serious operation.

1. First, if possible, begin this preventive action with a group of people who can support each other, although it may be conveyed individually as well. Act close in time and place to the predicted crisis, as at a hospital ward shortly after admission.

2. Arouse anticipatory distress by describing expectable stresses in such detail as to generate a clear response from the listeners but not too much anxiety. (How to modulate the evocative details to the level of the audience is not specified; presumably, one watches the reactions and judges whether one has gone far enough. Addressing a mixed audience of adults and children makes this a difficult decision.)

3. Offer ways that the listeners may master these expected stresses, including emphasis on the time-limited nature of the discomfort (when it is possible to do so—don't be deceptive).

4. Tell the listeners what they will be able to do themselves to gain relief and how they can get help from others—so that they will be active participants in the crisis, rather than passive sufferers. Aid family members and other friends in helping each other as well as the target person.

5. Raise the hope that the activity as well as the natural unfolding of events in the brief time period will lead to a successful outcome. Never deny or obscure the gravity of the situation.

6. Identify expectable confusion and distress as normal reactions of healthy people exposed to an inescapable predicament and not signs of any incipient psychological disorder.

Caplan (1989) discusses other methods and tactics in crisis intervention, which takes place during the crisis, whereas anticipatory instruction occurs before the crisis phase of a predictable problem. These additional methods are used to supplement the client's expectable reductions in cognitive, affective, or behavioral functioning as well as to offer material assistance as needed in mastering the challenge:

7. Conduct repeated short contacts during the buildup of the crisis period so as to satisfy the naturally increasing dependency needs of the clients.

8. At the height of the crisis, begin a strategic withdrawal of help while supporting the client and family's active confrontation of the challenge. During this time, provide needed information, help the clients focus on the present, find existential meaning in this set of circumstances as far as possible, and help the clients plan what to do.

9. Help the family members and friends communicate with each other, including the expression of negative feelings and ways to overcome them. Emphasize the normality of expectable upset feelings and counteract the blaming of self or others as a way to relieve tensions.

10. Help everyone—patient, family, and friends—bear the frustrations of unknown outcomes while trying to be supportive of one another. Warn clients of the dangers of expectable fatigue and the use of division of labor to reduce it. Rest periods for helpers are necessary.

11. Maintain hope but not false hope. Encourage the client and family and friends to be active so as to achieve a sense of mastery. Encourage seeking outside help when needed and counteract possible shame that equates asking for help with personal weakness. Remind participants of

I. The First Dimension

their precrisis identity as strong and effective people, and do not reinforce a crisis-eroded identity of weak helplessness.

5. Specific Cognitive Competencies: Coping With Stress

Competence refers, in the most general sense, to one's abilities to adapt to the human condition. Although this global meaning of the term is important to provide a context for discussion, it is the specific competencies that I focus on in this section. When a specific challenge comes along, how (with what personal, social, and physical tools) does one respond?

A class of responses may be labeled *coping*—although there is considerable disagreement over the term's meaning and domain. I use the term to mean conscious tactics that enable a person to deal with some stress or stren (Hollister, 1967). The conscious aspect distinguishes coping conceptually from defense mechanisms presumed to deal at an unconscious level to protect the ego from intrusions of unacceptable sexual or aggressive urges. Problem solving carries more of the sense of a planned adaptation, whereas coping seems to refer to natural or stylistic adaptation, that is, how the person typically responds to stress or strens.

Just because a person is healthy, wealthy, and wise does not mean that he or she doesn't have a lot of stresses (and strens) to cope with (Albino, 1984; Bloom, 1985; Compas & Phares, 1991; Cummings, Greene, & Karraker, 1991; Forman, 1993; Hawkins et al., 1989; Lazarus, 1985; Stolberg, Kiluk, & Garrison, 1986; Weissberg, Caplan, & Swo, 1989; Woolf, Lewander, Filippone, & Lovejoy, 1987). Life is composed of challenges, both internal and external to the system in question (Erikson, 1963; Evans, Jacobs, & Catalino, 1987; Felner, 1984; Little, Gaffrey, & Grissmer, 1991). Puberty involves internal hormonal stimuli; an attractive person of the opposite sex involves an external challenge to a heterosexual teenager. The same stimulus can be a stress to one person and a stren to another or to the same person at a different time or to the same person at the same time (such as wanting to approach the beloved but being too shy to do so).

Following the steps of Monat and Lazarus (1985, p. 3), I use the term *stress* to mean any internal or external challenge (or both) whose demands tax or exceed the adaptive responses that the given system can make (Selye, 1956, 1976). With this usage, Monat and Lazarus make clear that challenges are neverending in life. Most of the time most people face and resolve these challenges—indeed, some challenges represent delightful stimulation that adds zest to life. But at some times for all people, the challenges push the adaptive capacity to and beyond the limit. If supplementary resources and aid are not available, then the person may be overcome and die (Selye, 1956).

Stresses are additive. Holmes and Rahe (1967) and many others have pointed out that stresses (and strens) coming from a wide variety of sources accumulate to reach a threshold that may be used to predict untoward mental or physical sequelae. Holmes and Rahe's Social Readjustment Rating Scale has been widely used, criticized, modified, and expanded to fit special groups (see Luthar & Zigler, 1991, for a recent overview of this literature). One of the criticisms has been that the scale excludes context. For example, in a civilian prisoner-of-war camp in the Philippines in World War II, the death rate was below that expected for the equivalent small town in America, despite the great stresses on the inmates over a 4-year period. Speculative reasons for this finding included the collective morale at this camp (in contrast with other camps), the cultural values of the inmates, and individual strengths (Bloom & Halsema, 1983). The context and meaning of the stress must be considered. (See George & Gwyther, 1988; Unger et al., 1992, regarding other stressors, hazardous waste, and caretaking of the elderly, respectively.)

People develop a typical style of adapting—I term this the *coping style*. Lazarus and Folkman (1984) distinguish two aspects. The first is termed *problem-focused coping,* which refers to efforts to make such changes in persons, objects, or relationships so as to resolve the stressful challenge. This includes information gathering and efforts to think through problems and potential solutions—this is very much like problem solving as discussed previously. The second aspect of coping is termed *emotion focused* (or palliative), which involves thoughts or actions whose goal is to reduce the emotional effect of the stress, which typically shows itself in bodily or physiological disturbances. This emotional aspect of coping has some characteristics of defense mechanisms. It is useful to define coping as being constituted by both aspects, which makes it different from each separate component—problem solving and defense mechanisms. People tend to use both aspects in their typical approach to dealing with challenges (Lazarus & Folkman, 1984).

Lazarus (1984) points out that self-deception (which is like the primitive defense mechanism of denial) is sometimes useful as an initial form of coping, wherein the person is temporarily confused and unable to act constructively and realistically. What would have been an overwhelming stimulus may be dealt with gradually and more manageably, as long as the person does not continue to deny the reality of the challenge. Lazarus points out that we all live by our illusions—perhaps these are our typical modes of coping with reality—which may promote a higher state of contentment than we might have reached without them.

Coping style may be related to several other concepts relevant to primary prevention. Kobasa, Maddi, and Kahn (1982) identify a constellation of personal factors termed *hardiness* characteristic of people who do not succumb to illness in the face of great stress. These people have a stronger sense of meaningfulness and commitment to self, a more vigorous attitude toward life, and an internal locus of control. The term *resilience* is discussed later in this chapter (E.4). Resilience refers to both personal and situational factors that enable some people to prevail over difficult circumstances (Werner, 1989a; see also Libassi & Maluccio, 1986; Maluccio, Washitz, & Libassi, 1992).

Seligman (1975, 1991) presents a programmatic series of research studies and theory building that has important implications for primary prevention. In his first work, on learned helplessness, Seligman (1975) studied how laboratory dogs appeared to learn to be helpless, that is, how animals placed in painful situations from which there was no escape appeared to be unable to take simple and accessible maneuvers to escape from another difficult situation. The analog between these creatures and human beings who also find themselves in intolerable situations from which they appear unable to escape is uncomfortably close. It is also helpful in comparing the ways in which the laboratory animals must be vigorously aided to relearn how to escape. There may be some treatment ideas for women who appear to be stuck in abusive situations (see also Baruch & Barnett, 1980). Seligman's recent work (1991) on learned optimism is more relevant for primary prevention.

Seligman (1991) identifies internal mechanisms called *explanatory styles* that process information and make life decisions. He distinguishes three aspects of explanatory style, three cognitive dimensions that offer ways to promote optimism. I will identify the dimensions with a negative tag for ease of communication:

1. Personalization—"It's my fault": When bad things happen, some people habitually blame themselves; if good things happen, these people

tend to believe other people caused them. Optimists think just the reverse; they cause good things to happen, but other people cause bad events.

2. Permanence—"It is always going to be like this": People who give up easily think the bad thing that has happened to them is permanent; they use words such as *always* or *never*. When good things happen to them, they see these events as temporary. The other style—people who resist helplessness—think that bad things are temporary, whereas good things are permanent.

3. Pervasiveness—"It's going to undermine every aspect of my life": People who view bad events as catastrophes also tend to see this one problem as affecting all other events as well. Optimists, on the other hand, believe that good events will enhance everything, whereas bad events have specific causes and limited effects. Seligman (1991) says,

> A pessimistic explanatory style is at the core of depressive thinking. A negative concept of the future, the self, and the world stems from seeing the causes of bad events as permanent, pervasive, and personal; and seeing the causes of good events in the opposite way. (p. 58)

Cognitive therapy helps create an optimistic explanatory style, which is empirically linked with constructive outcomes. In a later section of this chapter (B.3), I modify Seligman's (1991) therapy proposals for primary prevention purposes. To anticipate this discussion, I will illustrate an optimistic approach to study behavior:

1. When one begins to recognize some negative thoughts flitting through one's consciousness, learn to dispute them with contrary and positive evidence. For example, these self-defeating thoughts—"I'm not going to do well on the test; I never do well on these kinds of exams; I know she always gives hard exams"—reflect the three dimensions of a defeatist explanatory style.

2. Dispute the defeatist style with positive facts on the same three dimensions—"I have done well in school for years; I have passed all kinds of exams; I have kept up with the class work and have studied amply for the test, and so there is every reason to believe I will do reasonably well." (There has to be some reality to one's positive thoughts—thinking how good one is will not, alone, enable one to pass a test.)

I. The First Dimension

3. Learn to make different attributions based on advanced planning and work: "I'm going to ace this class because I am interested in the content and I will arrange my time to keep up with lessons, and to study well just before the exam. This is the way I've always done well in school in the past, and I can do it again." (Again, make the reality of good study habits fit one's explanatory style.)

4. When inevitable doubts and worries arise—"Wow, this material is difficult to grasp"—learn how to distract oneself from depressing thoughts by constructive ones—"Everyone's in the same boat in my class and I have been studying more than most. I'll get it if I keep plugging away like I've always done."

5. It may be helpful to have a support group to aid in the reality of the task, as well as in the cognitive and affective states that occur during this time period. (Women's study groups have been used as a way to reject math anxiety—a learned defeatist style—in favor of a positive style; the mutual aid of the group gives substance to that mental state; see Tobias, 1978.)

From this diffuse arena of coping concepts, several main points are clear:

1. Challenges can be very useful and stimulating but they may also tax or overwhelm the individual's capacity to respond. This is especially true when negative challenges accumulate in short time periods or when chronic conditions persist for long periods of time. Positive challenges also accumulate and may counteract the negative. (More research is needed on this point.) Albee's (1983) general formula regarding factors related to the incidence of mental disorder includes coping as a major factor in reducing the potential problem. Many prevention programs are experimenting with training in coping skills as one way to increase resilience (Cowen, Work, & Wyman, 1992, p. 162; Parker et al., 1990), create resistance to helplessness (Meichenbaum, 1977), immunize against future traumas (Schwebel, 1992, p. 122), acquire health-enhancing habits (Albino, 1984), deal with homophobia (D'Augelli, 1993), and aid people in confronting chronic and acute stressors (Ellis, 1985; Moos, 1992). No uniformity in coping programs exists as of yet.

2. Substitute or compensating social systems may lend support or resources to enable the individual (or group) to resolve the challenge successfully. Few people cope with powerful challenges (stresses or strens) alone. Preventers should probably think of coping in its social context for a more realistic understanding of what primary prevention can do—

directly for stressed individuals or indirectly for support systems for these people (see Chapter 4).

3. People learn how to cope in their own way and develop a style for handling challenges. These coping styles may be hardy or foolhardy, resilient or not. We are at the beginning stages of learning whether or not we can effect hardiness or resilience in people who do not possess these traits naturally (see Parker et al., 1990, p. 32, on teachable attributes of resilience). It is clear that the sociocultural and physical environments are strongly involved in aiding or inhibiting coping behaviors. Indeed, changing personal coping styles and situational opportunities for coping in large numbers of persons are the core issues for current welfare reforms. Neither alone will be sufficient as the social work axiom—always view the person in continuous interaction with the environment—affirms.

4. The task-solving side of coping can probably be augmented through problem-solving methods. The emotional aspect of coping may also be modified, probably through modeling methods, techniques for managing anger, and existential grappling with solvable and unsolvable problems. Denial-like behaviors may be productive for the individual in the short run, however, so as to get organized to deal with the challenge. An emotional overload can interfere with rational problem solving.

5. It is possible to teach coping skills to people in advance of any need as a kind of psychological immunization, even though many of the real-world events such as war, earthquakes, or economic depressions are essentially unavoidable. Norman and Turner (1993) review McGuire's (1968) cognitive inoculation theory, in which weak exposures of aversive stimuli are given to build up resistance before a strong exposure occurs. Norman and Turner also describe Evans and Raines's (1990) social inoculation theory, in which students are aided in resisting social pressures and advertising that pushes drug use. (These are discussed in other sections of the book.)

B. Affective Aspects

1. Attitude Change

Many of the particular methods of prevention and promotion involve a general process called *attitude change*. The study of attitude change has

I. The First Dimension

been central throughout the 100-year history of social psychology, but only recently has this knowledge base been focused on primary prevention. Edwards, Tindale, Heath, and Posavac (1990) present a number of important chapters indicating the diversity of applications of the general knowledge base. I will present a brief overview of this extensive knowledge base, followed by some general principles for changing attitudes.

Attitudes refers to a complex set of factors by which an individual is cognitively aware of some event, has certain feelings (affects) about that event, and may get ready to act with regard to that event. The cognitive aspect involves beliefs without regard to their accuracy. The affective aspect represents an assignment of positive-approach or negative-withdraw feelings about a given event. The action component of attitudes is hazy. Early definitions of attitude referred to a predisposition to respond, a kind of mental set that preprogrammed the muscles and bones to act in a certain way. Because attitudes were not invariably connected with their corresponding actions, theorists had to establish conceptual linkages by which beliefs and feelings led to actions. (See, e.g., the Fishbein & Ajzen, 1975, and Fishbein & Middlestadt, 1989, theory of reasoned action, discussed in Appendix B.)

Another useful conceptualization breaks down the complex process of attitude change in terms of the communication components. McGuire (1968, 1984) distinguishes among the source, message, receiver, and channel factors and summarizes the research related to each component. Briefly, source factors refer to the expertise and trustworthiness of the sender of the message. Jaccard, Turrisi, and Wan (1990) summarize this factor by noting that source expertise can be enhanced by

> presenting the relevant credentials of the source (presented prior to the message itself), using a source who is attractive, familiar with the topic, and similar to the target population; having the source speak at a slightly faster-than-average rate, taking a position that is only moderately discrepant from that of the audience; and having the source dress appropriately, make good eye contact with the audience, and exhibit few signs of nervousness. (p. 129)

The message factors include types of arguments, message style, what is included and excluded from the messages, the amount of message material presented, the ordering of the message content, and the extremity of the position urged. An important part of the message delivery concerns the level of fear aroused. Fear generates immediate attention to the topic, but if the level of fear is too little or too large, the message tends to be ignored or avoided—and thus lost. Sometimes fears are dissolved in alcohol; Fisher and Misovich (1990) attribute college students' high AIDS-risk behavior despite high AIDS knowledge to the combination of drinking and unsafe sex. Positive appeals usually result in longer retention and consistency of behavioral compliance (Jaccard et al., 1990). Humor has been found to be useful for gaining attention and for retention, as long as it is related to the sender's message (e.g., a board of directors of a cigarette company is discussing ways to promote cigarette sales despite the overwhelming evidence on the harmful effects of smoking because "we're not in this business for our health").

Compliance-inducing strategies are important to primary prevention (Cialdini, 1984). Evidence suggests that a strategy is more successful if one begins with inducing small changes in the intended direction rather than large ones and then framing the persuasive attempts so as to make them appear to involve relatively low levels of effort and commitment (Jaccard et al., 1990, p. 131).

Receiver factors represent the third major aspect in McGuire's (1968, 1984) model. Individual differences are studied with regard to influenceability and compliance. For example, McKusick, Hoff, Stall, and Coates (1991) discuss differences in behavioral strategies for reaching heterosexual men or women and gay men. Schinke, Botvin, Orlandi, Schilling, and Gordon (1990) present strategies for preventing HIV infection among African American and Hispanic American adolescents, combining behavioral skills for problem solving, coping, and interpersonal communication with emphasis on ethnic pride. A meta-analysis by Bruvold (1993) discusses the relative effectiveness of four strategies to prevent smoking in adolescents—social reinforcement models are most effective, followed by affective education and alternatives approaches, with the pure information approach being least effective.

Influenceability and conformity reach their maximum around the ages of 9 to 12 and then decrease. Snyder and Rouse (1992) note that one can target audiences for AIDS messages based on the audience's perceived self-risk levels. For example, people who deny their risk for AIDS require more personally relevant messages with safe-sex strategies. People who are gamblers regarding AIDS risks need messages stressing the need for consistency in safe-sex behaviors and their fear of nonmonogamous sexual styles. People who panick need rational messages from trusted peers and

I. The First Dimension

respected (expert) sources. For the unthreatened who accurately assess their own low risk level, communications about AIDS should try to mobilize them to reach other people with the preventive message.

Channel factors refer to the various media by which messages are sent. These include printed forms (books, pamphlets), visual forms (TV, advertisements), and auditory forms (radio, personal conversation—especially with "opinion leaders," persons who filter information through to others). Obviously, some of these forms are more pertinent to certain audiences at certain times, such as the best time slot for TV (8:00 p.m. to 11:00 p.m., with large, heterogeneous audiences) or radio (the a.m. and p.m. commuter hours from 5:30 a.m. to 10:00 a.m., and 3:00 p.m. to 7:00 p.m., which have the largest and most heterogeneous audiences).

The art of designing a social action program is to align the elements from the major factors of source, receiver, message and channel in the optimal fashion, considering projected costs, benefits, and feasibility—all viewed in the context of the subject matter of the program. There are many forms of social influence, including education and propaganda, imitation, and induced compliance or conformity. These employ various strategies, from giving information, to arousing emotions as stimuli to action, and from providing models for problem solving to controlling punishments and rewards for the performance of defined or normative actions. They all have in common the intention of making changes in cognition, affects, or behaviors of targeted individuals or persons in certain social roles (Dorfman & Wallack, 1993).

Let me use McGuire's (1968, 1984) communication model in connection with an ecological-behavioral approach by Geller (1990) to address drunk-driving prevention. The scope of this problem is enormous: In 1985, about 43,800 people in the United States died in traffic accidents and 3.5 million others were injured; the estimated cost to the nation was approximately $69.5 billion in 1984. Two factors have been identified as contributing most to vehicle crashes: an excess of alcohol consumption and a deficit in the use of safety belts. Alcohol contributed to about half of all fatal vehicle accidents in 1985; more than half of all fatalities and 65% of all injuries could have been prevented by the use of safety belts. But driving-and-drinking continues, and the use of safety belts, even with state mandatory use laws, is less than 50%. Thus we have a significant problem requiring changes in individual behavior. How might this problem be approached through attitude change methods?

In Lewin's (1951) picturesque terms, attitude change involves unfreezing of one attitude set, moving it to another region of the person's life space or giving it a different value (say, from positive to negative), and then refreezing the more socially adaptive attitude set in place. The factors we have to work with from McGuire's (1968, 1984) model include the source of the attitude change message, the message itself, the nature of the receiver, and various channel factors. Let's look at some of the many innovative projects that Geller has conducted using these concepts.

In one study (Thyer & Geller, 1987), small stickers (1.5×2.5 in.) with the printed message "Safety Belt Use Required in This Vehicle" were attached on the passenger-side dashboard by 24 graduate students who kept track of belt use. In a 2-week baseline period, the mean use was 34%. For the 2 weeks with the sticker in place, use increased to 70%. When the stickers were removed, use dropped to 41%; a later replacement of the stickers engendered mean seat belt use of 78%. This simple ABAB single-system design permits the inference that the presence of the sticker caused at least part of the buckling-up behavior. Let's analyze this project: The source of the message was obviously the driver or owner of the car, the graduate student. The message was instructional, not fear oriented, but neither was it informational. Presumably, its presence announced the "rule of the vehicle." The receivers of the message were presumably young adult friends of the graduate students. The channel was the inside automobile space where the sticker was immediately visible to the passenger during daylight. At night, a light went on in the car, making it possible to read the sticker, although visibility was reduced. The continuing presence of the sticker is another factor to be considered. One can imagine how Thyer and Geller might have strengthened this project—by making the sticker larger and more visible, by changing the message to a stronger or more passionate plea to buckle up, by having the driver engage the passenger in a conversation about the sticker, and so forth. Each of these suggestions is a variant of one or more of the communication ingredients from the McGuire (1968, 1984) model.

Geller and his colleagues have engaged in a variety of other ingenious projects for the purpose of increasing use of seat belts. In one project, Geller (Thyer, Geller, Williams, & Purcell, 1987) had students "flash" vehicle occupants as their vehicles exited parking lots at a university campus; the flash read, "Please Buckle Up—I Care." Seat belt use more than doubled. In another project, Geller handed out 3×5 in. cards to airline pilots or flight attendants requesting that they make an announcement to the effect that, "Now that you have worn a seat belt for the safest part of your trip, the flight crew would like to remind you to buckle up during your ground transportation." Geller reports receiving cooperation from some airlines, although one distributed a memo to its staff specifying that they should ignore the request of the professor from Virginia Tech with the blue card.

Geller and his colleagues have provided educational programs in corporate settings that tripled safety belt use among blue-collar workers (Geller & Hahn, 1984). They monitored seat belt use on TV and circulated petitions that obtained 50,000 signatures from 36 different states requesting that popular stars be shown using seat belts. (Geller was invited to Hollywood to give a safety belt workshop to writers, producers, and TV stars for his efforts.) Geller and his colleagues conducted large-scale investigations at his college campus in which buckle-up pledge cards were given out. Signing the cards implied a commitment to buckle up for the whole semester. A portion of this pledge card could be detached as a slip for a raffle from prizes donated by local merchants.

In all these clever ways of unfreezing attitudes, moving, and refreezing, one can see sensitive use of the source of the message (e.g., the flight staff of an airplane), the message (e.g., it is the rule of this car that passengers use seat belts), the receiver (e.g., taking a public stand to commit oneself to use seat belts, seeking positive reinforcement in the raffle), and the channel (e.g., stickers, flash cards, verbal announcements). In each case, it would be possible not only to suggest how to increase the strength of the attitude change message, but also to determine at what cost and with what effect. Attitude-change methods require fine-tuning to fit given audiences at given times (Hawkins et al., 1991). It is not easy to change attitudes. See Walther (1986) on trying to change attitudes regarding wife abuse, Roosa and Christopher (1990) regarding sexual abstinence, or Katz (1960) on the ego-defensive functions of attitudes.

Ordinary social communication skills use the same factors. A skillful communicator makes the best use of himself or herself as the source, selects the message to be sent with care, varies the medium through which this message is delivered, and is attentive to the attributes of his or her audience— all to the end of communicating more effectively. People must learn these skills to be socially effective; these skills may be taught both promotively and as rehabilitation for people with social deficits (Gordon, 1970; Satir, 1983; Schinke & Gilchrist, 1984; Stark, Campbell, & Brinkerhoff, 1990).

2. Moral Reasoning,
Values Clarification, Character Education

People, everywhere, throughout history, have socialized their children so that the youngsters could eventually take their place as good citizens of their nation. This singular goal has been accomplished to a greater or lesser degree by various means. When social problems emerge and families appear not able to perform this task unaided, other institutions—schools, churches, or businesses—come forth to contribute to this socialization process.

An important part of socialization involves the instilling of morality—a set of ideas about right and wrong actions within one's society. Morality seeks to regulate people's relationships with one another and the behaviors that promote survival of the whole group. In this section, I survey three approaches to helping children experience moral development; I briefly mention the first two and focus in more detail on the third.

Industrialist Robert Owen (1771-1858) is well known for his reformations, beginning with the working conditions of his cotton mills and extending to the villages he set up for his workers and their families. He was guided by his philosophy that a person's social environment strongly influences his or her character. In his mill town, Owen rebuilt the social and physical environment to shape character. He built new housing for his workers and set up nursery schools (the first ever) where children played with real tools, not toys. He instituted adult education for workers and employed trained teachers (another innovation). He established a central store where quality foods and goods could be purchased at discount (a food cooperative principle for which he is an acknowledged innovator). He set up workmen's insurance systems and decreed shorter working hours and the removal of child workers from the mills (a radical idea at the time). He removed all forms of punishment in the community but manipulated the environment for paternalistic ends (e.g., he gave prizes and public praise for clean homes at a weekly voluntary inspection). In general, Owen created various social arrangements to encourage sobriety, industry, and civil contentment. Owen came to the United States to set up a utopia at New Harmony, Indiana, but it proved to be unmanageable. He achieved all this while making a handsome profit. He might have spread his reform gospel even further, except that he eschewed organized religion and estranged himself from the political powers (Butt, 1971; Morton, 1969).

I mention Owen as an introduction to an unrelated social movement 100 years later called *character education* that involved some Owen-like ideas that a planned social environment can help form a person's character. Specifically, this involved a set of methods to enhance "moral character" by the teaching of specific values (such as honesty and responsibility) through school methods such as class discussion, role-playing, games, and written exercises (Edelman & Goldstein, 1981; Zimmerman, 1983, pp. 225-226). Critics found that teaching these specific values amounted to indoctrination—although this is probably not the only indoctrination that goes on in schools.

An additional criticism of character education is that children were not aided to decide between conflicting values. This same problem, which can be termed *the relativity of values,* plagued another major movement in teaching moral development called *values clarification.* The approach also took place in a school setting where students were aided to problem solve by acquiring, clarifying, and applying their personal values to situations involving moral conflicts. Values clarification argues that values are relative to person, time, and place and thus values are essentially personal choices (Edelman & Goldstein, 1981, pp. 273-275). Zimmerman (1983, pp. 227) notes that teachers merely stimulate students to examine and clarify their own values—without challenging their inadequacies or their inconsistencies. Maintaining a "value-free" stance, the supporters of values clarification are in fact imposing a value—value relativity (Cooper, Munger, & Ravlin, 1980; Zimmerman, 1983, pp. 227-228; see Lockwood, 1978, for a critical review of values clarification).

The third approach to moral development has an elaborate and coherent theory and an empirically based method by which *moral reasoning—* the label for this approach—can be facilitated in schools and elsewhere. Kohlberg and his colleagues developed this model, which rejects the value relativity and the indoctrination aspect of the other two approaches. I will summarize Kohlberg's (1981, 1983, 1987) discussion.

Contemporary society is much conflicted about moral education, that is, how children should be taught the rules to decide between right and wrong actions in specific situations. One school of thought (the romantics, such as Neill, 1960) suggests that we need to let the inner good in children unfold and let the inner bad be allowed to be brought under control through an unconflictful and permissive environment, which will foster healthy development. We cannot and should not impose any values on children, except nonviolence toward others sharing this special environment. Kohlberg seems to be suggesting that this is the philosophical basis of values clarification.

A second school of thought, *cultural transmission,* views education as the communicating of culturally given knowledge and values from the past to the present generation. Whereas the romantic school is child centered and stresses the freedom of each unique child, the cultural transmission school is society centered and stresses the need for children to learn the rules of the established social order, usually by means of a strongly ordered curriculum (Kohlberg, 1981). Kohlberg seems to be suggesting this as the philosophical basis of character education.

The third type of educational ideology is called *progressivism* (after Dewey's pragmatic educational philosophy). Education is seen as "the work of supplying the conditions which will enable the psychical functions, as they successively arise, to mature and pass into higher functions in the freest and fullest manner" (Dewey & McLellan, 1895/1964, p. 207). This psychological development occurs by means of problem-solving experiences that challenge the child to develop both cognitively and emotionally. Children acquire moral rules as an active change in patterns of response to problematic social situations, not through the learning of culturally accepted rules in the abstract (Kohlberg, 1981, p. 54).

Kohlberg (1981) adopts Dewey's position in his cognitive-developmental theory of moralization. The important assumptions Kohlberg makes for his theory include the following:

1. There is a culturally universal invariant sequence of stages in moral judgment. Kohlberg (1981) cites his own research program in a half dozen countries (pp. 24-25), with people of different races (p. 111), religions (p. 25), and social classes (p. 111), to support this cultural universality assumption (see also Kurtines & Gewirtz, 1984, 1991; Zimmerman, 1983).

2. The sequential progression represents movement from a less adequate to a more adequate psychological state (Kohlberg, 1981, p. 85). Kohlberg assumes that children prefer thinking at the next higher moral or logical stage to thinking at their own stage or lower ones. This is what energizes people to move up in the moral stages. Kohlberg believes people reason at different levels at any given time. In a normal curve, the major area under the curve represents the primary mode of reasoning; the two tails of the curve represent the fact that people occasionally reason above or below this predominant stage of moral reasoning. Being aware of the

higher stage of moral reasoning may pull the individual into making this his or her preferred mode. This assumption of the attraction of the next higher moral level is essential to Kohlberg's theory. Under normal conditions, irreversible upward movement is normative, although a person need not achieve the highest stage (Arbuthnot, 1992).

3. Kohlberg's (1981) model focuses on the form of thinking, not the content; that is, Kohlberg is concerned with how one thinks or the reasoning process, not what one thinks per se (see also Shure & Spivak, 1988). The stages of moral reasoning that constitute the heart of Kohlberg's model are made up of different logical forms, each qualitatively different from the others.

4. Kohlberg (1981), like Dewey and Piaget before him, disavows the value-free or every-value-equal-to-every-other position (value relativism). A hierarchy of values is embodied in Kohlberg's three levels (six stages, two within each level). Each stage is a "structured whole," a total way of thinking that is not linked to particular contents of thought. (This is why the stages are viewed as universal—the contents may differ but the form of thinking stays the same.) Kohlberg identifies justice as the basic moral principle (p. 175) because it is obligatory and categorical and takes precedence over other considerations (such as law or welfare). Justice is content-free in the sense that it simply states that principles should be impartially applied to all (p. 176).

5. Kohlberg (1981) distinguishes between development in cognitive and in moral stages. Cognitive stages are more general and so a person has to move through (Piagetian) cognitive stages to be able to move through parallel moral stages. One must be cognitively mature to reason morally but one could be smart and yet not reason morally (p. 138). Yet Kohlberg asserts that psychological theory and normative ethical theory are isomorphic or parallel enterprises on the grounds that "the formal psychological developmental criteria of differentiation and integration, of structural equilibrium, map into the formal moral criteria of prescriptiveness and universality" (p. 180). For Kohlberg, the truth of this assertion lies in the fruits of predictions stemming from this parallelism—and Kohlberg has been successful in showing he can change moral judgments through his challenge method. Moral conflicts stimulate the person to experiment with alternative ways of reasoning, of which the higher forms are more satisfying. It is this assumption that offers a method to promote higher stages of moral reasoning.

Table 2.1 presents a summary of Kohlberg's (1981) six stages of moral reasoning by providing brief descriptions of the formal properties of the

Table 2.1 Six Stages of Moral Reasoning

Level A: Preconventional Level (Moral judgments made in accordance with Piaget's preoperational stage of cognitive skills)

    Stage 1: Punishment and Obedience—"Right" is obeying rules and authority (who are viewed only as having superior power over one), avoiding punishment, and not doing physical damage to people or property for egocentric reasons exclusively. The point of view of the other party or parties is not considered.

    Stage 2: Individual Instrumental Purpose and Exchange—"Right" is serving one's own needs and another person's needs insofar as a fair deal for a concrete and immediate exchange of benefits can be had—"you scratch my back and I will scratch yours." The point of view of other parties is recognized but also that it may be in conflict with one's own. "Right" is relative and must be negotiated through instrumental exchanges of services or through fairness, with each person getting the same amount.

Level B: Conventional Level (Moral judgments made in accordance with cognitive skills developed after the Piagetian period of concrete operations begins)

    Stage 3: Conformity through Mutual Interpersonal Expectations and Relationships—"Right" is playing one's role according to the expectations of others (and eventually, according to one's own expectations) by living up to rules just as one expects others to do toward oneself. (A golden rule limited to specific others, not people in general.) The point of view of specific others is central, so that shared agreements and expectations take precedent over individual interests.

    Stage 4: Social System and Conscience Maintenance—"Right" is doing one's duty by upholding the laws and order of society so as to maintain the welfare and survival of the group or society as a whole. The individual takes unto himself or herself this sense of duty (acting on the basis of conscience or one's own self-respect). The point of view of the system (society) is central, taking precedent over individual or interpersonal interests.

(continued)

I. The First Dimension

stages and how they characteristically act. Table 2.1 also includes the parallel Piagetian cognitive stages, beginning at the period of concrete operations, starting at about age 7, and running through about age 11.

The literature contains some interesting examples of Kohlberg's (1981) model of moral education as applied in treatment contexts (see Arbuthnot, 1992, on enhancing moral reasoning among antisocial youth). Let me

Table 2.1 Six Stages of Moral Reasoning (Continued)

Level C: Postconventional and Principled Moral Choices (Moral judgments made in accordance with cognitive skills developed after Piaget's formal operations period begins)

Stage 5: Social Contract—"Right" is making moral decisions based on principles that are (or would be) agreed to by all people (who are party to the social contract) in a fair society. One shows respect for the rights of family, friends, work associates, and others as part of this social contract. The individual is concerned that laws and duties are based on a rational calculation of overall utility—"the greatest good for the greatest number." Persons at this level find it difficult to reconcile the conflicts between the moral and the legal points of view.

Stage 6: Universal Ethical Principles—"Right" is following a universal ethical principle that all humanity should follow. Particular laws are valid because they rest on these principles—such as the equality of human rights, respect for the dignity of human beings as individuals, and treating humans always as ends, not means. When laws violate such principles, one acts in accordance with the basic principles of justice (as in principled civil disobedience).

SOURCE: Kohlberg (1981, pp. 408-412).

offer a brief heuristic example regarding the prevention of sexually transmitted diseases in adolescents. The basic strategy using Kohlberg's model is to direct a communication/action program at a youth corresponding to his or her level of moral reasoning, usually in some peer group context in which the participating youths are at different moral levels. The discussion of either case material or real moral conflicts should ideally proceed at about half the level where the client is and half in the next higher stage. The discussants must become thoroughly involved for optimal effect. Some theorists believe that the social context, a just community of equal members participating in question defining and decision making, most facilitates moral development (Arbuthnot, 1992; Higgins, 1991).

Level A: Preconventional

Stage 1: Punishment-Reward. Convey information that engaging in unprotected sexual activities will lead to outcomes that are detrimental to oneself—pain, sickness, sterility, and, in case of AIDS, death. (This information should be personalized, as in the cognitive-behavioral model described in Chapter 1.)

Stage 2: Interpersonal Instrumental Behavior. Convey personalized information that sexual activities must involve both protection and fun for self and other—"You satisfy my sexual desires and I'll satisfy yours; you protect my health and I'll protect yours."

Level B: Conventional

Stage 3: Conformity to Mutual Interpersonal Expectations. Convey personalized information that sexual activities require one to be concerned about one's partner and living up to that partner's expectation of being nice ("good boy," "good girl"). "I will do unto you as I would have you do unto me in regard to safe sex."

Stage 4: Social System and Conscience Maintenance. Convey personalized information that one should do one's duty regarding safe sexual practices toward one's partner for the sake of the group and society. This is what one's conscience (having taken into oneself the values of one's family, neighbors, and culture) tells one to do.

Level C: Postconventional

Stage 5: Social Contract. Convey personalized information that everyone agrees that safe sex is the right way to act for the good of society and for the partners involved. This not only shows respect for the partner but is for the greatest good for everyone.

Stage 6: Universal Ethical Principles. Convey personalized information that all sexual acts should involve equality between the persons involved—one should not merely be a means only for the other's satisfaction, but sexual acts, like all others, should be conducted in respect for the partner's intrinsic value as a human being, an end in himself or herself.

These abstract statements would then be used as guides to a specific interventive program, starting at the highest level of moral discussion the individual has attained.

I. The First Dimension

It should be noted that this theory has been criticized on many grounds, including that it may be relevant only to (instrumental-oriented) males because females take as their highest value the notion of caring, not an abstract justice (Gilligan, 1982). Others note that it is hard to replicate Kohlberg's (1981) research because of the measurement tools and of faults in the model itself. This theory has proved to be a heuristic for other research, however, and thus permits testing of its conceptual network and value assumptions (Arbuthnot, 1992; Hay, 1994).

3. Instigation of Hope, Promotion of Optimism

Hope is a little-studied phenomenon (Peterson & Bossio, 1991) but it is omnipresent in the real world and thus must be considered as a method in relation to preventing individual problems and promoting individual goals. In the common language sense, hope adds a sense of confidence to the mere wish that something desired will happen. In looking at the world through "rose-colored glasses," one is massaging reality (Munoz, Snowden, & Kelly, 1979), not denying the obvious problems of reality (Taylor & Brown, 1988) but looking at reality in a particular way that is self-satisfying and possibly helpful to some degree.

When hope is combined with action, a separate term, *optimism,* can be used to emphasize this difference. Seligman's (1991) important programmatic studies in helplessness and optimism share the adjective *learned*—meaning that in some significant way, people may contribute to their own feelings of helplessness and optimism. As I discussed earlier in this chapter, learned helplessness is a general giving-up reaction that follows from the belief that whatever one does won't achieve the desired goal, whereas learned optimism is the opposite reaction (Seligman, 1991). In fact, Seligman offers only negative definitions of optimism, such as a set of skills on how to talk to oneself when one suffers a setback. It is possible to offer a positive definition of optimism based on Seligman's theory and research, however: Optimism is a style of engaging or adapting to the situation that follows from the belief that what one does can have the effect of achieving one's desired goal or making the possibility of achieving that goal more likely.

A longitudinal study by Peterson, Seligman, and Vaillant (1988) explored the style of explanations of bad events in a group of 99 men at age 25. The authors found, overall, that men who used optimistic explanations for bad events at this age were healthier later in life than men who used pessimistic explanations for the same events. The relationship peaked at age 45 and fell off somewhat by age 60.

Scheier et al. (1989) report similar findings regarding the beneficial effects of optimism among bypass surgery patients. Optimism (defined by responses in the Life Orientation Test) was associated with making a better recovery 6 months later, which included return to work and resumed recreational, social, and sexual activities. (Connect these findings with the discussion of anticipatory instruction [this chapter, I.A.4], where knowing the worst is combined with hoping for the best.)

Seligman (1991) cites a large number of studies and stories that support the concepts of learned helplessness and learned optimism. Some of these are correlational studies; there is a lingering question as to the nature of the phenomena involved and the direction of causality: Exactly what is learned optimism? Do healthy people become optimistic or does optimism cause health? Or is the relationship reciprocal and complex, possibly involving other factors not yet identified? Studies are needed to continue to untangle the threads of this important concept; in the meantime, it is certainly worth experimenting with strategies for promoting hope and optimism. To add to the mystery, read Cousins's (1979) amazing recovery from a severe illness.

The constructionist perspective offers a rationale for hope or optimism as having causal efficacy. As one perceives the world in a way one wants it to be, the individual moves toward helping to construct that world so as to achieve that objective—to the extent that he or she can affect it. One's expectations set an expectation in others about that objective and they respond to initiatives as if they were self-fulfilling prophecies. People's responses to one's actions further act to confirm the movement toward the hoped-for event, and so the circle of reciprocal expectations continues. (This may be one basis for the effectiveness of assertive actions. See section E.2 in this chapter.)

Hope does not occur in isolation. Ripple and her colleagues (1964) describe a study employing a Hope/Discomfort Ratio, which suggested that clients had to have a sufficient degree of both discomfort and hope for effective outcomes—discomfort to make them want to change the problem and hope to provide the direction and aspiration for that change. If either were missing, the client did not do as well in attaining the goals.

The limit of hope may be expressed in the folk expression "hope against hope," that is, wishing for an objective even in the face of expectations

Table 2.2 Dimensions of Cognition

Dimension	Pessimists	Optimists
a. Permanence	Habitually believe that bad events will last a long time	Habitually believe that defeats are temporary setbacks
b. Pervasiveness	Believe that bad events will undermine everything they do	Believe that the causes are confined to this one situation
c. Personalize	Believe that they are at fault in causing the bad event	Believe that the defeat is not their fault

SOURCE: Adapted from Seligman (1991).

that it is very unlikely to occur. This may be a one-in-a-million shot, but at least it is not "hopeless." Such hope keeps alive the efforts of the individual and others to achieve some goal. Even if we fail, there is the satisfaction that we did all that we could do to the end. Keeping hope is keeping the faith, a sharing that transcends any one loss.

No-hope situations, like learned helplessness, usually result in inactivity—little effort to accomplish one's objectives. It may be that giving up hope speeds the terminal processes, which under difficult conditions may be a relief from suffering. Discussions of euthanasia do not have much place in a book on primary prevention, except to say that voluntary euthanasia seems to involve substituting a positive although negating goal (seeking to die) for another negative although life-affirming goal (relief from intractable pain). Attaining one's freely chosen goal, negative or positive, may be our ultimate freedom and hence an ultimate human value (Downing & Smoker, 1986; Hathaway & Pargament, 1991).

In summarizing this section, I would like to present a brief adaptation of Seligman's (1991) methods of promoting learned optimism, expanding my earlier discussion:

1. There are three dimensions of explanatory styles—that is, the cognitive structures, which mediate challenges of the external world and one's behaviors in dealing with the challenges. In effect, Seligman (1991) identifies two types of explanatory styles, the pessimistic and the optimistic, each of which is defined in terms of three dimensions of cognition, as shown in Table 2.2.

2. Two other factors strongly influence optimism, especially in children: being depressed (which is probably associated with pessimism) and having bad events really happen (this is independent of our cognitive images of ourselves and our world). For depression, cognitive therapies (Beck, 1984; Ellis, 1974) seem to be satisfactory; they follow the steps described below for promoting optimism. Bad events (death of parent or sibling, divorce, relocation of family) are usually out of the hands of people; nonetheless, everyone must adapt to them. Again, a social-cognitive approach seems the best available (see Stolberg, 1988, on prevention programs for divorcing families). Life is a mixture of events and personal styles; the point of learned optimism is to move forward to promote a desired orientation to life.

When a bad event occurs, an optimist characteristically employs an explanatory style—that is, a cognitive mind-set—in which he or she thinks the bad event is temporary, limited to this given event, and with many possible causes other than himself or herself. This explanatory style saves the person from stress and mobilizes energy toward constructive goals in this situation. In the face of a bad event, a pessimist characteristically thinks it is permanent and pervasive and he or she is personally at fault—an explanatory style that leads to destructive actions, a kind of self-fulfilling negative prophecy.

When a good event occurs, an optimist characteristically thinks it is permanent and pervasive and he or she had a personal hand in causing the outcome. Again, this explanatory style provides an advantage for the optimist. On the other hand, a pessimist believes the good event is temporary, limited, and caused by something other than his or her own actions. This likely leads to destructive actions.

3. Given the possibilities of depression and major untoward events, the core strategy for optimistic adaptation follows an ABC4DE model (note the differences between this and Ellis's, 1985, similarly named therapy model):

A = Adversity (some bad event occurs, such as a bad grade on a test or being called a bad name by peers)

B = Belief (the explanatory style—either the pessimistic or the optimistic cognitive style as described above, using the three dimensions of permanence, pervasiveness, and personalization)

C = Consequence (either some negative emotion one feels about oneself regarding the bad event or some positive emotion regarding that event)

D1 = Distract (stopping negative thoughts [see Chapter 3, II.A.3], break out of the negative mind-set)

D2 = Dispute the factual evidence of the situation; vigorously seek alternative interpretations—this is the heart of the method by which one interprets a situation as being temporary, limited to this one case, and with many possible causes

D3 = Distance oneself from the pessimistic orientation—beliefs are not necessarily facts (or the full story)

D4 = Decatastrophize—the implications are rarely as dire as pessimists believe

E = Energize oneself toward the optimistic orientation; persevere in this optimistic belief; make the most of one's talents and situational resources; optimism is a self-fulfilling prophecy because it constructs and creates the reality that one seeks—to the extent that it is possible to bring about that goal

C. Behavioral and Skill Aspects

1. Learning Theories

It will be helpful to review briefly some general learning principles that may be useful in the discussion of all three applications to primary prevention—operant, respondent, and social learning (Bandura, 1986; Skinner, 1953; Wolpe, 1958).

Learning refers to the relatively stable changes that occur in a person's behavior that take place in the course of psychosocial experiences and are not produced by genetic or chemical causes. Kanfer and Phillips (1970) distinguish several components of the psychosocial experience that become points of preventive intervention. My modified Kanfer and Phillips formula states that stimuli (S) act on the individual (I), who responds (R) and thus receives contingent (K) consequences (C), which start the cycle all over again, that is, the consequences become the new stimuli. Thus the formula S-I-R-K-C will enable one to locate the emphases that different learning theorists make of this process. The Pavlovian or respondent conditioning focuses on the first three symbols, the Skinnerian or operant learning emphasizes the last three, and the social learning considers all these elements, especially the role of social models and the cognitive processes of the individual.

The stimuli (S) can be external social or physical events, or internal thoughts, feelings, or tissue changes of which the individual may be unaware. (This means that the individual may be the stimulus for his or her own change by means of future "hopes" and "goals" that initiate actions thought to lead to those ends. Likewise, biochemical changes unknown to the individual may impel that person toward seeking food, sex, or sleep.)

The individual (I) is viewed developmentally, even though behaviorist theorists do not put forward a universal stage conception of human development (Thyer, 1992). The person's life experiences produce quantitative and qualitative changes in that individual, reflecting the unique set of stimuli and consequences. So the meaning of stimuli differs for people at different ages or at the same age with different life experiences. The response (R) refers to externally visible actions, internal thoughts, and feelings that are reported by the person concerned or physiological changes of which the person may or may not be aware.

The terms *consequence* and *contingency* are related. A consequence (C) is the response the world makes to one's own responses. A person who raises her hand at an auction has *ipso facto* made a bid on that antique vase. A person who raises his hand in class will likely be called on. This leads to Skinner's (1953) fundamental idea of a reinforcer, a consequence that makes the preceding response more likely to recur.

A more complex form of consequence is called *rule-governed behavior*. This occurs when reinforcement happens over many instances. The pattern among these instances is learned. For instance, if one has followed instructions and positive outcomes have transpired, then one learns the pattern or rule in these series of experiences. The individual eventually learns that following instructions per se leads to desired outcomes. This provides a basis for certain kinds of moral and social behavior, which are essentially rule-governed behaviors (Thyer, 1992).

The contingency (K) is the pattern of the relationship between one's response and the consequence. One pattern is called *continuous*—every time a person raises her hand at an auction after everyone else has stopped raising theirs, those antique vases are hers. Another pattern is called *intermittent*—sometimes when a person raises his hand in class he will be called on but not always (depending on how many others have done so for a particular question). The intermittency may be based on regular sequences (for example, the teacher calls on the person every other time) or based on an irregular sequence (the teacher calls on people in no particular order for no apparent reason). Or the intermittency may be based on a timed sequence (the individual is called on every 10 minutes whether or not he has his hand up at the time).

The behaviorists note that all one can do with behavior is to increase it, decrease it, or keep it at about the same level. This fundamental, if arid, statement directs all behavioral interventions: There are two basic ways to increase behavior and three to decrease it. Increasing behavior can be accomplished by positive reinforcement and negative reinforcement. Decreasing behavior can be made to occur through positive punishment, negative punishment, and extinction.

Positive reinforcement is any consequence that follows a response such that the response is made more likely to recur. Nothing is intrinsically reinforcing, so one must wait and see how the person responds, but generally speaking, pleasant stimuli (candy, compliments, attention) act as positive reinforcers.

Negative reinforcement involves the removal of an unpleasant stimulus if a desired behavior increases. (A mother will stop nagging her son if he cleans his room.)

Behavior can be decreased, according to the behavioral model, if *positive punishment* (or an *aversive* consequence) is used—that is, an unpleasant stimulus is presented if an undesired behavior is exhibited—or *negative punishment* (or *response cost*) is employed—that is, a desired stimulus is removed when the person performs some undesired behavior. (Every time a child leaves her room a mess, it will cost her some of her free time to stay home to clean it up.) A final way to decrease a targeted behavior is by extinction, which involves the removal of any consequence to an undesired behavior. One instance of *extinction* is a "time-out" procedure, in which the offending individual is removed from the presence of others for a short time to cool off. Neither positive nor negative consequences occur to the person in time out, and the behavior in question stops for lack of any kind of response from others. (Not giving an aversive response means that none of the negative concomitants of punishments occur—the individual exhibits brief compliance and possibly returns to the offending behavior when surveillance is removed. See Goldstein, 1983; Swizer, Deal, & Bailen, 1977.)

To apply the learning model to primary prevention, one must distinguish two actions that eventually have to be performed in tandem: predicted problems to be prevented and goals to be promoted. I will modify the conventional steps in behavior modification (Gambrill, Thomas, & Carter, 1971) to fit this primary prevention context, as shown in Table 2.3.

Table 2.3 Steps in Behavior Modification

A *Targets (Undesired Events)* *to Be Prevented*	B *Goals (Desired Events)* *to Be Promoted*
1. Identify events in the present situation that are viewed as leading to a predictable problem. This is the preproblem state.	1. Identify desired goals that currently do not exist. If possible, select goals that are alternatives to the existing (preproblem) states and are incompatible with them.

2. Functionally analyze the probable controlling conditions that will likely lead to the preventable problem:
    Who are involved?
    What are they doing?
    To whom? Where and when?
    This involves looking at antecedent, concurrent, and consequent events related to that predictable problem: What consequences reinforce this undesired train of events? How can one plan to change these consequences?
	2. Functionally analyze the probable controlling conditions that will likely lead to the desired goal:
	    Who are involved?
	    What are they doing?
	    To whom? Where and when?
	    This involves looking at antecedent, concurrent, and consequent events related to the desired goal: What events would encourage this desired goal to emerge? How can one plan to bring about these change conditions?

3. Act so as to prevent the predicted problem (A2). Also, conduct concurrent monitoring.	3. Act so as to promote the desired goal (B2). Also conduct concurrent monitoring.

4. Match the results and the objectives, both the prevention of the predicted problem and the enhancement of the desired alternative, so as to know when the primary prevention services can be terminated.

5. Maintain a successful preventive or promotive effort, which often involves activating the natural reinforcers of the desired set of events (and the natural inhibitors of the undesired set of events that have been prevented) so that the overall outcome can be maintained after the helping professionals have left the scene.

Each of the columns in Table 2.3 can be read separately, but the spirit of primary prevention is to combine columns—not only to prevent an untoward event but also to promote a desired one in its place. These are two separate sets of activities, but they are dovetailed in that the alternative events of the one may be the main events of the other.

Examples abound. Consider the parents of a 2-year-old who is showing signs of throwing temper tantrums. This is a predictable problem for some 2-year-olds, for which a diversionary behavior, such as getting the child to listen to a story, is an alternative goal. Or consider the parents of a young child who is being encouraged to become interested in reading. The parents are spending large amounts of time reading to the child, including when the child is being unruly, which diverts the child's attention toward more sociable directions. Now imagine that these two examples are about the same parents and child. This joint prevention and promotion is a more complete form of primary prevention and succeeds not only in preventing a predictable problem but also in promoting a positive objective that is incompatible with the problem.

So pervasive is positive reinforcement that almost every example provided thus far employs some kind of reward for desired preventive behavior and probably a kind of extinction of undesired ones. Positive punishment is rarely used in primary prevention. Behavior modifiers have an axiom of practice that can be used in primary prevention as well: Catch the client behaving in the desired manner and reinforce that behavior. This includes behaviors that are even slightly in the desired direction—people can't be dissolute all the time. The empirical research on the thousands of examples of behavior modification studies is generally very positive and offers much for primary prevention.

Respondent or classical conditioning (see Pavlov) is not nearly as commonly used in primary prevention as are operant or social learning models, but there are some interesting examples, such as the study by Early (1968), who applied classical conditioning to influence classmate behavior toward social isolates (children that the others did not choose as someone they wanted to sit near). By pairing positive words such as *funny* and *friendly* with the isolates, under the guise of a memory test, Early found that the conditioning produced positive responses toward the isolates by their peers, as well as improved social behaviors by the isolates themselves.

Table 2.4 Risk of HIV Infection for Heterosexual Intercourse in the United States

Risk Category of Partner	One Sexual Encounter Risks Contracting AIDS	500 Sexual Encounters Risk Contracting AIDS
HIV seronegative, no history of high-risk behavior, using condoms	1 in 5 billion	1 in 11 million
HIV serostatus unknown, not in any high-risk group, not using condoms	1 in 5 million	1 in 16,000
HIV serostatus unknown, in high-risk group, not using condoms	1 in 50,000	1 in 160
HIV seropositive, not using condoms	1 in 500	2 in 3

SOURCE: Hulley and Hearst (1989, p. 63).

With regard to examples of social learning theory or social cognitive theory (Bandura, 1986), again many of the exemplars in primary prevention employ this model to guide their practice, from svelte exercise trainers helping their gravity-challenged clients, to a sweater-wearing president urging his fellow citizens to conserve energy by dressing more warmly. See Appendix B for an overview of the social cognitive model and associated references.

One final example illustrates the combination of learning principles applied to promoting AIDS-risk reducing behaviors (Catania et al., 1994; Coates, 1990). That people knowingly engage in life-threatening behavior is not new; the assumption is that the payoff is preferable to the threat, even among persons who are intelligent and well informed. But with AIDS, the odds are quite clear. Hulley and Hearst (1989) offer the estimates of risk of HIV infection for heterosexual intercourse in the United States in Table 2.4.

These data tell us that the greater number of sexual encounters with high-risk status partners (i.e., homosexual men, intravenous drug users, blood product recipients, heterosexual partners of infected individuals, and newborn infants of infected women)—with or without using condoms—the greater the chance one has of contracting the AIDS virus. These authors propose the following behaviors to reduce the risk of HIV infection, in decreasing order of priority:

- Avoid sexual intercourse, even with condoms, if partner is HIV positive.
- Choose a partner who has no high-risk behaviors, past or present.
- Test for HIV antibodies when in doubt of HIV status.
- Employ measures that reduce risk: use condoms with spermicidal cream; avoid anal intercourse; avoid sexual intercourse if genital lesions are present. (p. 65)

One of the more successful programs to prevent AIDS occurred in San Francisco's gay community. Many interventions were introduced, although not all with adequate evaluation. Let's look briefly at these programs from the lens of behavior decision making described above.

The events viewed as leading predictably to AIDS are unprotected sex, particularly anal sex, with multiple partners in places involving casual encounters (where protective devices and orientation might be lacking). The desired goals were various behavior changes alternative to the pre-problem ones and incompatible with them, such as protected sex with few partners in locations where safer sex is supported. The functional analysis of these preproblem and desired goals identified who was doing what with whom, along with the important preventive axiom that the desired alternative to be substituted for the preproblem behavior must be equally (although perhaps differently) reinforcing and that the partners must know this and be motivated to act on this knowledge.

The prevention program was active along many fronts, involving advocating major role models, enlisting the support of settings where gay people gathered, providing candid and direct information, and emphasizing the equal but alternative joys of safer sex. The social context (the gay community in this case) was supportive of the change, rather than forcing individuals to break ranks to act in a protective manner. Provision of resources (condoms) and instructions on their effective use was widespread. (The Swiss, who have the highest rates of AIDS in Europe, originated a condom distribution plan that emphasized "hot rubbers," eroticizing what were ordinarily dull wrappers; see Kapila & Pye, 1992. Also, Switzerland was the first nation to mail a candid information booklet on AIDS to every household, an action later copied by many other nations.) Positive feedback was provided to reinforce the continuing desired actions further.

Results appeared to show significant reductions in risky behavior as the gay community took up the change as part of its own survival. In due time, rates of venereal diseases in general decreased, as did the rate of those testing HIV positive. Recent reports of younger gay people, who are not yet part of that gay community, beginning the cycle of unprotected sex, however, mean that other forms of incentives must be devised to provide the kinds of reinforcements to engage in safer sexual behaviors (see Bandura, 1989a; Catania et al., 1994, on prevention of AIDS).

2. Social Skills Training

Two broad categories of skills training are pertinent to these discussions. One involves social or life skills training, which is illustrated in the work of Schinke and Gilchrist (1984; see also Botvin & Tortu, 1988; Patrick & Minish, 1985). The other broad area involves physical skills that are needed in going through everyday life—sewing a loose button, fixing a dripping faucet, putting up storm windows, and the like. Social or life skills require one set of experiences; physical skills demand another.

Both kinds of skills fall within the domain of primary prevention, but for different reasons. Life skills enable one to maneuver effectively through the social waters, avoiding conflicts and obtaining one's fair share of the good things of life. Physical skills enable one to deal with the physical environment as it supports human growth and development and to make life a little more comfortable and convenient. Obviously, there is some overlap (see Young & Adams, 1984, on the development of social and physical skills in 4-H club members), but it is useful to contrast them.

In calling attention to the six major components of Schinke and Gilchrist's (1984) life skills training program, I will be mainly reminding readers of what I have already discussed (or anticipating topics in later chapters). It is the combination of these components that makes up the life skills training model. As such, this discussion also fits in what I will later call holistic or multifactor approaches to primary prevention. Here are the six components:

1. Information: Schinke and Gilchrist (1984) focus on adolescents but their point is applicable to any age group. People are in need of information relevant to their life pursuits. Such information must be age appropriate and individualized. I discussed the general educational mode earlier in this chapter (I.A.1) and the need to individualize any educational effort as described in Schinke et al. (1979). Professionals in primary prevention

need to learn how to communicate in a wide variety of forms and how to make use of repetition, simplification, and dramatization to get their message heard and remembered. (See also Chapter 2, I.B.1, attitude change; Chapter 4, III.D.3, mass media; Blum, 1983; Cole & Cole, 1983).

2. Problem-solving skills: Schinke and Gilchrist (1984) suggest that training in basic problem solving will enable people to make their way through the inevitable tangle of social events by anticipating consequences of multiple possible behaviors that can be used to accomplish some objective. This topic is discussed in Chapter 2, I.A.2. (See also Shure & Spivak, 1988; Srebnik & Elias, 1993.)

3. Coping: Schinke and Gilchrist (1984) note that coping adaptively requires people to anticipate and prepare for stressful situations. I add that dealing with strens (i.e., strengthening situations) also requires coping skills. By coping openly and rationally, people may not only be effective in the social world but also reflect on their mastery experience, which adds to their sense of self-efficacy when it comes time to deal with new challenges (see Chapter 2, I.A.5, coping; Chapter 2, I.E.1, self-efficacy).

4. Communication: By communication, Schinke and Gilchrist (1984) mean the full range of verbal and nonverbal exchanges of information presumed necessary in effective adaptation. I discussed this in the section on attitude change (Chapter 2, I.B.1), with reference to McGuire's (1968, 1984) communication model and interpersonal communication (Englander-Golden, Elconin, & Satir, 1986; Gordon, 1970). Professionals are trained in active listening skills (Bloom, 1990); the point is to provide training to clients in these same skills for active listening because these skills are useful in every social interaction.

5. Self-instruction: Schinke and Gilchrist (1984) describe self-instruction as "verbal mediation through covert instructions to oneself" (p. 15). This permits internal control over one's behavior (i.e., by one's private speech to oneself). I will discuss this topic more fully in Chapter 3, II.A.3, on self-instructional training, but the practices promoting optimism share some of these self-instructional ingredients (see Chapter 2, I.B.3, hope and optimism).

6. Support systems: The last component of Schinke and Gilchrist's (1984) model involves social groups that are presumed to mediate life stresses and to facilitate growth-enhancing experiences. These topics are discussed in Chapters 4 and 5 (see also Deering, 1993; Srebnik & Elias, 1993).

The important point in calling attention to the Schinke and Gilchrist (1984) model and to its empirical study (Kirkham & Schilling, 1990) is that although individual components can be successfully implemented, one must also consider the combination of components for a more effective outcome. This is another restatement of the configural equation described in Chapter 1.

To take an example, consider how one might aid an adolescent seeking his or her first job (thus without prior direct work experiences). Such a promotive project would involve (a) providing the youth with information about the job market, (b) communicating with the teenager about objectives for working but also modeling how to listen actively and present oneself assertively, (c) teaching problem solving in the sense of trying to figure out what the job calls for and being able to demonstrate relevant talents and experiences, (d) providing instructions on reminding oneself how to present oneself and how to respond to interrogations, (e) teaching how to cope with possible setbacks, and (f) providing a support group to facilitate role-playing experiences or to provide succor for given outcomes. Each discrete portion of the job-hunting experience has some specific trainable skills, but these pieces are best seen as coordinated into a whole package of skills training. Such a life skills model is applicable to a wide range of developmental circumstances (Azrin & Besalel, 1980).

I want to address the question of systemic learning of a whole complex set of instructions. Ivey and Authier (1978) present a technique called *microcounseling* that might be applicable here. In microcounseling, the complex learning task is broken down into discrete components—such as the various tasks involved in successful interviewing, like posture, eye contact, and reflecting feeling and content. Then each component or natural set of components is specifically taught. The sequencing of these lessons involves practicing all the preceding lessons as one approaches a new assignment. Thus by the end of the program, all the pieces are learned to identified criterion levels; they are further learned (overlearned) in the context of one another. This microcounseling approach could be applied to a set of primary prevention practices within a configural context. Each component would have to be defined specifically in terms of what constitutes satisfactory performance. Then sets of components would have to be trained in the context of one another. This contextual learning may impose strains that learning a given component separately does not produce. But contextual learning is exactly what living is all about. Step by step, additional prevention practices are combined until the whole set of them can be activated effectively at one time. The art of training involves constructing the most effective order and combination in teaching the parts so as to achieve mastery of the whole.

Another approach to complex learning is borrowed from Bandura's (1986) social learning model. This calls for the learner to observe others similar to himself or herself doing the whole complex set of behaviors in a context similar to the learner's. This provides the learner with a full moving picture, a holistic learning experience where the pieces are already combined in a life situation. Then, working backward, the learner can master each component while having in his or her mind's eye how this component fits into the whole. Having this overview makes putting the components together easier to do (see Chapter 7).

With regard to the second major type of skills training, that of physical skills, few guidelines or documented procedures exist. A host of examples enable me to offer some beginning statements, however. For instance, where do children learn how to change light bulbs, fix a running toilet, or build shelves for a closet? They learn such skills by watching adults do these things and by being given apprentice-like experiences. Sometimes these experiences may come at school through ordinary instruction, but mostly they are learned informally and without much fanfare. They may not be learned, however, if opportunities or teachers are not available. The not-knowing becomes a predictable problem. Here are some beginning principles:

1. All people with at least ordinary levels of intelligence and physical dexterity can master any physical skill if they have appropriate training experiences combined with a healthy self-efficacy regarding needed physical skills (Bandura, 1986). Putting a shelf in a closet requires some beginning skills with a tape measure, screwdriver, and the like. These skills will be combined in a new way for the shelf-installing challenge, especially if the learner has seen how a "master builder" has done such a job before.

2. The apprentice must be enabled to learn how to perform the activity, either vicariously or directly, including receiving corrective feedback regarding the actions constituting the skill (or set of skills). Not every nuance will be picked up in ordinary observational learning; the student must be aided to focus on critical steps in the process.

3. Depending on the task and the level of competency of the learner, the teacher may provide some cognitive context of understanding for the

actions. These become skill principles—such as always making three measured marks on a piece of wood to ensure that the cutting line will be straight. Otherwise, the learning is by rote and may be limited in generalizability.

4. The student must be exposed to some practice experiences or the vicarious learning will dissipate. The more practice, the more facile the individual will become in dealing with these and like situations. Indeed, problem solving may become an enjoyable experience in its own right, a challenge that motivates the do-it-yourself project person, although necessity is another driver of the application of physical skills. Trial and error is another method, but it is slower, more painful, and more wasteful in comparison with apprenticing experiences.

Being able to master the ordinary challenges of everyday life provides a foundation for advanced skills as well as a sense of self-efficacy and self-esteem. To paraphrase an old saying, a society that neglects the teaching of either social skills or physical skills is likely to have people whose relationships and houses don't stand up to the tests of time.

D. Physiological and Biological Aspects

1. Nutrition

People need certain amounts of nutrients on a regular basis to protect them against diseases, to sustain health, and to enable them to engage the opportunities in life. Hunting and gathering for these supplies have given way to shopping in grocery stores for the majority of Americans, yet the task of obtaining necessary nutritional elements—not too little, nor too much, in an optimal manner—has evaded many (Agras et al., 1989). Poverty means that the nutritional needs of large numbers of people require special support, such as the food stamp program aiding 25 million Americans (in 1992), school breakfast and lunch programs, and food services for the elderly (Ellis & Roe, 1993) and other special groups. Children who are not fed appropriately are less alert, more prone to sickness, and do not learn well (Birch, 1972; Birch & Gussow, 1970). Adults experience similar problems (Chernoff & Lipschitz, 1988).

Obesity has its hazards (Forster, Jeffery, Schmid, & Kramer, 1988; Jeffery et al., 1993; Striegel-Moore & Rodin, 1985; Stunkard et al., 1985).

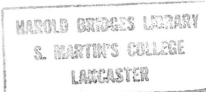

Former Surgeon General C. Everett Koop has established a campaign called "Shape Up America!" to encourage the more than 30% of the population who exceed desired weight standards to lose weight (starting with small weight losses of 5 to 15 pounds) and to exercise more (beginning with 15 minutes of walking a day increasing gradually to near capacity exercising at least three times a week). Burros (1994) quotes the former surgeon general that 300,000 deaths a year are caused by obesity, which means disproportionately heavier use of the health care services by overweight people.

Americans have been subjected to dietary recommendations of a questionable nature for more than a century (Goldstein, 1992), but in the past 25 years, important advances have been made in understanding the relationship between diet and health (Institute of Medicine, 1991) and lifestyle (U.S. Department of Agriculture and U.S. Department of Health and Human Services, 1990). There are three major challenges for nutritionists as honest health promoters:

- What kinds or groups of foods should we be eating?—the challenge of dietary guidelines
- How much of these foods should we be eating?—the challenge of the food guide pyramid
- What is in each food that is healthful or not healthful?—the challenge of food labeling

Let's look at each in turn for its current status and preventive or promotive efforts.

Dietary Guidelines

Dietary guidelines provide the most general directions for how to eat so as to be reasonably healthy, assuming that "we are what we eat," meaning that if one eats healthful foods (and exercises and deals with stress), then one is likely to be healthy. Obviously, health is not that simple for everyone at each life stage, but the assumption is useful as a point of departure.

I report here the dietary guidelines for Americans from the U.S. Department of Agriculture and U.S. Department of Health and Human Services (1990), augmented by recommendations of the Surgeon General of the United States (1988), indicated by square brackets. I will add some further observations, indicated by parentheses, that will connect diet with other lifestyle activities:

1. Eat a variety of foods.
2. Maintain healthy weight. (Balance food intake and physical activity to maintain appropriate body weight.)
3. Choose a diet low in fat, saturated fat, and cholesterol. (The intake of fat and cholesterol can be reduced by substituting fish, poultry without skin, lean meats, and low- or nonfat dairy products for fatty meats and whole-milk dairy products; by choosing more vegetables, fruits, cereals, and legumes; and by limiting oils, fats, egg yolks, and fried and other fatty foods.)
4. Choose a diet with plenty of vegetables, fruits, and grain products. [Increase consumption of whole grain foods and cereal products, vegetables (including dried beans and peas) and fruits.]
5. Use sugars only in moderation. [Those who are particularly vulnerable to dental caries (cavities), especially children, should limit their consumption and frequency of use of foods high in sugars.]
6. Use salt and sodium only in moderation.
7. Drink alcoholic beverages only in moderation. [No more than two drinks a day, if at all. Avoid drinking any alcohol before or while driving, operating machinery, taking medications, or engaging in any other activity requiring judgment. Avoid drinking alcohol while pregnant.]

These few fundamental principles are as abstract as they are important. Ordinary shoppers need more help in selecting and preparing foods, which leads to the second challenge (Rogers et al., 1994).

Food Guide Pyramid

After considerable struggle among interest groups on how to present the idea of how many of what kinds of foods to have each day, the government produced a food pyramid that visually and through words describes six major food choices. At the top of the pyramid—its smallest unit—are fats, oils, and sweets, to be used sparingly. The next layer of the pyramid has two sections, each involving 2 to 3 servings a day of (a) milk, yogurt, and cheeses and (b) meat, poultry, fish, dry beans, eggs, and nuts of all types. The third layer involves still larger numbers of servings each day: (a) the vegetable group, with 3 to 5 servings a day and (b) the fruit group, with 2 to 4 servings a day. The base of the pyramid, with 6 to 11 servings a day, consists of bread, cereal, rice, and pasta.

I. The First Dimension

Table 2.5 How Often to Eat Certain Types of Food

Food Group	Eat Often	Eat Sometimes	Eat Seldom (Small Amounts)
Proteins	Chicken breast (without skin)	Chicken drumstick, thigh, breast with skin	Fried chicken thigh, wing with skin
Milk	1% low-fat milk products	2% low-fat milk products	Processed cheese, soft or hard whole milk cheese
Fruits and vegetables	All fresh fruits and vegetables (except ones listed in other columns)	Dried or canned fruit in own juice	Pickles, coconut, potatoes, au gratin or scalloped
Grains	Whole-grain breads and hot cereals, rice, bulgur, air-popped popcorn, pasta	Muffins, heavily sweetened pancakes, waffles, egg breads	Donuts, Danish pastries, buttered popcorn

This is helpful, as many people recognize food groups and can modify their behaviors accordingly. Various groups have taken this food pyramid a step further by noting that some foods may be used often, sometimes, or rarely ("Are You Eating Right?" 1992; *Nutrition Action Health Letter,* 1995). Table 2.5 provides an example of how often to eat certain types of food.

Food Labeling

Merely having a pattern of foods that "are good for you," "sometimes OK for you," and that you should "eat only once in a long while" is only part of the problem of disseminating information on nutrition. "Natural" or "low fat" must be defined and regulated so that consumers can have a better chance of knowing what they are buying ("Better Food Labels—At Last," 1993; Rudd & Glanz, 1990). Groups with special nutritional needs require additional strategies for coping with the flood of commercialism in marketing foods. (See Archer, 1989, regarding persons with AIDS, and Venters, 1989, regarding a family-oriented approach to preventing heart disease.)

Needs such as these led to the Nutrition Labeling and Education Act of 1990. Consumers now can get important information at the point of purchase as the basis for selecting among brands as well as types of food in relation to percentage of daily requirements (for a 2,000 calorie diet). Specially indicated are the critical features in one's diet: the total calories a food provides and the percentage of these calories that comes from fat. Saturated fat (the bad kind) is distinguished from total fat. Cholesterol and sodium (salt) are indicated, as are total carbohydrates (further distinguished in terms of dietary fiber and sugars) and protein—all these in terms of percentage of daily requirements (for the 2,000 calorie diet). Major vitamins and minerals are also indicated. This is an enormous amount of information that is to be connected with one's overall needs and resources.

However helpful all these major dietary changes have been, there is still the underlying question of how to get ordinary shoppers to use this information wisely in planning and preparing their "daily bread." Zarkin, Dean, Mauskopf, and Williams (1993) make some projections on the potential health benefits of these nutrition label changes over the next 20 years and present a range of 40,000 to 1.2 million life-years gained, either end of the scale being an enormous public health benefit at relatively low cost. Whether or not these labels are used, and used wisely, remains to be studied. Experience with alcohol warning labels for adolescents does not show substantial changes in behavior 1 year after they appeared on bottles, according to research by MacKinnon, Pentz, and Stacy (1993). Innovative delivery of nutrition messages may be needed (Barratt et al., 1994; Gomel, Oldenburg, Simpson, & Owen, 1993).

2. Lifelong Exercise

Lifelong exercise regimens are simultaneously preventive, protective, and promotive (Berger, 1983/1984, 1986; Berlin & Colditz, 1990). Exercise involves exerting pressure on muscles to make them work harder and thus become capable of harder work. Muscle mass increases with exercise; continuous exercise is required to maintain that mass. All forms of motion against resistance constitute *exercise,* but the term is usually restricted to intentional and repetitive movements in certain sectors of the body. Exercise in the sense of movement against resistance occurs throughout life, but the activity must reach a certain threshold before growth occurs.

Modern society has many pressures toward inactivity, with cars to take the place of walking, convenience machines to take the place of housework, and industrial equipment to take the place of physical labor. Few are willing to give up these modern devices, so the challenge of exercise is to find enjoyable ways of moving one's muscles against resistance beyond the critical threshold and to continue to do so frequently on a regular basis so as to benefit from its contributions. For example, vigorous regular exercise is said to reduce the chance of having a heart attack by 35%, which is more than the 30% reduction attributed to stopping smoking (Goldstein, 1992, p. 88). Exercise also is said to reduce the severity of such an attack among middle-aged and older individuals (Biegel, 1984). Smith (1988) describes studies showing that exercise prevents bone atrophy. Moreover, exercise is said to reduce psychological tensions; deVries and Adams (1972) demonstrated that walking 15 minutes (with a heart rate of 100 beats per minute) has the same effect in reducing tension as a tranquilizer (meprobamate). And inevitably, exercise is said to enable older people to have sex lives like those of younger people—claims that have been made for over 100 years (Goldstein, 1992).

Despite the faddish nature of some of these claims, there appears to be reasonable evidence to support them, and current medical policy is to endorse exercise for persons of all ages. A multibillion dollar industry has grown up around these exercise programs. Even though only a small fraction of people who buy exercise machines, clothing, and shoes actually use them for their intended purpose, exercise is here to stay. I will try to sort out the lean strategy statements from the fat.

Mayer (1975) notes that lack of physical activity is the major factor explaining obesity, another unwelcome by-product of modern living styles. Intensive physical activities have the effect of decreasing body fat, which results in the increase of muscular tissue (see Burros, 1994).

Biegel (1984) describes research supporting the positive relationship between physical fitness and mental achievement for any given level of intelligence. The research also notes that regular exercise, in combination with other good living habits—such as a balanced diet, not smoking, and getting adequate sleep—can help increase life expectancy by as much as 11 years for men and 7 years for women.

The combination of good muscle tone, reduction in tensions, knowledge of beneficial health effects of exercise, and closer approximation of culturally supported height and weight norms should be linked to improved self-image (Katlin & Goldband, 1980). Positive self-concept, in turn, may be linked with better interpersonal relationships. The major message from all these sources is exercise as if your life depended on it, but enjoy exercise over your lifetime. Regular exercise regularly leads to a synergistic effect physically, mentally, and socially.

Given this background, a number of principles guide exercise programs. The following statements are adapted from Biegel (1984) and Haskell (1985) to be relevant for people of all ages:

1. Exercise must be within the person's current capacity, without great discomfort. The person should be urged to exert beyond the present range of physical skill, but not so much so as to be dangerous or harmful. The cliche "use it or lose it" may be needed for peak athletic achievements but is definitely inappropriate for maintaining good health (Haskell, 1985, p. 121).

2. Exercises should be planned as a group and should provide progressive exertion of muscles to develop strength and endurance. This progression may be composed of increasing intensity of the activity or increasing duration at the same level of effort. Each change is made after the body adapts to the previous demands made on it. Knowledge is available on exercising specific groups of muscles at a time.

3. All exercises should involve a warming-up period—rhythmic activity of muscle systems to be exercised and increasing intensity to the tolerance range, that is, the range where the existing level of physical fitness meets the next higher level of demand.

4. Periods of vigorous activity should be alternated with periods of lesser activity. Higher levels of physical fitness involve increased proportions of vigorous exercises compared to lesser activities. There should be a brief cooling-down period.

5. There are limits of physical fitness. Olympian levels are for few people; optimal levels are relevant to everyone. What is optimal depends on personal potentials. Norms are often suggested (e.g., RAF exercises). These norms become goals to be approximated over time with regular and progressive steps that challenge the body and mind to work a little harder. This optimal level achieves the best working order of the physical portion of the human being. An individual's natural limits must be honored; exceeding them for long may be detrimental.

6. There is a psychological dimension to physical exercise that enables people to initiate and maintain a lifelong exercise program (the "healthy

mind in a healthy body" ideal). There are psychological limits that the individual (and his or her coach or physician) needs to recognize and honor. Progressive experiences will aid the individual in recognizing both physical and psychological limits. The emphasis in lifelong exercise is not on outer limits of skill and endurance as much as on continuous and enjoyable exercise of the body as partner to a healthy mind and a vital soul.

7. Adherence to the regimen in these progressive exercises is difficult in the face of the many alternatives of contemporary life. Past experiences with exercise influence self-efficacy, which in turn encourages continuing adherence. Exercise program characteristics may also improve the rates of adherence (Arnold, 1981; Haskell, 1985).

8. Safety factors should be observed in all exercises to reduce accidents and injuries. For example, orthopedic injuries in joggers are very common and costly. Care should be taken in selecting appropriate supportive equipment and in learning what one's body can and cannot do (Goldstein, 1992).

Various kinds of exercises and sports activities have been rated as to their contributions to promoting fitness. Many are useful in promoting fitness but differ in what facilities or accessories are needed. Overall, walking may be the best form of exercise because it costs nothing (but time), can be done in all weather, and requires no accessories (except shoes that are good for walking, i.e., that support the foot appropriately).

The highest cluster of activities in terms of contributing to physical fitness (cardiorespiratory endurance, muscular endurance, muscular strength, flexibility, and balance) are jogging, bicycling, swimming, skating (ice or roller), handball (squash), skiing (cross-country or downhill), basketball, tennis, calisthenics, and walking. (Golf, softball, and bowling contribute less than half as much to physical fitness as those just mentioned.) The same pattern exists for exercises contributing to general well-being (weight control, digestion, and sleep).

Not mentioned on this list is dancing, which can also be a good exercise because it involves a continuous movement of large muscle groups in the body. Creative movement, as in a program for the aged involving a variety of movement activities often accompanied by music that is designed to encourage spontaneity and self-and-body awareness within a social setting, is widely used in nursing homes and senior centers. Likewise, "arm-chair exercises" are helpful for those with severe limits of physical strength and agility. A person seated comfortably in a chair is instructed to wave or bend his or her hand, arm, foot, leg, or other body part in various short sequences, producing a pleasing and stimulating motion. Sometimes these exercises are accompanied by music or participation in imaginary situations (conducting an orchestra) to sustain motivation.

The overall questions are how to embed exercise within an ordinary schedule of daily routines and how to keep it there year in and year out. Exercise is enjoyably self-reinforcing in that it improves muscle tone and self-image. Like other significant activities, it belongs as part of everyone's everyday routine, individualized to fit the person's situation and family situation (Venters, 1989) or when traveling (Weinhouse, 1987).

In recent times, exercise has become chic, with stylish clothes, expensive exercise facilities, and personal testimonials. One should not minimize the commercialization and popularization of lifelong exercise; it may be the necessary ingredient to keep people moving energetically and happily throughout their whole lives. In fact, primary prevention may have much to learn from the success of this area for applications to less compelling methods and areas. (See Danish, 1983, and Danish et al., 1990, 1993, on the role of sports in competency and development.)

In closing this topic, I want to cast a dark shadow that applies to every area of primary prevention: If health-promotive activities are so good and so much fun, why don't all people engage in these wonderful activities all the time? This is a complex question, similar to the one Weinstein (1987, 1989) addresses—how to understand and encourage self-protective and promotive behaviors. Motivations are complex. Certainly the preventive and promotive message is a strong one but competing messages and pressures are often stronger. The siren call of the fast-food industry, the couch potato syndrome, and messages that evoke the response "Don't tell me there is something else I like that I have to give up in order to be healthy" conspire to operate against lifelong exercise and other beneficial actions. My response to this general question is to ask whether enough of the configural components have been seriously considered in designing a primary prevention program. Our limitations of vision and energy probably interfere with understanding the full dynamic picture and making suitably full and dynamic programmatic responses. We must make healthy alternatives as appealing as their competitors, in addition to whatever contributions to health these may have.

I. The First Dimension

3. Immunization and Vaccination

People can become immune to certain diseases either by a natural process (*natural immunity*) or by an artificial means (*vaccination*). In each case, an infectious substance enters the body, which reacts to this substance by producing antibodies that attack and destroy it. In natural immunity, that infectious substance might be a disease such as measles, in which case the person gets the symptoms of measles and also produces the antibodies that eventually destroy the measles. The person is left with the antibodies that will destroy any future invasion of measles before any symptoms occur. In vaccinations, a dead or harmless form of the infectious disease is introduced into the body. Antibodies are formed but with few if any symptoms of the disease itself. Vaccinations leave the person with protective antibodies should he or she experience a future invasion of the disease.

Some of the most thrilling developments in medicine have come in the form of vaccinations for fatal diseases such as smallpox, poliomyelitis, and diphtheria. Smallpox has been wiped out for all practical purposes through the use of vaccination; most other major infectious diseases are now within control given suitable inoculations of children. New vaccinations are being developed that, like the old ones, will strengthen the individual to defend himself or herself against certain diseases.

But diseases return when societies let their guard down (Albritton, 1978) or under new circumstances, such as seen in the rise of tuberculosis in the face of the AIDS epidemic and impoverished living conditions. Furthermore, protective vaccinations are more common in certain areas of society, whereas in others—usually poor inner-city areas—large numbers of children do not receive vaccinations (Hutchins et al., 1993). This is incredibly shortsighted on the part of decision makers, as the costs of caring for victims of disease are enormously higher than preventive care. Even when free vaccinations are available through public health auspices, there is often a lack of parallel educational efforts to encourage parents to make use of the resources (Stehr-Green et al., 1993; Vickery & Fries, 1980).

Table 2.6 portrays the common vaccinations and times to receive them. Preventive shots for the flu are also available, particularly for vulnerable people such as the elderly. Again the challenge is how to enable all persons in need to learn about the value of these preventive measures and to

Table 2.6 Common Vaccinations

Age	Vaccine
2 months	DTP (diphtheria, tetanus, and pertussis [whooping cough], poliomyelitis
4 months	DTP, poliomyelitis
6 months	DTP
15 months	Measles, mumps, and rubella (German measles)
18 months	DTP, poliomyelitis
4-6 years	DTP, poliomyelitis
14-16 years	DT (diphtheria and tetanus)

SOURCE: Kunz and Finkel (1987).

facilitate obtaining them in an effective manner. Travelers also need protective shots for certain diseases found in foreign lands that are not common to the United States (Weinhouse, 1987). The Centers for Disease Control has an information service that presents up-to-date information for travelers (for a recorded message, call 404-332-4565).

As Albritton (1978) points out, the measles immunization program in the United States is cost-effective: $1.00 in program costs gains $10.34 in program benefits, calculated from lives saved, retardation prevented, and school days and work years saved. But Albritton and others point out that diseases move in cycles, both in terms of building up epidemic levels and in the responses people give (or do not give) to them. We tend to grow lax when there is no epidemic, and we become hyperactive as the epidemic escalates. Public health workers have to figure out ways of institutionalizing immunization procedures so that they become passive events required of everyone, such as laws requiring immunization to attend school. Active strategies must also be applied, solving how to change people's attitudes and behaviors in the direction of seeking and obtaining timely immunizations. Currently, high proportions of inner-city youths lack basic immunizations, which puts them at a health risk, which affects their educational status, which affects their employment status, which affects their ability to pay taxes. Recognizing this vicious cycle is a benefit of the systems perspective, because the understanding may enable one to take preventive measures to break the cycle.

In suggesting principles for encouraging inoculations among at-risk populations, I will draw on the configural perspective because there are

I. The First Dimension

likely to be many factors pulling parents or guardians of children away from taking advantage of free inoculations:

1. Whenever possible, try to embed the inoculation program within a larger social context, such as requirements for entrance to kindergarten or Head Start programs. This legal or administrative action creates other gatekeepers for children's health in addition to parents and puts pressure on many persons to put forth the efforts to have children inoculated. The existence of laws does not guarantee compliance with the laws (Cummings, Pechacek, & Shopland, 1994; Rigotti, Stoto, Bierer, Rosen, & Schelling, 1993), but it does orient public thinking (see also Chapter 5, IV.D.3).

2. Assume that parents or guardians would be cooperative in getting their children inoculated if they had the relevant information, motivation, and support. The information must be delivered where the need exists, often in poor areas where good communication vehicles may be lacking. One example of sensitive communication is the use of videotapes in the waiting offices of public welfare, social security, and similar places where people wait to be served. Sensitive and lively media productions that are repeated may be a useful way of conveying information simply, through role models similar to the client population (see discussion on attitude change, this chapter, I.B.1). Pamphlets might be available to back up the videotape. Telephoned computer-generated reminders might also be useful (Stehr-Green et al., 1993). Local (ethnic) newspapers, church announcements, or neighborhood circulars might be other ways to communicate with relevant populations.

3. The information must be at the reading and comprehension level of the intended audience (Alcalay, Ghee, & Scrimshaw, 1993; Meade et al., 1994; Snyder & Rouse, 1992). It should be presented in a series, before the charted vaccination times emerge and again at the suggested time of vaccination. Such information may be included with other child-rearing materials, such as the Pelican series that provides developmental information from birth to school age (Kelly, 1982).

4. The information must be motivating, which means both not blaming parents who have been unable to have their children inoculated for various reasons and positively encouraging parents with regard to the action involved, the supports available, the benefits to the child, and so forth. Cultural meanings of inoculation must be incorporated into the

messages, including alleviating the fears an uneducated parent has with regard to injecting diseased materials into his or her young child. It may be helpful to have indigenous workers move through the community explaining the situation and the process to others based on their own experience with inoculations.

5. Parents who are impoverished economically may have hidden costs to having a child receive "free" shots, such as the costs of getting to the clinic, taking off work, or bringing along other children if child care is not available. Innovative ways of taking the clinic to the people may have to be used, such as traveling bus clinics or storefront clinics. Yet parents are the ultimate gatekeepers of their children's health and they must take responsibility for these actions. We are at the beginning of thinking on how to promote such responsibility. Social scientists must move ahead in this area before repressive authoritarian methods are used.

E. Holistic or Multifactor Approaches

1. Perceived Self-Efficacy

Bandura's (1986, 1989a) social cognitive theory is presented in Appendix B and is discussed at different places throughout this book, but in this section, I want to emphasize one idea, *perceived self-efficacy,* as an example of a master concept that brings together many personal and interpersonal aspects that permit a fuller understanding of human behavior, particularly in the context of primary prevention.

To provide some background, I first must distinguish self-efficacy from self-esteem. Carl Rogers, writing over a half century from the 1930s to the 1980s, emphasized the self as the concept that provides the core to understanding human behavior. What is the nature of human nature? Rogers envisioned people as experiencing several basic forces: the tendency toward self-actualization, the countertendency to have conditions of worth imposed by significant others onto the self, and the resulting struggle of becoming what one has the potential to be. Central to this argument is the development of the self-concept, an awareness of one's own physical and psychosocial being and functioning, particularly in relation to others' views of this self and the values that are attached to these perceptions (Meador & Rogers, 1984, p. 158). Rogers not only developed this conceptual model over time, but he also constructed ways to measure change in the self during therapy. He also added considerably to training the professional self to be genuine, accurately empathic, and to hold unconditional positive regard for the client. These tenets have become the core of every helping professional practice.

Yet Rogers's view of the self was very global. Rogers's therapeutic methods of encouraging the natural tendencies of the individual to unfold through an encouraging but benign environment appeared to limit his interest in the use of specific active ingredients of the self and how to affect those aspects in a preventive or promotive way. Indeed, except for a global sense of the goal of a self-actualizing individual, Rogers's work is little used in primary prevention (Mecca, Smelser, & Vasconcellos, 1989).

On the other hand, Bandura's (1986, 1989a, 1989b) theories address the same issues on the nature of human nature but provide the conceptual tools for a proactive primary prevention. Bandura's initial interests in learning theory focused on the role of the stimulus model and what individuals could learn directly or vicariously from that social stimulus. More recently, he has refocused his interests on the human agent and, in particular, on the role of that person's perceived self-efficacy, which is the person's perception of his or her own ability to perform a specific action (not a global sense of self or self-esteem). These self-efficacy beliefs may be self-aiding or self-hindering as people go about their daily activities. In effect, people predict how events will transpire for them and what part they personally play in negotiating these events successfully (see Seligman, 1975, 1991, on learned helplessness and learned optimism; Chapter 2, I.B.3). As Bandura (1989a) writes,

> [People] who have a high sense of efficacy visualize success scenarios that provide positive guides for performance. Those who judge themselves as inefficacious are more inclined to visualize failure scenarios that undermine performance by dwelling on how things will go wrong. (p. 1176)

Self-efficacy beliefs influence levels of motivation, as reflected in what people choose to do, how much effort they exert, and how long they persevere in some endeavor. Bandura (1989a) remarks on Gertrude Stein's invincible self-efficacy that allowed her to continue submitting poems to editors for 20 years before one was finally accepted. The muses frequently work overtime for people who have a strong sense of self-efficacy.

Perceived self-efficacy also influences people's selection of environments, such as avoiding situations and activities believed to exceed their coping capacities (Bandura, 1989a). Research has indicated that self-efficacy beliefs affect career decisions; the more efficacious people judge themselves to be, the wider the range of career options they consider open to them and the better they prepare themselves educationally for these different occupations (Bandura, 1989a; Betz & Hackett, 1986; Lent & Hackett, 1987).

Bandura (1989a) notes that people use forethought as a way of adapting to the environment. This constitutes purposive behavior and the setting of goals. This is like Rogers's position on free will—people can influence their futures. But unlike Rogers's theory, Bandura's triadic formula of person, environment, and behavior means that free will is limited by the environment or, rather, is expressed in interaction with the forces exerted by the environment. Thus as with the configural equation, Bandura identifies the reciprocal determinism of the person (i.e., cognitive and affective aspects), the person's behavior, and the environments in which these events transpire: Each affects and is affected by events from the other two components.

Bandura's conceptualization about influences of self-efficacy provides primary prevention with explicit directions for enriching this master concept. Self-knowledge about one's efficacy (accurate or not) is based on four sources of information, which become the four points of entry in helping to raise perceived self-efficacy:

1. Goal-attaining performances that are authentic and specific mastery experiences contribute greatly to perceived self-efficacy (Bandura, 1986, p. 399). A person's own efforts that accomplish goals in a given area raise that person's self-appraised efficacy, whereas repeated failures lower it. Thus the primary strategy is to create real success experiences in natural contexts. After a strong sense of self-efficacy is developed, occasional experiences of failure are not likely to change a strong positive sense of one's capabilities. There is no one-to-one correspondence between positive performance and perceived self-efficacy. Rather, self-efficacy is an inferential process weighing the contributions of one's ability and contextual matters. Through planned experiences, however, one can influence performance attainments; this becomes the key to strengthening self-efficacy. For example, school work can be constructed on a no-fail basis by

I. The First Dimension

dividing tasks into manageable competency-based units that accumulate to overall success on meaningful portions of work. (This was the basis of Skinner's, 1953, work on programmed learning—mastery and immediate feedback on small steps toward learning a complex task.)

2. Vicarious experiences of others performing successfully may increase one's own self-efficacy. One learns both how to do the action as a whole and whether or not certain behaviors are rewarded or punished. Vicarious learning is especially important in complex behaviors. Again, primary prevention has many possibilities for presenting vicarious experiences in meaningful ways, from the mass media (Maccoby & Altman, 1988) to positive peer group experiences (Kelly, St. Lawrence, Brasfield, & Hood, 1989; Schinke & Gilchrist, 1984).

3. Verbal persuasion from others that one has the requisite skills and knowledge increases self-efficacy but not as much as the previous two sources. As with communication, its effectiveness depends on the the message, the sender, the receiver, and the channel (McGuire, 1968). Thus, natural influencers, such as parents, peers, teachers, and employers, may be enlisted and trained in the lifetime effort of encouraging people to practice efficacious behaviors.

4. Reading one's state of physiological arousal may also lead to an increased sense of self-efficacy, as being "up" for the task. That is, one judges that one has the capabilities and the skill to accomplish the task based on internal feelings. Paralyzing feelings, however, whether or not they are accurate, may adversely affect one's perceived sense of efficacy, even though the task itself may be seen as highly important. (McAuley & Courneya, 1993, review the place of self-efficacy with regard to adherence to exercise and physical activity and offer suggestions to improve adherence using the Bandura model.)

Thus the concept of perceived self-efficacy combines a person's perception of cognitions, affect, and physiological states and behaviors in the context of some social task. In Bandura's (1989a, 1989b) theory, *self-efficacy* is a critical term influencing many outcomes. By planned influences of self-efficacy, one has a directive for producing desired outcomes in primary prevention. This is truly a case of helping the client help himself or herself. Four conceptual entrance points, and their combinations, exist by which to influence self-efficacy so that clients can be aided in preventing predictable problems and achieve desired goals. (For illustrated applications of the self-efficacy concept, see Bandura, 1989b; Chambliss & Murray,

1979; Flora & Thoresen, 1989; Lawrence & McLeroy, 1986; Lustig, 1994; Manning & Wright, 1983; McAuley & Courneya, 1993; Roper, 1991; Schilling et al., 1989, 1992.)

2. Assertiveness and Resistance Training

Assertive behavior is viewed as a golden mean between the extremes of aggressiveness and passivity (Bloom, Coburn, & Pearlman, 1975). Derived from a clinical tradition (Wolpe, 1958), assertive behavior has been applied to normal populations in community contexts. In terms of primary prevention, assertiveness training helps individuals become aware of their real thoughts and feelings and then communicate them directly, honestly, and appropriately so as to attain desired goals without infringing on the rights of others. Being assertive in justifiable situations means that people become able to rid themselves of self-defeating or overly antagonistic behaviors while adding to their own self-respect and some control over their lives. Thus assertiveness involves thoughts, feelings, and actions of one person vis-à-vis another person or persons. Because it involves three dimensions of the individual, I am including assertiveness training in this holistic or multidimensional category.

People, particularly women, are socialized into passive and dependent roles that carry the expectation that they should always put the interests of others ahead of their own interests (see Friedan, 1981; Osborn, 1991). At the same time, these women are expected to learn tricks such as coyness or pretended helplessness to get others to do as they wish without having to say so in direct language. These tricks preserve the passive-dependent role while obtaining some of the desired objectives. This results in a dishonest lifestyle that often diminishes the person's self-esteem beneath the social expectations of passive servitude. Women also learn to be sensitive and caring (Gilligan, 1982); these are desirable traits that should not be lost as one learns to assert one's real feelings and ideas (Bem, 1975/1985).

Consciousness raising is a phrase used in contexts in which oppressed people are aided to understand the nature of their oppressed circumstances, even when it involves fur-lined cages—these are still cages. Of course, oppression has many ruthless dimensions, particularly when it is embedded within the official laws of the land (Freire, 1990). Attempts to overcome oppression may be dangerous. As victims and facilitators meet together to examine ordinary life situations, they come to realize the nature of how commonly accepted patterns of life came to be. This sets the stage for making changes.

Assertiveness training is a particular form of dealing with personal and social oppression. Although it is not intrinsically a "women's issue," I will focus on women and children in this example. Assertiveness training goes beyond consciousness raising "by preparing women to act on what they recognize as problems" (Bloom et al., 1975, p. 17). All people, especially women in a sexist society, have the right to be treated with respect, to be listened to and taken seriously, to get what they pay for (including information from helping professionals), to set their own priorities, to make mistakes, and to say "no" without feeling guilty (Bloom et al., 1975).

Children and adolescents are in a similar bind in having to learn to say and do things that they would rather not do in deference to people with power over them. They may achieve one objective (e.g., staying on friendly terms with the other person) while losing another (e.g., sticking up for one's rights). These "games" people play are manipulative and self-dishonest attempts to gain short-term benefits while ultimately losing basic self-respect and self-control. For example, a friend might put pressure on a person to join her in drinking or shoplifting—with the implied or stated price of her friendship if the other refuses. The basic issue of assertiveness is how to say "no" when a person honestly wants to say "no" without breaking up the (presumably valued) friendship.

Englander-Golden and her colleagues (Englander-Golden, Elconin, Miller, & Schwarzkopf, 1986; Englander-Golden, Elconin, & Satir, 1986) have developed a role-play situation for 5th to 8th graders called Say It Straight (SIS). This school-based program teaches pupils to resist group pressures regarding alcohol and drugs through assertive/leveling communications (Satir, 1972, 1983). SIS training gives students the opportunity to explore reasons and feelings involved in situations when they have said "yes" to some request when they really wanted to say "no." Students employ Satir's (1972) body-sculpting techniques of creating postures that express feelings (such as getting on one's knees as one attempts to placate another) so as to get a vivid physical experience of what they are doing to themselves psychosocially. Then they learn through group interaction to be aware of their real feelings and to be sensitive to the feelings they invoke in others. Ultimately, they learn to make and communicate constructive decisions based on their true feelings given the realities of the social context.

The Englander-Golden research reveals some important points: Some ways of responding to other people's pressure plays lead to undesirable reactions. For example, changing the subject as a response to a friend's social pressure leads to anger and frustration in the receiver and feeling scared and stupid in the sender. (A: "Come over and smoke a joint with me." B: "Did you see that new program on TV?" A: "Yes, but are you going to come over?") Likewise, giving excuses results in feelings of powerlessness and low self-esteem in the sender; moreover, this kind of response is almost always followed by further pressures. Superreasonable responses often produced name calling in the receiver. (A: "Smoking causes cancer in rats." B: "I'm not a rat, you jerk." (Englander-Golden, Elconin, & Satir, 1986).

Only when these youngsters send or receive assertive leveling communications do they report feeling respect for themselves and the other person (Englander-Golden, Elconin, Miller, & Schwarzkopf, 1986; see also Evans & Raines, 1990; Hansen & Graham, 1991; Yates & Dowrick, 1991). Assertiveness training is also used with people who have aggressive tendencies (Huey & Rank, 1984). Note the parallels between assertive/leveling communications and the core professional interviewing skills of accurate empathy, warmth, and respect and genuineness that Rogers describes.

Results of the SIS training show positive prevention outcomes (lower alcohol-related and drug-related school suspensions), whether or not it is combined with other school prevention programs (Englander-Golden, Elconin, Miller, & Schwarzkopf, 1986).

Let me offer a brief summary of the basic ideas of assertiveness training that extend to many life situations:

1. One must come to understand the situation one is in, as to whether it is or is not a problem. Many women like being housewives and caretakers of their children (and elderly relatives). Other women do not find this fulfilling. However, no one can impose this decision on another person. Each must decide for himself or herself if a problem is present. Consciousness-raising groups or reading materials often supply relevant information.

2. If one accepts a given life situation as problematic, then the next issue is to decide whether or not to change it. Again, this is a personal

decision. One may choose to live with a difficult situation as the lesser of two evils. For example, to choose to be independent is risky and generates much anxiety for some. For others, the possibility creates positive excitement.

3. If one decides to make a change in some aspect of one's life, then one must analyze the forces that currently make this situation as it is to understand what has to be changed to make the situation better. There will be some positives as well as some negatives in the existing situation (e.g., some material protectiveness as well as some social put-downs and lack of self-respect). Some of the forces holding the problematic situation in place are of one's own making, such as irrational beliefs (e.g., "I have to be perfect; everyone must like me all the time"—these beliefs are irrational because the costs of attaining these impossible states far exceed the presumed benefits). People have been socialized to believe these ideas; they must now be trained to rethink them and change their views: "It would be nice if people liked me, but I neither can please everybody all the time nor want to spend my time that way" (Ellis, 1985).

4. Because nonassertiveness is self-perpetuating, people must find a way to break out of the cycle without bursting the social setting in which the events take place. Exercises in gradual assertive efforts are preferable to explosive outbursts that are likely to generate stiff resistance. Gradual assertive behaviors help the learner clarify legitimate requests, lower the anxiety one feels in making such changes, and state them clearly and honestly.

Bloom et al. (1975) offer a number of exercises in beginning assertive actions, such as imagining a successful assertion for a legitimate objective that doesn't violate the rights of others, sending covert messages of self-encouragement, and consciously relaxing so one can say what one feels. During the interaction with the other person, the assertive individual listens carefully and lets the other person know that he or she is heard and understood. In addition, the assertive person lets the other person know how she feels and what she wants. The assertive person must stick with this message, tactfully, without rancor, but firmly. The combined message and the medium of its delivery are the core of assertiveness. Here is a checklist guiding assertive actions (modified from Bloom et al., 1975, pp. 181-182):

1. Clarify the situation and focus on the issues. What is my goal and how do I want to accomplish it?

2. What do others do that sets up this situation, and what do I usually do to avoid asserting myself or trying to change it?
3. What are the costs and benefits of change? What would I give up and what would I gain by the change?
4. What is stopping me from asserting myself? If it is holding irrational beliefs, then what can I do to replace them with rational ones? If it is being culturally conditioned to perform certain roles in certain ways, what can I do to overcome this so that the needed activities get performed in some suitable way?
5. If I am anxious about asserting myself after a lifetime of not doing so, what can I do to reduce this anxiety (such as joining a support group or reading self-help books)?
6. Do I have all the relevant information I need about the situation—from all sides of the question? This involves listening to the other person's side and letting that person know I understand him or her, but also that I tell that person how I feel and what I want in this situation.
7. Act! Chances are that reasonable assertions will be responded to reasonably. But even if the reaction is hostile, recognize my own strengths and the rightness of my assertion. Practice with others helps make assertiveness smooth. The support of others makes the transition to an egalitarian life situation more bearable.

Social Resistance Training

Social resistance training is used in a variety of contexts, especially in connection with assertiveness training. It deserves explicit discussion because it expands one aspect of assertiveness to a distinctive tactic. For example, Botvin and Tortu (1988) are quite explicit in training youths to resist social influences aimed at getting them to drink, use drugs, or otherwise be involved in harming or harmful behaviors. They couch this resistance training in a Life Skills Training program that involves general social and problem-solving skills.

As developed by Evans and his colleagues over a long period of research (Evans et al., 1978; Evans & Raines, 1990), young persons are alerted to the social concern that they will soon face, such as being pressured to smoke or drink so as to be "part of the gang" or "grown-up" or to rattle the cage of adolescence. The real risks are discussed, but the emphasis is on making one's own choices and not being suckered or bullied into doing things one does not want to do. Training in knowing how social pressure works—either how mass advertising manipulates consumers (Davis, 1987) or how peer pressure works—supplies the young person with ways of resisting, if he or she so chooses. Knowing the general techniques of advertising renders these techniques less harmful. Knowing what one's friends may urge one to do enables one to anticipate and practice methods of responding in advance (Englander-Golden, Elconin, & Satir, 1986). Thus resistance training involves some anticipatory socialization, some basic education, and some social skills training, all in the context of learning how to make mature choices that get the person what he or she wants without offending others in the process.

Elder et al. (1993) describe a longitudinal study in the prevention of tobacco use among junior high students that involved refusal skill training. This training was combined with other prevention methods and was delivered by college undergraduates in a variety of ways, including one-to-one telephone calls and classroom interventions. Results over 3 years were both favorable and cost-effective. Research by Ellickson, Bell, and McGuigan (1993), however, included a skills training component in resisting drugs; after 6 years, these authors found no difference between the experimental and the control groups. A number of major differences between these two studies could account for the opposite results; I mention them only to emphasize that every method must be evaluated within its own context; one cannot assume success because a method has been successful elsewhere.

1. Resistance training generally takes place in group contexts, mobilizing group norms involving collective and public information about the kinds of pressures to which individuals and groups will be subjected.

2. Resistance training reinforces the value position of self-choice rather than victimization by social pressure. This is a content-free value position; it simply asserts that the individual has the right to make this decision free of unwanted social pressure. Role-play enables young people to experience the kinds of tactics that bullies and others might use and how the young person can defend himself or herself. Group brainstorming is helpful here, both for ideas and for the social support to resist pressure.

3. Resistance training offers the opportunity for the maturing of personal values, such as regarding the nature of friendship (involving sharing of feelings and ideas, not the forcing of actions). Again, seeing humane values expressed in groups provides the opportunity for young people to move ahead in their moral development (Kohlberg, 1981).

4. Resistance training helps young people recognize the need to say no or yes, as they themselves wish, while at the same time maintaining contact with

people whom they value as friends. As the research of Englander-Golden and colleagues (Englander-Golden, Elconin, Miller, & Schwarzkopf, 1986; Englander-Golden, Elconin, & Satir, 1986) shows, there are ways of communicating with intimate associates without turning them off as friends. This provides a personal sense of empowerment without necessarily losing valued friends.

3. Affective Education

The term *affective education* includes a wide variety of practice methods that seek to change the way people feel about themselves and others. This is seen by some theorists (Bronstein, 1984; Group for the Advancement of Psychiatry, 1989) as a basic aspect of children's general education, coequal with cognitive and behavioral developments. It is also seen as a neglected aspect in formal training, even though everyone admits that feelings or emotions are a part of every human action and development. Whether or not awareness of feelings should be "taught" (formally) in public schools is a smoldering issue in many local school districts around the United States, where calls to return to the "3 Rs" (i.e., basic cognitive education without "frills") may be tied to voter revolts against higher local taxes.

Feelings develop over time (Bloom, 1984; Group for the Advancement of Psychiatry, 1989; Knollmueller, 1993), just as do cognitions and behavioral skills. But it seems as if maladaptive feelings are all too easily generated, leaving the person with burdens that may develop into problems in living (a more neutral term for mental disorders). Thus affective education becomes a primary prevention concern of vast potential. Affective education is not another term for psychotherapy; rather, therapy is needed precisely because a person's emotional life did not develop in a healthy and functional manner (Guerney, 1988).

Affective education is a term of a thousand names, none of them particularly explicit or adequate. I present here a brief summary of a number of terms that have been used to some degree interchangeably with affective education, using Cooper et al.'s (1980) review of this literature as a guide. Note that affective education makes use of formal contexts, such as the school classroom, to obtain its goals, but little modification would be required to apply these ideas in churches, unions, and even in the workplace (Colan et al., 1994; Felner et al., 1994; Kline & Snow, 1994). Writers have advanced various ideas about affective education

I. The First Dimension

under diverse labels: *human relations education, mental health education, values education, psychological education, behavioral sciences education, psychoeducation,* and *affective education,* among other terms. In general, the goal is to have children and youth understand their (and other people's) psychological functioning more fully and to apply this knowledge to everyday interactions.

Affective education is delivered through a variety of approaches. Listing these approaches (from Cooper et al., 1980) conveys how diverse and unrelated the methods are even though they share some version of the general goal described earlier (Durlak & Jason, 1984; Jason et al., 1984):

- Large group discussion (Glasser, 1969), in which the teacher facilitates a nonjudgmental consideration of what is important or meaningful to class members
- Confluent education (Brown, 1971), the process of introducing experiences that assist students in understanding their emotions, attitudes, and values as related to cognitive subject matter
- Small group discussion (Bessell, 1972), in which children sit in a "magic circle" for semistructured discussions and activities presumed to improve self-confidence, social interaction, and awareness of feelings
- Growth and development areas, such as sex education or self-care for "latchkey children" (Colan et al., 1994)
- Comprehensive curricula for personal and interpersonal adjustment, which target different grade levels and include books, puppets, tapes, and activities around age-related affective issues (Baenen, Stephens, & Glenwick, 1986; Shure & Spivak, 1988)
- Values clarification curricula, which seek to evoke value ideas and principles from discussions around stimulus situations; the group leader does not impose "the answer" on any value offered (see this chapter, I.B.2)
- Moral education (Kohlberg, 1987), discussed in detail in section I.B.2 of this chapter
- Awareness of others (McPhail, Ungood-Thomas, & Chapman, 1975), which involves real-life "situation cards, tapes, or films" designed to stimulate awareness of other people's feelings and values
- Psychological curriculum (Weinstein & Fantini, 1970), which involves experiential teaching procedures related to development of a sense of identity, a sense of potency, and a sense of connectedness (self-help and consciousness-raising groups seem to have similar goals, as do worksite prevention programs) (Colan et al., 1994; Felner et al., 1994; Foote et al., 1994)
- Behavioral science curriculum (Cooper & Seckler, 1973), which is focused on the behavior of the students themselves and conflicts in the classroom as

a vehicle for learning about problem solving. For example, Ellis's (1985) Living School situation embeds children in a total context of self, social, and academic learning.

- Communication and group process skills (Gordon, 1970, 1974), which include skill training on how to listen and communicate effectively and without rancor for parents, teachers, and children. Butler, Rickel, Thomas, and Hendren (1993) present a program to build competencies and reduce stressors in adolescent parents by means of a peer advocate who models a trusting relationship and effective use of community resources; Gordon (1977) extends this idea to people in leadership situations in the business world.
- Causal understanding of behavior (Ojemann, 1972), in which students are taught how to think about what produces a given behavior
- Decision making and problem solving (Spivak & Shure, 1974), which is described in section I.A.2 of this chapter
- Self-control curriculum (Fagan, Long, & Stevens, 1975), which focuses specifically on skills for confronting, making, and acting on difficult decisions (see the discussion of social resistance training in the preceding section)
- Enhancing self-concept and self-esteem (Canfield & Wells, 1976; Coopersmith, 1976), which involves aiding children to develop self-concepts as effective learners; these curricular materials may also aid students to learn about their personal strengths. There are many adult versions of these topics, such as the California Friends Can Be Good Medicine promotion (see Hersey, Klibanoff, Clyburn, & Probst, 1982; Mecca et al., 1989; Roppel & Jacobs, 1988; as well as the various types of social support groups that are discussed in Chapter 4).
- Life-space interview (Morse, 1968), which involves "emotional first aid" by working through a critical incident or problem that happens in the class situation (see also Ellis, 1985, p. 68)

Cooper et al.'s (1980) list includes general and specific approaches, one-shot programs, and well-developed studies and some sensible as well as some faddish approaches. Whether or not it is possible to teach affective or psychological understanding in sufficient depth to be of any practical value over a lifetime requires further study (Elias & Clabby, 1984).

Hansen, Johnson, Flay, Graham, and Sobel (1988) found no preventive effect of an affective education program on multiple substance use among 7th grade students. On the other hand, Malow, Wets, Corrigan, Pena, and Cunningham (1994) assessed whether a psychoeducational program designed to reduce HIV-risk behavior among recovering drug abusers, as compared with a standard information service, was effective.

These authors found that after a 6-hour small group intervention, experimental participants showed significantly enhanced self-efficacy, condom use skill, and sexual communication skills as compared with the controls. Psychoeducation has also been used in other treatment contexts (Baenen et al., 1986; Wallace, 1989).

In summary, I suggest that each specific subtype of psychoeducational program be considered on its own merits and on an experimental basis, because there is no clear picture of the effectiveness of the method in general. In addition, one might consider other active approaches, such as wilderness programs and even sports, for helping affective development (Blumenkrantz & Gavazzi, 1993, p. 206; Danish, 1983; Danish et al., 1990, 1993).

4. Resilience

Resilience refers to the fact, as Garmezy (1971) so neatly expresses it, that sometimes healthy children emerge from unhealthy settings (p. 114). This fact pushed its way into the scientific consciousness from many researchers working independently in many places around the world. It took the field of primary prevention a long time to recognize this concept's centrality and importance. Primary prevention developed in the shadow of treatment and amelioration of existing problems—that is, in the shadow of pathology. Early workers in primary prevention chose to work on preventing predictable problems (pathologies), probably because they themselves were trained in treatment fields that were dedicated to dealing with illness and disease.

Eventually, the full meaning of primary prevention—as prevention, protection, and promotion (see Chapter 1)—emerged to guide research and practice (Cowen, 1985; Geismar, 1971; Segal, 1986). Then followed a serendipitous finding—that some children apparently thrive under harsh conditions—which was recognized as an important fact worthy of further study. The concern changed from interrupting the natural course of events for children who ordinarily would not thrive, to studying the factors related to resilient children who did thrive. Once we knew what these resilient youngsters had going for them, we might be able to duplicate these things for all children.

A number of early voices in this area defined the field and have kept the fires of imagination glowing brightly (Anthony, 1974; Anthony &

Cohler, 1987; Cowen & Work, 1988; Cowen, Wyman, Work, & Iker, 1995; Garmezy, Masten, Nordstrom, & Ferrarese, 1979; Hauser, Vieyra, Jacobson, & Wertleib, 1985; Luthar & Zigler, 1991; Rutter, 1987; Werner & Smith, 1977, 1982, 1992; and others). The sum effect of their efforts has been to reveal the complexity of the concept. Reviewing the literature on resilience is an awesome task—more than 100 variables have been linked, in one study or another, with resilience (Bloom, 1996). Benard's (1992) insightful analysis on fostering resilience in children and youth offers a comprehensible introduction to methods of promoting resilience.

Benard (1992) adopts an ecological-systems perspective in noting that children are embedded in families, which are connected to schools and to the community at large. One cannot look at only one piece of this social fabric because—and this is critical to the configural approach of this book—a check and balance system exists among individuals, families, schools, peer groups, and the institutions of the community: When there is a problem in one sector, other sectors may step in and help achieve balance in the developing individual. Primary prevention has two chief ends: to enable the persons at risk to help themselves and to ensure that some other sector in the social system will be there to step in as needed—before problems occur.

Benard (1992) reviews the literature to identify what empirically supported factors have emerged that might help foster resilience in children at risk—and, by implication, all children. She summarizes the attributes that characterize the resilient child, the factors within the family that provide protective support for resilience, the characteristics within the school that enable children to be resilient, and the attributes of the competent community—one that supports its families and schools to encourage resilience. In listing Benard's categories, I refer to other places in this book where I have offered summaries of relevant primary prevention practices.

Characteristics of Resilient Children

1. Social competence: This involves having social skills relevant to working, playing, loving, and expecting well. Variables include responsiveness, flexibility, empathy and caring, communication skills, a sense of humor, and the like (see Chapter 2, I.A.5, I.E.2).
2. Problem-solving skills: This includes the ability to think abstractly, reflectively, and flexibly to recognize alternative options and likely outcomes (see Chapter 2, I.A.2).

I. The First Dimension

3. Autonomy: This term covers a broad territory of variables such as self-efficacy, internal locus of control (Rotter, 1982), impulse control, and related ideas. A useful concept relevant to living with a dysfunctional family is "adaptive distancing" (Berlin & Davis, 1989; see Chapter 2, I.E.1).

4. Sense of purpose and future: This concept points to a person's belief that he or she has a healthy expectation of the future, some goals to be attained, supported by an achievement motivation, hope, and hardiness (see Chapter 2, I.B.3).

Protective Factors Within the Family That Promote Resilience

1. Caring and support: Evidence is clear that if a child has the opportunity to establish a close bond with at least one adult (not necessarily a parent) from whom he or she receives appropriate attention in the early years of life, this becomes a major predictor of resiliency in that child (see Chapter 4, III.A.3). This person may be a parent, grandparent, relative, even an older sibling; teachers, ministers, or neighbors may also serve in this vital capacity (Sheline, Skipper, & Broadhead, 1994; Silverman, 1989).

2. High parental expectations: This involves parental attitudes that express the view that the child has the potential for a successful future and thus hold high expectations for the child's behavior (see Chapter 3, II.E.4; Chapter 5, IV.B.1).

3. Encouragement of children's participation in the family: Part of the high expectations include valuing the children as participants in the family's activities. When children are given chores, even at a very early age (proportional to their capacities), the message is that they are contributing members of the family. This gives the child the opportunity to participate meaningfully in the life of the family (see Chapter 4, III.B.2).

Protective Factors Within the School—Teachers

Benard (1992) reviews the large number of studies indicating ways in which schools (especially through warm and effective teachers) can encourage resilience in children.

1. Caring and support: Teachers may provide a buffer against problematic family or community conditions, as well as offer positive growth experiences (strens; see Chapter 4, III.A.3; Chapter 5, IV.C.2).

2. High expectations from the school and institutional support: This factor points to the power of the educational institution as a whole to foster the well-being of disadvantaged children if strong academic emphasis is given, with clear teacher expectations and support along with varied resources

through which to achieve learning goals (see Chapter 2, I.A.1, I.A.4, and I.A.5).

3. Youth participation and meaningful involvement in the school system: Having responsible roles within their own educational experience teaches children lessons beyond the pure academic. Children who are treated responsibly tend to react accordingly and not experience alienation from this major aspect of society (see Chapter 3, II.C.4).

Protective Factors Within and Beyond the School—Peers

I distinguish the peer aspect of the school environment from the academic structures because of the importance of peer groups in the lives of children (and adults) and because peer groups overlap schools, neighborhoods, and other institutional settings. The major function of peer groups relative to resilience is the caring and support that may be present to buffer children at risk from harsh family or community influences and may stimulate their constructive growth and development. Peers may also stimulate each other to higher levels of expectation and performance. Peer groups may reinforce antisocial values and actions as well (see Chapter 4, III.A.1, III.A.3).

Factors Within the Community

1. Caring and support: The "competent community" promotes the social networks and social cohesiveness to provide the support for a lifetime of growth and development. This includes the availability of key resources such as health care, housing, education, job training, employment, and recreation (see Chapter 5, IV.C.1, IV.D.2).

2. High expectations by the community of its young citizens: Social norms have a powerful effect on the behavior and values of youth. By valuing youth as a community resource and by providing resources to enable them to participate, the community creates the expectations that youth will become successful citizens (see Chapter 5, IV.D.3).

3. Opportunities for participants: Meaningful opportunities in social and economic tasks generate heightened self-esteem, enhanced moral development, and social competence. When youths perceive that there will be decent occupational positions that they can qualify for, given appropriate training, this provides one basis for bonding with that society (see discussion in Chapter 2, I.C.2, on social skills). Having youth help others may be even more helpful to the helpers in the long run (see Chapter 4, III.A.1). Many important studies of resilience have sought to identify what seems to

I. The First Dimension

produce (or lead to) effective and contented citizens, even among those who start life with many problematic conditions lined up against them. This is a rich and provocative literature and may be the leading edge of theory, research, and practice during the last decade of the 20th century. This concept appears under many labels—resilience (Rutter, 1979, 1987); invulnerable child (Anthony, 1974; Anthony & Cohler, 1987; Garmezy & Masten, 1991; Garmezy, Masten, & Tellegen, 1984); vulnerable but invincible (Werner, 1989a, 1989b); superkids (Kauffman, Grunebaum, Cohler, & Garner, 1979); stress resistant (Hauser et al., 1985); and ego resilient (Block & Block, 1980), among others. All have in common the search for health-producing factors in individuals, families, peer groups, schools, churches, social institutions, communities, states, and nations that enable some children to thrive where others fail. Much work needs to be done in this area to understand the notion of resilience, to put its empirical correlates into some meaningful conceptual network, and to translate this into effective primary prevention practices (see also Beardslee, 1989; Fonagy, Steele, Steele, Higgitt, & Target, 1994; Garmezy et al., 1979; Herrenkohl, Herrenkohl, & Egolf, 1994; Neighbors, Forehand, & McVicar, 1993; Work, Cowen, Parker, & Wyman, 1990; Wyman, Cowen, Work, & Parker, 1991).

3
METHODS OF PRIMARY PREVENTION

Dimension II. Decreasing Individual Limitations

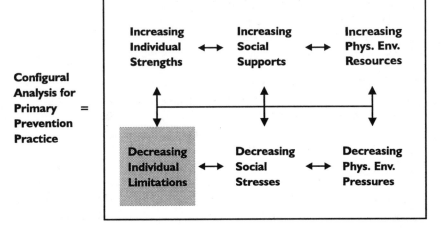

Configural
Analysis for
Primary   =
Prevention
Practice

| Increasing Individual Strengths | ←→ | Increasing Social Supports | ←→ | Increasing Phys. Env. Resources |

| Decreasing Individual Limitations | ←→ | Decreasing Social Stresses | ←→ | Decreasing Phys. Env. Pressures |

Time Frame

Figure 3.1. The Configural Equation

This chapter continues the discussion of primary prevention practices related to the individual, focusing on personal limitations that have to be reduced or eliminated. As with Chapter 2 (on personal strengths), this chapter is to be used in combination with the chapters on sociocultural and physical environmental strengths and limitations in a configural or systems approach to primary prevention.

Dimension II. Decreasing Individual Limitations
A. Cognitive Aspects

     1. Cognitive Reframing or Restructuring
     2. Anticipatory Coping
     3. Self-Instructional Training: Thought Stopping and Thought Starting
  B. Affective Aspects
     1. Defense Mechanisms: Denial
     2. Stress Inoculation
  C. Behavioral and Skill Aspects
     1. Risk Reduction, Accident Prevention, and Safety Promotion
     2. Reducing Self-Harmful Behaviors
     3. Reducing Behaviors That Harm Others
     4. Behavioral Rehearsal Through Role-Playing
     5. Relapse Prevention and Booster Shots
     6. Reducing Prejudice and Discrimination
  D. Physiological and Biological Aspects
     1. Diagnostic Screening
     2. Genetic Counseling
     3. Relaxation Training
  E. Holistic or Multifactor Approaches
     1. Trends in the Prevention of Substance Abuse
     2. Stress Management
     3. Prevention of Problems Associated With Job Loss
     4. Parent Effectiveness Training

II. The Second Dimension

This chapter addresses the second facet of the configural analysis: decreasing individual limitations or weaknesses. In Chapter 2, I defined personal limitations as referring to any aspect of the person that interferes with adapting effectively to inner or outer challenges. Limitations are not necessarily the opposite of personal strengths. Each is independent of the other. In many instances, however, adding to a person's strengths will at the same time decrease his or her limitations and vice versa.

I use the same format in this chapter as in the preceding one, reporting methods used to reduce limitations in a person's cognitive, affective, behavioral, or physiological and biological aspects or in multiple factors viewed as a unit. From the configural perspective, no specific technique is viewed in isolation; rather, most human concerns require a variety of techniques at several levels of the configuration.

The general hypothesis guiding this book is reflected in the configural equation that appears at the head of each chapter. Specifically, it asserts that primary prevention goals are more likely to be achieved by increasing the interactive strengths of individuals, sociocultural supports, and resources from the physical environment in combination with reducing the interactive individual limitations, social stresses, and pressures from the physical environment.

A. Cognitive Aspects

1. Cognitive Reframing or Restructuring

The terms *cognitive reframing* or *restructuring* convey a general strategy that involves aiding persons at risk to change their regular way of viewing a situation so as to prevent the emergence of a significant problem. Reppucci, Revenson, Aber, and Reppucci (1991) conducted two studies that point out the unreal optimism among adolescent smokers as compared with their nonsmoking peers. Smokers do recognize the increased risk of various illnesses due to smoking, but they do not apply this knowledge strictly to themselves. One implication of this kind of research is that before any preventive or promotive program can be introduced to adolescent smokers, we may need to help them reframe or restructure their attitudes and understanding about the risks involved and the direct connection to them personally.

In general, a cognitive perspective predisposes the way one has of taking in information (selectively) and interpreting the information (to suit or bias one's needs, regardless of the reality) so as to guide one's behavior (which may result in reduced effectiveness proportional to the biased view of reality from which one acts). Reframing this cognitive perspective to be more open to the reality of one's situation should result in better decisions and outcomes.

Consider the wide range of situations that might involve restructuring to be more attentive to reality. Persons making any number of important transitions from one social context to another might benefit from the reframing of ideas and events. Felner and Adan (1988) describe a junior high to high school transition program designed for what is often a challenging experience, in which youths may either push forward in their development or deteriorate by showing decreased academic performance, increased absenteeism, and greater susceptibility to substance abuse and delinquency (Roesch, 1988). Felner and Adan helped junior high students cognitively restructure what to expect at the high school and how to cope with new demands, rather than initiating prevention programs on improving grades, reducing absenteeism, or training for resistance of substance abuse per se. The focus was more general in helping new students restructure their perceptions of the physical and social environments. It is important to note that this program also restructured the school environment itself into educational units to keep the new students together, rather than letting them get lost in the crowd. I will discuss various kinds of social and physical environmental interventions in the following chapters. (See also Baker & Butler, 1984; Gerrard, McCann, & Fortini, 1983; Gilchrist, Schinke, Snow, Schilling, & Scnechal, 1988.) Thus one can view personal reframing and social and physical restructuring as parallel activities that are interactive and that may complement one another.

Lutzer (1987) provides direct reframing instructions by means of an educational and peer support group for mothers of preschoolers at risk for behavioral disorders. These mothers were "diagnosing" their children incorrectly because they lacked knowledge of developmental norms and characteristics. Lutzer formed small support groups that were used to reframe these issues and then conveyed relevant information. Lutzer lists a number of approaches to parent education, all of which offer some ways to restructure parents' cognitive perspectives on a potential problem, such as disseminating information and teaching communication and self-management skills.

Anderson and Quast (1983) address their version of restructuring to young children of alcoholic families. Such children must have a good grasp of the realities of their situations, so the investigators provided a cognitive-behavioral intervention (based on rational emotive therapy) that successfully developed the children's sense of self-competence by means of a self-counseling method. (See also the discussion on resilience, Chapter 2, I.E.4.)

Reframing may be useful in such contexts as the prevention of unwanted pregnancy. Gerrard et al. (1983) conducted a study that showed that a cognitive decision-making process could differentiate effective from ineffective contraceptive practices. The results of this study were applied in a second investigation by using a cognitive-restructuring technique. Information was presented to participants in a lecture and then through a group discussion a week later.

Tadmor and Brandes (1984) conceptualized cognitive restructuring in a type of crisis intervention involving perceived personal control in a sample of women giving birth by Caesarean method, a known high-risk group for emotional problems. Anticipatory instructions were given to the mother to reduce emotional dysfunction and to increase bonding with the newborn. As with the Felner and Adan (1988) study on high school transitions, the Tadmor and Brandes study involved restructuring the hospital environment to provide more support in the birthing process. (See also Roskin, 1982, and Williams, 1989, who both deal with issues of transition of immigrants, and Adelman, 1989, on learning disabilities.)

Elias (1993), Wright (1993), and others have pointed out how a videotape, *An Ounce of Prevention,* may be used to provide students and others with a primary prevention perspective, as contrasted with the dominant medical-pathology perspective widely used in the helping professions. In Chapter 4, I discuss the enormous potential mass media have for primary prevention, in part because viewers' cognitive views of the world are modified.

To generate specific recommendations for cognitive reframing or restructuring, it may be helpful to review the following facts: Stress includes both physical tenseness and accompanying unpleasant thoughts and feelings. Physical and mental relaxation are designed to reduce physical tension, whereas cognitive and affective methods are used to reduce stressful thoughts and feelings. Each kind of stress reduction probably augments the others. Moreover, any physical or psychological response is both an individual and a social event—for example, feeling tension on the job involves both personal feelings and social roles. Every stressful situation likely involves a configuration of factors, which suggests that dealing effectively with personal stresses also involves dealing successfully with social stresses and vice versa.

Meichenbaum (1985) notes that cognitive restructuring makes clients aware of the part cognitions and emotions play in generating and maintaining stressful situations (p. 58). Using Beck's (1984; Beck, Rush, Hollon, & Shaw, 1979) approach to cognitive therapy, Meichenbaum lists several kinds of problematic conditions suitable for reframing:

- Negative, self-defeating, stress-engendering, absolutist thoughts, such as "I'm not as good as others," "life has no meaning," "I let them down; it is my fault"

- Stereotypic thoughts involving the words *must, should, always,* and *never* (Ellis's, 1974, list of irrational beliefs would fit here, e.g., "I must be loved by everyone," "I must be perfect in all possible respects," "There is a perfect solution for every problem.")
- Overgeneralizing or selectively focusing on one part rather than dealing with a whole situation
- Seeing catastrophes in ordinary stresses

Thus reframing and restructuring involve the following steps:

1. The preventer should identify stress-producing thoughts of the four types listed above: negative, absolutist thoughts; stereotypic thoughts; overgeneralizing or selectively focusing; or catastrophic thinking.

2. The preventer should help the client reframe these ideas, for example, reframe absolutist statements as hypotheses to be tested in everyday life. Repeated reality testing should help clients to see this portion of the world in new ways. For instance, change "life has no meaning" to "life has some meaning, the meaning I give to it through my actions." The client must learn to turn certainties into possibilities, in which it becomes possible for the person to influence or control events. Phrases such as "I must" become "I would prefer"; "I can't" becomes "I may find it difficult." Thus, if a problem-solving technique fails to attain its objective, the outcome is simply unfortunate, not tragic, and the person has the energy to try again. With regard to overgeneralizing or selectively focusing on one part rather than the whole situation, help the client keep a sense of proportion about the stressful situation. A poor grade on a quiz is not failure in the course (or in one's sense of self), but it is also not something to be ignored as meaningless. Quizzes are feedback mechanisms and should be used to redirect the student's energies in learning (or learning how to learn). Likewise, with making mountains out of molehills, the challenge for the client is to keep a sense of proportion by putting the event into proper perspective.

3. Once the client has been helped to reframe stressful ideas into manageable challenges, then the client must learn to do this independently of the practitioner. What was a cooperative process of reframing particular stressful situations is modified into the general approach to reframing so the client is ready for any stressful situation that comes along. As part of the general primary prevention perspective, in addition to reframing a

negative thought, one should also counterpose (or reframe, if necessary) a positive thought to take the place of the negative one.

4. Relapse prevention (discussed later in this chapter) is another ingredient of reframing, because it is likely that the client may initially experience the same conditions that led to the problematic situation in the first place. By considering possible events, cues, feelings, and the like that may move the person back to the original problematic situation, the preventer may be able to assist that person to avoid these signals for setback. Even if there is a minor setback, it is worthwhile in analyzing what didn't work. Thus a failure experience can be turned into a learning (relearning) experience.

2. Anticipatory Coping

Anticipatory coping is a close relative of anticipatory instructions (discussed in Chapter 2, I.A.4); the differences lie in whether one focuses on increasing individual strengths or decreasing individual limitations. Instructions may lie more exclusively in the cognitive area, whereas coping may blend into feelings and actions as well. The preventive activity of anticipating a potential stress seeks to reduce the predictable problem by doing damage assessment and crisis planning before the problem occurs. The theoretical basis for this seems to be that having some rational plans, useful skills, and stored resources available in case of a chaotic emergency situation is the best way of reducing the potential damage (Gillespie & Banerjee, 1993).

Consider first-aid training. The assumption is that some physical health emergency (and its inevitable emotional stress) is going to occur—to someone, somewhere, sometime. There is probably no one who goes through life without being a victim of or a party to some medical emergency; training is given to large numbers of citizens from all walks of life to prepare them for whatever events occur. The classic first aid training (American Red Cross, 1979, 1993) instructs the "first aider" in thinking about the whole situation in which one or more persons (self or others) are injured or suddenly take ill. (Most of the focus in first aid is on treatment of existing emergency problems; I will emphasize the preventive aspects where possible.) Prompt action saves lives and reduces injury and emotional distress. There are certain classes of urgent actions— rescue from a dangerous situation, blockage of breathing, severe bleeding,

II. The Second Dimension

poisoning—and there are situations that do not require haste. First aid is not medical treatment; it involves actions taken before professional help can be attained. Training classes review types of potential problems—wounds, shock, specific injuries, water accidents, poisoning, drug abuse, burns, exposure, and sudden illnesses such as stroke and heart attack, to name some. No one person is likely to experience all these calamities but anticipatory training allows one to think ahead of what to do and how to do it, should such a calamity occur.

In the larger sense, a review of classic first aid may be generalized into principles of anticipatory coping, thinking in advance of problems how to prevent the untoward events from occurring or how one will act so as to reduce the subsequent trauma. Classic first aid not only trains the mind—to understand the nature of the many classes of potential problems—and the hands—to conduct emergency rescues and transfers and to tie the legendary Red Cross bandages—but it also trains one's attitudes toward reducing accidents. Thus it is a quintessential preventive strategy combined with crisis training.

Gillespie and Banerjee (1993) present an organizational model of prevention planning and disaster preparedness; I discuss this topic further in Chapter 6. I offer here some extensions of their model with reference to individual preparedness: What general ideas can be offered regarding anticipatory coping?

1. On a periodic basis, say once a year when paying income taxes or whenever one is making an important life transition, mentally perform a systems check for potential problems and strengths. Changing jobs? (Or is your occupation in jeopardy of changing around you?) What are the factual and emotional implications? Are there some new characteristics you would like to add to your personality as you present yourself in the new setting? Looking for a new place to live? What are the factual and emotional implications? Found a new potential friend? What are the factual and emotional implications? It is a fair assumption that every subsystem will be affected by a major untoward event or a potentially very positive event; the more central or vital the risk or the potential, the more immediate and intense should be the preventive or promotive effort.

2. For each new challenge (or the absence of any challenge where there should be some), check out these implications for each aspect of the life configuration—persons, groups, social-cultural contexts, physical envi-

ronments. Remember that the strength of the configural equation (Chapter 1) is that one subsystem may be used to offset limitations in another subsystem. To gain the full advantage of the interactive (and supportive) effects of the components of the configuration, one must be aware of the possibilities and the risks. Gillespie and Banerjee (1993) provide a model of organizational disaster preparedness; a parallel model may be relevant to individual participants:

a. awareness of the possible risks or potentials leads to
b. assessment of the nature of these future events, both the cognitive and the affective, which activates
c. knowledge about how to deal with existing events preparatory for future events, which leads to
d. planning or turning general knowledge into specific strategies that eventually become
e. personal action, which reopens the entire cycle as a person becomes aware of new possible risks or potentials

3. The major issue for anticipatory coping is how to stockpile resources (strengths, goodwill, concrete reserves) for unknown problems. The general answer is to have such resources in all sectors of one's life and to be able to move them around as needed.

a. One must build up one's sense of personal efficacy (see Chapter 2, I.E.1) so that should a setback come along, one has the intelligence to understand the situation, the skills to do what needs to be done, and the motivation to adapt appropriately.
b. One should become part of strong primary groups that will be able to provide buffering of life's stresses and resources to help one adapt (see Chapter 4, III.B).
c. One should become part of a viable employment situation and community, as far as possible, that could offer support as needed and through which one could offer support for others (see Chapter 4, III.C).

And so on, through the other components of the configuration. In the course of ordinary life, people tend to make friends, obtain work situations in viable communities, and so forth. What people generally do not do is to prepare emotionally or be aware of the emotional resources they have to draw on in emergencies. No one enjoys looking at possible problems:

II. The Second Dimension

Is there talk of layoffs at work? Are some good friends thinking of moving away? What are the actual possibilities (those one can deal with as part of problem solving)? What are the emotional possibilities? These too require some advance coping methods:

a. What options are possible for a given situation? (If a good friend moves away, would it be possible to write letters? Visit? Call? Find substitute friends?)

b. What are the possible emotional and factual consequences of each option? (Will talking by phone allow both friends to engage in meaningful conversations? Would they get right to the heart of the matter faster? Will a new friend require more energy and time to cultivate than it would be worth? Would a new friend have some unique strengths?)

Thinking about these issues in advance may enable a person to anticipate various scenarios, the consideration of which may make the chaos of the possible future events easier to comprehend and deal with appropriately.

3. Self-Instructional Training: Thought Stopping and Thought Starting

This topic includes a number of methods of thinking and talking to oneself so as to prevent a predictable problem, to protect an existing state of healthy functioning, and to promote a desired state of affairs. Different terms are used, with emphases that move from mostly cognitive to mostly affective: thought stopping and starting, imagery rehearsal, and stress inoculation (the last of which is discussed in the section on affect in this chapter).

Sometimes healthy people get into habits of perseverating about unpleasant things, making themselves increasingly unhappy as well as being unable to start productive problem solving. A simple procedure for temporarily breaking out of the unproductive mode of thinking is called "thought stopping" (Cormier & Cormier, 1979). In thought stopping, when one is aware of beginning to perseverate about some unpleasant and unproductive thought, then one says to oneself, "Stop it!" (This can be emphasized by saying this out loud, where appropriate, by snapping one's fingers, or enacting any physical action, such as getting up and moving around, adequate to get one to focus on the break-off command.) Breaking into one's perseverating unpleasant thoughts is relatively easy; staying away from them for a longer period of time is more challenging.

To thought stopping, I add the parallel notion of "thought starting." Not only must one break out of unproductive thoughts; one must enter into productive ones in their place. Just as thought stopping can benefit from some priming, so can thought starting. Rimm and Masters (1974) recommend "assertive thought starting" to interrupt anxiety-producing unproductive thoughts and to move toward productive ones. Even when the risks are real, one can generally assert that one has had the experience of handling such challenges before. (This might be in the form of mastery experience in perceived self-efficacy—see Chapter 2, I.E.1—or anticipatory coping—see Chapter 3, II.A.2.) Thus one begins the thought process on what one can do, or has contemplated, to deal with the current challenge.

Let me offer the following strategy statements on preventive thought stopping and thought starting:

1. When one has an unproductive or unpleasant idea come to mind about which one starts to perseverate, one must break out of unproductive patterns of thinking by physically or verbally interrupting the negative thought. (This is thought stopping.)

2. Immediately, one should try to substitute a positive thought in its place. Two paths lead toward this goal: involving the affective tone of one's thoughts (the pleasantness or unpleasantness of the thought), and involving the cognitive message (how productive or unproductive the thought is). Thoughts and feelings probably occur simultaneously, but for this strategy, I will distinguish them.

3. Regarding the affective tone of thought starting: One can get into a generally pleasant mind-set by thinking (vigorously) of some positive thoughts—"This is a beautiful day; I enjoy seeing . . . snow, rain, blue skies." This strategy is like systematic desensitization, in which a person counterposes a stronger pleasant thought in place of the anxiety-raising stimulus. It would be wise to select a positive thought at a higher level of intensity than the negative one it seeks to replace. For example, at a basic level, one can contemplate a dinner at a friend's house this weekend; at a higher level, the family celebration at Thanksgiving; higher still, the excitement one anticipates about a planned trip to New Zealand.

The pleasant thought-to-be becomes compelling and is capable of being developed through ordinary cognitive processes. If one has neither read about nor been to New Zealand, however, then imagining a vacation there would be hard to sustain. The pleasant thought-to-be should not be of the "impossible dream" type, as these are too hard to believe and may not keep one from the unproductive thought (see relaxation techniques, Chapter 3, II.D.3, and keeping the problem in perspective, Chapter 3, II.A.1).

Another kind of affective thought is about oneself, such as a self-affirming thought that says "I can do it" (Rimm & Masters, 1974); "I have useful experiences in this topic area"; or "I am a person of worth." Or more picturesquely, as seen printed on a T-shirt, "I may not be perfect, but parts of me are very good." This in effect denies the negative implications of the unpleasant thought but does not address the cognitive content as such.

4. With regard to the cognitive part of thought starting, whether or not one employs a positive tone of the thought-to-be, one can substitute a cognitive topic on which one can generate some productive ideas. Life is filled with potentially productive topics, which can also be at various levels of intensity. For example, one might think about the reading for one's next class; at a higher level, preparing the short exercise for that class; at a still higher level, outlining the term project for that class. It would probably be wise to select a solvable productive thought so as to have a successful experience in the thought-starting process—"What materials do I need to do that exercise?" Other potentially productive thoughts—"What am I going to do when I grow up?"—may be too much to handle and cause as much discomfort as the unproductive thought. Once a productive idea is being energetically considered, it is difficult to think simultaneously of the original disturbing thought.

5. It may also be useful to review a previously successful problem-solving effort that is similar to the one at hand, both for the remembrance of the success (which contributes to one's positive self-efficacy for this kind of work) and for considering previously successful solutions that may be modified in the new situation.

6. Self-reflective reinforcement is useful at the conclusion of a successful thought starting. This reinforces the idea that one has control over one's mental life and can make it take one wherever one wishes to go—"Say, that was a rather creative solution, if I do say so myself!"

7. There are occasions in life when it is difficult to dream away a serious event, such as a death in the family and an economic downturn—the list is long. Thought stopping and starting are intended for lesser scale events, but mourning must eventually end and economic depression requires eventual activity if one is to surmount it. This technique is not Pollyannish—positive

thinking does not make everything positive. Rather, it enables one to turn toward constructive feelings, thoughts, and actions as the occasion requires. People must deal with significant life transitions, large and small; social customs and rituals facilitate this. Thought stopping and starting are the spark plugs.

Meichenbaum (1977) suggests a training procedure in self-instruction in which an adult trains a child. I will modify this procedure in terms of this book:

1. An adult model performs a task that is relevant to the challenge the child is facing. The adult talks to himself or herself out loud: defining the problem, focusing attention on correct responses, correcting errors, and providing self-reinforcement. (Connect the Shure & Spivak, 1988, interpersonal problem-solving process at this point—What is the problem? What alternatives exist to solve the problem? What are the probable outcomes? Which one should I select as the best alternative?)

2. The child then performs the same task while the adult gives verbal directions. (Corrections are made verbally to a criterion of performance. Reinforcement is given for adequate performance.)

3. The child next performs the task while talking to himself or herself out loud, that is, giving self-directions just as the adult model did. (The level of performance should meet minimum standards. If not, the adult should provide verbal corrections until that standard is met. This provides the opportunity to teach error-correcting self-statements. Also, the adult may remind the child to self-reinforce correct performance.)

4. The child then whispers the instructions while going through the task, including these basic self-instructional categories: defining the problem, focusing attention on the problem and one's responses to it, correcting errors, and providing self-reinforcement.

5. Finally, the child performs the task entirely through private speech.

B. Affective Aspects

1. Defense Mechanisms: Denial

In classic psychoanalytic terms, *defense mechanisms* are viewed as unconscious adaptive strategies that reduce anxiety emerging from instinctual forces (sexual or aggressive) seeking expression, which are, in turn, resisted by the conscious and socialized portion of the individual. A price is paid for this reduced anxiety, because the mechanisms force various distortions of reality onto the ego, from outright denial of that reality to various kinds of projections and reversals of fact and feeling.

Coping mechanisms, on the other hand, may be viewed as conscious adaptive mechanisms that seek to solve problems (especially ones involving strong feelings). Coping mechanisms are not necessarily rational in that some forms of conscious coping distort reality. But coping skills can be learned and corrected and so have clear implications for preventive and promotive behaviors.

Although few scientists currently uphold psychoanalytic principles, there are instances where people appear to perform what may be considered nonrational behaviors. Consider, for example, the discussion by Schechter, Vanchieri, and Crofton (1990) on the reasons women do not make use of mammography—"a low-risk, quick, and painless procedure" to detect breast cancer, for which all women 40 years and older are at risk. (Breast cancer can be treated successfully if detected early enough, although some of the options of treatment require choices that may involve physical disfigurement.) The reasons Schechter et al. provide for this lack of use include lack of perceived need (as reported by women in focus groups who had neither symptoms nor family history of breast cancer); lack of physician referral (it has been estimated that more than 80% of women would get a mammogram if referred by their physician); and personal procrastination (due to fear, inconvenience, expense; see also King, Rimer, Seay, Balshem, & Engstrom's, 1994, study of differential ways to encourage women to come in for annual free mammograms). The point is that some set of factors—rational but also nonrational or unrecognized—may be holding these people back from obtaining lifesaving—but sometimes body-scarring—preventive services. This complexity requires us to look more carefully at defensive maneuvers.

Lazarus (1984) argues for the adaptive function of denial, especially in situations where it is impossible to exert control by oneself. Denial is used in a transactional sense, rather than in a typical psychoanalytic sense of an unconscious defensive distortion. Denial in this conscious sense can be used to protect oneself, perhaps by permitting a gradual assimilating of the meaning of the situation and thereby marshaling one's energies to deal with the problem. My Scottish social work professor related a story of the time she first encountered an air raid attack in World War II. She remembers very clearly how she hunted around for clean clothes to put on so as to help pull people from the rubble. She interpreted this, in retrospect, as to take a few moments to escape the horror she was about to witness and come to her task gradually so as to be in control of herself. Whether this is unconscious or transactional is a matter of definition.

In any case, denial can mean detachment, rationalization, and even self-deception to make the individual feel better, maintain feelings of hope (see Chapter 2, I.B.3), and preserve a sense of self-worth. (Siegel's, 1986, famous book, *Love, Medicine, and Miracles,* links a loving orientation with self-healing and makes use of a mixture of nonrational hope and denial.) These feelings of hope and denial operate at what Lazarus and Folkman (1984) call "emotion-focused coping," which seeks to regulate emotions, not to solve problems that are causing the stress. (The latter is the focus of Lazarus and Folkman's second category: problem-focused coping.)

The point of noting the possible workings of defense mechanisms, in addition to conscious coping mechanisms, is that sometimes we "rational animals" need to take a holiday from our exclusive rationality because it serves a useful function in the larger configuration of our lives. We need to be both rational and nonrational at times throughout our lives—to work and to love, as Freud expressed it.

Consider the obverse of this topic: Why do people decide to take care of themselves? Weinstein (1987) presents an intriguing introduction to the study of protective behavior by examining what precautions people take to avoid various kinds of hazards. He introduces several theories for protective behavior and then explores research in health, crime, injury, and natural disasters. Then he attempts to find some commonalities among research in these diverse areas. The individual as decision maker appears throughout the anthology. This is something like the health belief model described in Appendix B of this book—that people tend to weigh the severity of the perceived threat, the likelihood of getting the problem, and the effectiveness of the preventive service. But even when these factors all seem to be present and supportive of preventive actions, not everyone acts to protect himself or herself. Why? The following considerations are drawn from Weinstein:

1. Short-term versus long-term considerations: People may be mainly governed by short-term outcomes, especially when the future harm may

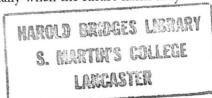

never happen to them. (Even though there are **40,000** or more automobile deaths each year, chances are slight that one of these will be you or me. So many people do not buckle their seat belts, the primary source of protection.)

2. The complexity of the decision-making task: Although information may be provided about the nature of a risk, such as the ingredients of various processed foods (see Chapter 2, I.D.1), it is a complex task to weigh all the information regarding the specific foods one eats in a day to optimize one's nutritional intake. It is difficult to be fully rational given the available information.

3. Social models and social pressure: People may fail to take preventive precautions because of the sociocultural context in which these challenges take place. (Three thousand young people start to smoke each day, not because they are ignorant about the effects of smoking by and large or because they love the taste of tobacco, but because their peers, parents, or role models are smoking and various external factors are pushing them to smoke.)

4. Wrongheaded preventive suggestions: Weinstein (1987) points to a painful fact: Some helping professionals have promoted excessive and sometimes silly actions under the banner of primary prevention. The consumer is right to reject these suggestions, but it may be difficult to identify the excessive from the effective.

To suggest steps in nonrational thinking sounds ludicrous, but perhaps I may be forgiven by the content of these proposals:

1. To be fully human is to be aware of one's full range of feelings, including those of fear, hostility, rage, sexuality, and the like. This does not mean that one gives into these feelings but, rather, one takes stock of the whole situation by being aware of the shadowy side of one's life (Jung, 1957). Energy is locked in these subterranean feelings; becoming aware of them means that one may tap into these energies to address the surface problems. If this sentence seems murky, it is. But it is also the kind of insight that many therapists have come to independently and so it deserves serious consideration and testing.

2. Being human also means being aware of the sublime feelings and ideals that are a part of the personality. People are rarely angelic for long periods of time because it is difficult to earn a living while being angelic

(cf. Melville's *Billy Budd*). Being aware of one's capacity for love, humor, and compassion also provides energy that can be tapped for everyday living or dealing with life crises (Siegel, 1986; Sorokin, 1954).

3. As a hypothesis, consider the usefulness of being able to absorb the meanings of both antisocial and altruistic feelings so as to be able to use the energies behind these extrarational states when dealing with life's problems and potentials. One must put these energies at the disposal of one's rational self, not to be a goody-goody conformist, but to engage the more vast areas of the self and environments toward a socially valued goal (Adler, 1959). Transactions among the rational, the nonrational, and the situational are ongoing objectives for the person who is fully using his or her potential (Bandura, 1986). As such, these speculative ideas may have preventive or promotive value.

2. Stress Inoculation

This section presents an overview of Meichenbaum's (1985) work on stress inoculation training with its sensitive and sensible advice to practitioners, but interested readers are urged to study this important work directly (see also Blythe & Erdahl, 1986; Janis, 1983; Mahoney, 1974).

Stress inoculation training (SIT) is a general term referring to an integrated set of helping procedures that begins with a conceptual perspective on stress and coping. A dozen specific operationalized tactics are then described, which must be combined in individualized ways to fit a particular client's situation. These tactics are arranged in three major phases.

1. Conceptualization phase
   a. Establish a collaborative relationship with the client and significant others where appropriate.
   b. Gather information about the stress-related problem in its situational context.
   c. Clarify client expectations and formulate short-term (or intermediate) objectives and long-term goals.
   d. Educate the client about the transactional nature of stress and coping—both personal and situational factors must be considered.
   e. Combine the client's description of particular stress factors with conceptual models from the literature, yielding a comprehensible practice model that may be used tentatively to guide practice.

II. The Second Dimension

  f. Anticipate possible client resistance and nonadherence to the SIT and help the client plan ways to reduce these possibilities.

 2. Skills acquisition and rehearsal phase
  a. Tactic: Relaxation training (see p. 167 of this book)
  b. Tactic: Cognitive restructuring (see p. 105)
  c. Tactic: Problem-solving training (see p. 30)
  d. Tactic: Self-instructional training (see p. 112)
  e. Tactic: Denial (see p. 115)

 3. Application and follow-through phase
  a. Tactic: Imagery rehearsal (see p. 105)
  b. Tactic: Behavioral rehearsal, role-playing, and modeling (see p. 145)
  c. Tactic: Graduated in-vivo exposure (see p. 62)
  d. Tactic: Relapse prevention (see p. 147)
  e. Tactic: Follow through (see p. 121)

(This is how I interpret Meichenbaum's SIT as both an integrative framework and a cafeteria of possible tactics. Because many items from this cafeteria of tactics have already been presented, I simply note in the above list where Meichenbaum's tactics are discussed in more detail.)

Meichenbaum's presentation proceeds in this fashion:

1. Preliminaries: Meichenbaum (1985) defines stress as a transaction influenced by both the person and the environment such that the demand taxes or exceeds available resources and thus threatens the person's well-being (p. 3). Coping is defined as the behavioral and cognitive efforts to master, reduce, or tolerate internal or external demands emerging in the stressful transaction (p. 3). The general psychological model from which Meichenbaum is working, a cognitive-behavioral framework, suggests that people can change their cognitions so as to reduce harmful emotions and behavior (Ellis, 1985; Silverman, 1988).

2. Given these preliminaries that set the stage for the stress inoculation, Meichenbaum suggests that the six steps of the conceptual stage flow in the order presented, with feedback loops throughout. The overall objective of the conceptualization phase is to form a collaborative relationship with the client so as to work together on the identified problem and goals.

3. The skills acquisition and rehearsal phase probably begins with a form of relaxation training so as to demonstrate to the client that some aspect of his or her world is under the client's control. (One cannot be

both physically tense and physically relaxed at the same time, so by learning how to relax deeply, one can learn to master graduated pieces of stress-producing experiences; Wolpe, 1958.)

Then, depending on the given situation, the practitioner might suggest either cognitive strategies or behavioral methods, each of which may also include self-instructional methods. Or in situations where these stress-reducing tactics do not work, the practitioner might enable the client to use denial for self-protective purposes (Meichenbaum, 1985). When doing nothing will not affect the stressful outcome, then clients have little to lose by being detached, or rationalizing, or deceiving themselves so as to maintain some degree of hope or a sense of self-worth and not to get overwhelmed. As Reinhold Niebuhr's victim states, "God, grant me the strength to change what I can, the courage to tolerate what I cannot, and the wisdom to know the difference" (quoted in Meichenbaum, 1985, p. 75). Some skills—cognitive or behavioral (or emotional denial)—will be selected as best fitting the client in Phase 2, possibly including self-instructions.

4. Eventually, these rehearsed skills will be moved into the third phase, application and follow-through. Again, the cognitive (imagery rehearsal) or the behavioral skills are applied as best fit the situation, and these will be enacted in graduated in vivo or in vitro exposures. These exposures constitute the actual application of the prevention plan.

Whichever applications are selected, they will likely be followed by relapse prevention (discussed in Chapter 3, II.C.5) and follow through; relapse prevention anticipates problems maintaining even a successful preventive effort, whereas follow through recognizes that problem solving is a continuous process that goes on beyond the clinical setting and must be carefully generalized and integrated into the clients' real-life world.

C. Behavioral and Skill Aspects

1. Risk Reduction, Accident Prevention, and Safety Promotion

The prevention of accidents is a never-ending battle against the easy way of doing things. It is easier to leave a bottle of pills on the counter

II. The Second Dimension

than to put it away for safe keeping. It is easier to leave a cupboard unlocked than to bother locking and unlocking it whenever you need cleaning supplies or a hunting rifle. Accidents, including deadly ones, are an easy reach away.

Accident Prevention

Guiding principles for accident prevention incorporate many of the themes from primary prevention. Although many of the things that can prevent accidents involve active strategies—that is, what an individual has to do consciously to protect him- or herself, such as putting the pill bottle away after each use—it is also possible to arrange events to obtain passive prevention—such as having all medicine jars produced with child-proof lids. Passive strategies, which build protective social or physical changes into the situation, are preferable to active strategies, where feasible, simply because they are "on guard" even when we are not thinking about accident prevention. This is especially true with infants (Trinkoff & Parks, 1993) and children and other people who because of their limited mental functioning are unable to understand and use active strategies. Passive strategies, such as banked highways that help drivers automatically compensate for curves in the road, seat belts, and air cushions, are also useful in routinized situations where otherwise able people may not be alert.

Accident prevention is intrinsically a person-in-setting activity. One must think about the structure and function of objects in settings in combination with the structural and functional capabilities of people in those settings to prevent accidents and promote purposive experiences. In the bathroom, one must think about slippery tubs, electrical appliances near water, breakable glasses—and the people who may use these objects. In the kitchen, one must consider sharp knives, hot stoves, and the risk of things falling—and the people who may be in the vicinity. At the job site (Shi, 1993), on the playground, or on the road, each setting has a particular configuration of person-and-environment patterns that constitute risk and protection regarding accidents.

An interesting example of accident prevention on the job is the study by Fox, Hopkins, and Anger (1987) on open-pit mining, a very hazardous job situation. When safety rules and devices were in place and accidents rates did not fall, the management arranged to offer tokens redeemable at nearby stores for clearly specified safe behavior. Families were informed

II. The Second Dimension

about these tokens; inevitably, they put pressure on the family workers to be safe so as to get the tokens as well as bonuses for extended safety records for individuals and work groups (which brought group pressure for safety to bear on the situation). The safety records were carefully monitored, a very important part of primary prevention research. Results were reported to be strongly positive: The workers benefited by being free of injuries, the families redeemed merchandise with the tokens to enjoy with their healthy family members, and the mining company's medical and insurance bills were reduced. This example of a token economy has broad implications for other forms of accident prevention, in a personal or familial situation as well as on the social-institutional level. Benefits for the whole configuration far outweighed costs of the token economy.

A basic rule for accident prevention and safety promotion is to counterbalance each negative prohibition and sanction with a positive directive and reinforcement. Much of child rearing consists of teaching children what should not be done—"Don't stick a hairpin in the electrical outlet . . ." —even if one gives a reason for this action—". . . because you'll get a shock and your fingers will be burned." We must work harder to think about positive alternatives—"Let me show you what happens if we wrap this wire around this magnet just so . . ." The pit mining example illustrates how positive reinforcements were arranged both close to the site of the problem and in the workers' family context, counterbalancing the inherent dangers of that mining situation—"Don't neglect to wear your helmet . . ."—even with a perfectly good reason—". . . because you may get bopped on the head." Thinking and planning are required to develop such cost-effective arrangements—"If you remember to wear your protective gear, then you won't get injured and you'll get bonus coupons, both of which will make your family very happy." Some family members might also add, "Keeping healthy will also reduce company medical costs, which will help maintain the company and your job situation."

Whereas each anticipated hazard has one or more potential countermeasures, many safety measures are also restrictions of human action and freedom (Etzioni, 1979). The question becomes, How much safety is to be purchased at the price of how much limited activity? We could make highways 99% safe by restricting speeds to 5 miles an hour, but these laws would not be received favorably, perhaps even by the 40,000 people who might otherwise be killed annually in automobile accidents. The public must be convinced of the seriousness of the hazard relative to the costs involved in reducing that hazard. This is not a purely rational calculation, as seen by the popularity of roller coasters, bungee jumping, and other fear-inspiring experiences. One does not talk in the evening of how safely one skied down the snowy mountain trails that day. We need research on the nature of preventive tradeoffs, how much security is purchased for how much cost, regulation, and monitoring (Crawford, 1978; Weinstein, 1987).

Safety habits decay over time and refresher courses, multiple reminders, and "booster shots" (Chapter 3, II.C.5) are useful. Young children (and probably everyone) are forgetful of activities that have no apparent reinforcement, and it is challenging to instill and maintain safety rules in youngsters (Dannenberg, Gielen, Beilenson, Wioson, & Jaffe, 1993; Garbaino, 1988; Peterson, 1984; Peterson, Farmer, & Mori, 1987; Peterson & Mori, 1985, 1986). Adults presumably incorporate safety notions in their working memories and have the added advantage of painful personal experiences and others that prompt remembering—most of the time. But even adults need reminders, which unfortunately puts preventers who use conventional methods in the position of being nags. The art of clever prevention reminders is underdeveloped, although the old antismoking posters and the newer safe sex posters have shown some brilliant starts. (My favorite: In a provocative Garden of Eden pose, Eve offers Adam a cigarette; he replies, "No, thanks, I'd rather have an apple.")

Design considerations are an important part of accident prevention, such as air cushions in cars, handrailings on stairs, and protective shoes for joggers. Packaging may be equally important, such as the "hot rubber" condom packages, the "be kind to your Mother Earth" T-shirts, and the like. I'll discuss these considerations specifically in a later chapter on the physical environment and the part it plays in primary prevention.

Safety Promotion

Consider safety promotion, the intentional efforts to obtain healthy states in contrast to untoward alternatives that arouse our curiosity. (See Gaboury & Ladouceur, 1993, on prevention of gambling among adolescents, and Volberg, 1994, on prevention of gambling among adults.) Also, especially for children and adolescents, there is the lure of the forbidden, testing limits (one's own and society's), and escape from the boredom of the ordinary routine. Some activities are risky without the participants' knowing it, as when children play hide and seek in the woods with shiny three-leaf vines all over the place.

Safety promotion in part involves making people excited about what they already have (e.g., good health) or what they could have (e.g., better health). It may involve raising fears about what could befall them; this is easier for known hazards, such as poison ivy, but it is much more difficult for unknown hazards, such as the wasps' nest hidden in the garage. It may involve arguing (probably fruitlessly) about the evils of what unhealthy alternatives a person may be considering.

Preventers have to be realistic about their crusades. There clearly are strong attractions to various untoward behaviors. For example, the attractions of smoking are part chemical addiction, part social participation, and part desired psychological response, whose immediate effects carry much more weight than do threats of distant pain. And how will one know what he or she is missing without trying it? These and other attractions present stiff competition for the would-be preventer who has to offer (a) alternative equal or superior experiences in the here and now; (b) knowledge, attitude change, and social skills for refusing the allures of the forbidden; and (c) hope for a continuing pleasurable future without the untoward consequences of the unsatisfied temptation. Preventers have done their best with knowledge, attitude change, and social skills for refusing the allures of the forbidden (beginning with Evans, 1976), have barely tapped into alternative equal or superior experiences in the here and now (a strong beginning was made by Cohen, 1975), and probably can't do much about hoping for a continuing pleasurable future without the untoward consequences of the unsatisfied temptation. My suggested principles of social promotion are intended to be provocative, because there is not much to offer that is substantially helpful:

1. Messages that take into consideration both sides of an argument probably have more persuasive power for relatively educated listeners than a one-sided communication. For example, take one of the widely printed messages, "Surgeon General's Warning: Cigarette Smoke Contains Carbon Monoxide." Here, the nation's highest public health official makes a scientific statement that is legally required to be printed on the offending object; it requires that users read the message and understand the hazard

II. The Second Dimension

named. Repetitions of this message appear by the millions. Yet when is the last time you read one of these messages? I could find no research evidence that these warnings were effective. (To the contrary, legally required warnings may actually absolve cigarette producers from consumer damage suits.)

Pro/con messages are difficult to construct. Consider this charming message: "Although some people think that smoking keeps you from gaining weight, it is definitely the case that smoking gives you stinky breath. Kissing a skinny smoker is like licking out a butt-filled ashtray." There is some evidence that people who stop smoking do gain some weight, but weight gain is a complex matter, and there is no direct causation between stopping smoking and gaining weight. Only excess calories cause weight gain. The stinky breath argument hits the socially sensitive teenager (and others) directly where it hurts and the weak humor of licking out an ashtray probably adds to the insult. But dedicated smokers can counter this with toothpaste slogans, breath sweeteners, and other commercial myths. So the struggle for the heart and lungs of people goes on.

2. Preventers must offer comparable alternatives to whet the appetites of the tempted. Cohen (1975) suggests many alternatives for the different types of gratification that drug users presumably seek. His suggestions are still timely, such as the physical highs produced by jogging, mountain climbing, and swimming; the social highs produced by happy intimate friendships, involvement in active clubs, and having viable and interesting work opportunities; and the psychological highs of yoga, religious experiences, or social activism on behalf of others. In addition to these somewhat exotic alternatives, current researchers are developing combinations of opportunities and incentives for youths to bond with and get committed to a conventional social order so as to assist people in making safety-promotive decisions (Hawkins & Weis, 1985). Conventional social norms are extraordinarily powerful if young people are given a fair chance of participating in them free of economic, ethnic, and gender discriminations. Exotic alternatives are also important, especially for those who are bored by the routine of the conventional. Preventers must make use of both ordinary and extraordinary social events. Let me illustrate this with a never-fail interest—sex.

Table 3.1 presents an adapted selection from the "Safer Sex Menu" (Hong, 1992). This one-page handout addressed to college students (but

Table 3.1 Safer Sex Menu

Appetizers

Talking to each other about safer sex (choice of English, Spanish, French, or Chinese)

Listening to music and/or dancing together

Stroking . . . or playing with each other's hair

Back and shoulder massage, foot rubs, and body rubs while still dressed (perfume or aftershave, optional)

Undressing each other . . . (with a side conversation on the humor of fashionable clothing)

Showering or taking a bubble bath together, dry with fluffy towels

Kissing, licking, or fondling your partner's body (except for genitals)

Main Entrée (Dieter's Delights)

Putting a latex condom on yourself or your partner, then posturing before a full mirror (laughing permitted)

Stroking, caressing, and fondling your partner's body, investigating odors au naturel (including genitals)

Rubbing your penis/clitoris against healthy unbroken skin on your partner's body, avoiding ejaculations or contacts with your partner's body openings, accompanied by soft music

Mutual or simultaneous masturbation to orgasm with your hands (with or without condoms, with no exchange of semen or vaginal fluids)

Desserts

Licking whipped cream, jelly, chocolate syrup, or honey off your partner's body, except for unprotected body openings

Soaking in a hot tub or whirlpool bath

Eating breakfast, lunch, or dinner in bed

SOURCE: Hong (1992).

with much wider potential) begins with the idea of abstinence as fasting—the most effective method regarding sexual risks. Most people do not fast, however, and so alternatives are suggested: "Our Health Chef suggests some delectable options for exciting sexual encounters between you and your partner which will reduce the risks of unwanted pregnancy, HIV infection, and other sexually transmitted diseases." The virtue of this menu is that it presents very erotic but relatively safe alternatives to the pervasive eroticism that people engage in frequently (Coates, 1990, on safe gay sex; Catania et al., 1994, on heterosexual minority condom use). What the

"Safer Sex Menu" does not do is provide some nonsexual alternatives, such as vigorous athletic activities (jogging, tennis, swimming, and even dancing), or intellectually stimulating mutual activities, such as going to a play, movie, museum, or cultural attraction or attending some spiritual activity together. One must generate and anticipate the idea of a mutually enjoyable context to enjoy any interpersonal activity, from sex to community service. Working together on a personalized safer sex menu comprising athletic, intellectual, and spiritual or cultural activities would be as helpful as using the menu.

3. Social promotion is something like the religions that generate the specter of sin and damnation and then offer redemption and absolution. The specter of AIDS and venereal diseases is connected with unsafe sex, whereas the absolution of these horrors is to be obtained merely by abstention, safer sex, or whatever is the current wisdom.

I would like to offer the following analysis of posters as being a lively tool for social promotion. Imagine a poster with a headline across the top: "Some people eat out every night." This draws on one's (middle-class) experience to assume this means at a restaurant. But the body of the poster shows an old woman sifting through a garbage can. You've been had—by your middle-class assumptions and the stark and brutal reality before you. You can't deny it or the strong feelings of guilt you may feel. Fortunately, at the bottom of the page—you have to look hard to find it—is salvation, the way to assuage guilt: "Give to charity." This is a United Way poster that breaks into the middle-class, self-constructed isolation from the world of poverty. The poster has to be strong, clever, and honest to get beyond the wall of indifference. Indeed, the last line reads, "Someone is waiting for you to give to the United Way"—a personalized message, for both the giver and the receiver.

This poster embodies many of the basic principles in the art of promoting a good cause:

a. Catch the audience's attention with a brief statement or question that is relevant to that audience, personalized where possible.

b. Present a visual image that is arresting and memorable, that will stick in a person's mind beyond the moment's viewing, and that creates tension for the viewer.

c. Resolve that tension by offering a personal way for the individual to respond.

The level of the response must be proportional to the content at hand, a few dollars to charity or a few years of your life in the military, as in the famous World War II poster, "Uncle Sam wants You! . . ."—with the finger of a serious-looking Uncle Sam pointing directly at the viewer (and it appeared to move as the viewer moved to the left or right)—". . . Join the army."

Consider May and Hymbaugh (1989), who developed a large-scale fetal alcohol syndrome (FAS) prevention program for Native Americans and Alaska Natives throughout the United States. Their central task was to provide information to pregnant women in these groups on the detrimental connection between drinking and birth defects in babies.

Young, low socioeconomic status women are particularly difficult to reach through mass public education. Although the overall rates of FAS among Native Americans are no different from the general population of the United States, in certain tribes the rates are very high, for cultural reasons.

> For example in some tribes such as the Pueblo, a low percentage of the women drink, but drinking women are often ostracized which increases the severity of their alcohol abuse and FAS. In others, such as some Plains tribes, FAS risk is caused by a higher percentage of drinking women and a greater prevalence of abusive-drinking patterns in the overall tribal population. (May & Hymbaugh, 1989, p. 509)

After learning what existing FAS programs were presenting, May and Hymbaugh (1989) developed FAS prevention materials sensitive to the cultural groups they were addressing, including well-crafted posters and brochures. Let's examine two of these: In Figure 3.2, the eye-catching statement at the top of the page stirs up ethnic pride ("Being Indian . . . ") and the hope of any parents-to-be ("having a normal healthy baby . . ."). This is connected with the direct instruction ("Don't drink"). The large central picture portrays in aesthetic if abstract form a man and woman looking at a papoose in a cradle board. The background represents the open landscape of Arizona or New Mexico. The traditional clothing is recognizable to the local peoples in any of the 20 Pueblo tribes in this area. At the bottom of the picture are further instructions on having a healthy baby. This poster takes a positive approach to the FAS message; brochures are available that spell out the fearful messages of birth defects

BEING INDIAN IS HAVING A NORMAL HEALTHY BABY...*DON'T DRINK*

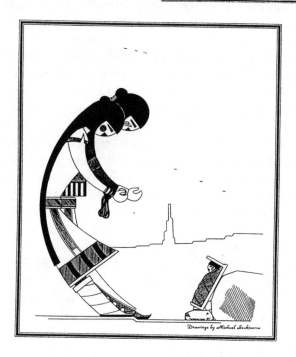

BE CAREFUL WITH YOUR BODY WHILE PREGNANT, FOR IT IS ALSO YOUR BABY'S HOME. THIS WILL HELP THE BABY FOR THE REST OF HIS/HER LIFE.

For more information contact:
National Indian
Fetal Alcohol Syndrome Prevention Program   2401 12th Street, N.W.   (505) 766-2873   FTS-474-2873
All Indian Pueblo Council   Albuquerque, New Mexico 87102   (505) 766-5969

Figure 3.2. Poster 1. Used with permission.

and deformities. Another poster (not presented here) presents similar written messages but changes the large figure to an attractive pregnant Alaska Native. Figure 3.3 presents another approach: A strong "Warning!" statement at the top, with a central figure (a pregnant Navajo woman about to take a drink) enclosed in the universal symbol for

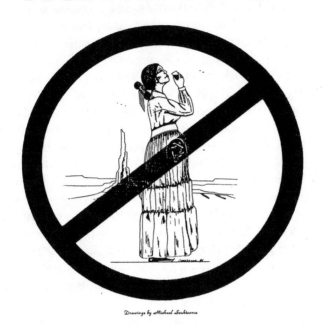

Figure 3.3. Poster 2. Used with permission.

something prohibited, followed by information at the bottom that directly spells out the connection between drinking and FAS. It also gives an address for more information. This is a classic poster design, which contributed to what was probably a very cost-effective project (May & Hymbaugh, 1989, p. 515; see also Alcalay et al., 1993, who designed prenatal care messages using posters, brochures, radio songs, and a calendar for low-income Mexican women so as to promote prenatal health education).

4. The last general principle for social promotion is that preventers need to construct an array of strens, those growth-promotive experiences, for every level of the configuration. Nature seems to conspire to offer temptations at each of these levels; preventers cannot do less. Moreover, a central organizing theme should offer an opportunity to pull the various pieces together. Let me give one example of this, which I borrow and generalize from the work of Hatcher (1990): the "great lover" concept.

Is there anyone in his or her secret heart of hearts who does not want to be a great lover? So the only question is, How? The basic ingredients of being a great lover involve personal, interpersonal, social, and cultural factors: being sensitive to the feelings of the beloved; never forcing sexuality onto someone; using an array of pleasurable techniques with skill and finesse; always using protective devices to prevent unwanted pregnancies and venereal diseases; and so forth. One can insert any number of good preventive or promotive lessons into the great lover concept, where they will join with other good practices to form a self-satisfying and socially useful cluster of positive behaviors. As a general approach to reducing individual limitations (or increasing individual strengths), the great lover model may be widely adapted: the great neighbor, the great parent, the great student. . . .

2. Reducing Self-Harmful Behaviors

People inflict harmful stresses on themselves, knowingly or not. When these harmful behaviors are knowingly inflicted, the situation is considered disordered behavior, such as the person who cuts himself or herself purposely. On the other hand, a much larger number of persons knowingly inflict harmful behaviors on themselves—such as smoking or drinking to excess or while pregnant—without these common actions being considered disordered. These latter behaviors are much more destructive and costly than the acknowledged disordered behaviors, but such distinctions are a matter of sociocultural definition, not merely sociomedical definition.

Type A Behavior

In the category of harmful self-behavior that has tacit social approval, if not encouragement, is what is termed *Type A behavior*. This distinctive class of common actions has been identified as a risk factor for coronary heart disease over and above the risks imposed by age, systolic blood pressure, serum cholesterol, and smoking. The Type A behavior pattern is characterized by a number of features: A Type A person is typically alert, work oriented, impatient (in the extreme), and chronically hurried. He or she shows aggressiveness, competitiveness, ambitiousness, and adrenal arousal (Chesney, Frautschi, & Rosenman, 1985, p. 323). There is some evidence that reducing the Type A behavior pattern will reduce serum cholesterol and blood pressure, although more conclusive research is needed to document that altering diet, physical activity, or serum cholesterol significantly reduces coronary heart disease risk. But it is important to add that making these modifications in Type A behavior may lead to a subjective sense of well-being and life satisfaction (Venters, 1989).

Methods of preventive actions do not seek to change a Type A person into a Type B person (who lacks the negative characteristics associated with Type A behavior). Rather, the objective is to reduce the coronary heart disease risks Type A behavior carries (Chesney et al., 1985, p. 325). To achieve at least short-term changes—the long-term effects are not yet known—Chesney et al. suggest the following:

1. Perform self-observation using a log of critical incidents that aroused anger, frustration, or time urgency. Presumably, this would enable the person (or professional helper) to figure out how to change the environmental pressures, the psychological orientation toward those pressures (I discussed this in Chapter 2, I.A.1), or both.

2. Perform self-contracting, in which the individual specifies what he or she is going to do in what situation. (I would add, for what intended result.) "I will avoid rushing at work by walking at a more relaxed pace to prevent my heart from pounding."

3. Model how successful people combine the desired outcome (such as productivity) without the impatience and aggressiveness of Type A behavior. It is not necessary that the persons being modeled be aware of their role, merely that they are accessible for observation.

4. Relax the muscles. Relaxation to help reduce excessive adrenal arousal, particularly when combined with an awareness of its effects (as in biofeedback; see relaxation tactics, Chapter 3, II.D.3).

5. Deal with hostility. Excessive impatience and competitiveness often produce hostility. The major insight from primary prevention on hostile

II. The Second Dimension

or aggressive behaviors is that people readily take alternative means to obtain desired goals when such means reduce the risk of punishment, which the hostile action would likely generate (Azrin & Holz, 1966; Bandura, 1986; Cairns et al., 1991; Fagan et al., 1975; Gordon, 1989). Thus, with Type A behavior, it may be possible to find alternative, often contextual, means to the same end. For example, if driving in crowded traffic sets a Type A person off, then mass transit or carpooling might be acceptable changes, as would adjustments of working hours to avoid heavy traffic.

6. Use group-oriented methods to assist in modifying Type A behavior, partly because role models are available (if only the group leader) and partly because members can role-play and gain support for newly emerging social skills and reducing the Type A person's often rigidly individualistic style. I will take up this discussion in the next chapters.

Prevention of Smoking

Smoking is identified as the most preventable of the fatal self-harming behaviors. It has proved to be a stubborn enemy, probably because of its addictive nature in combination with effective product promotion (Davis, 1987; Flay, 1987; Glynn, 1989) and cultural traditions such as being "adult," cool, macho, sexy, or thin. Attempts to aid people to stop smoking (or never to start—an interestingly different problem) have been numerous. There is a chemical approach—nicotine patches that release minute quantities of the drug into the skin, reducing the physical need to obtain it through smoking. There are psychological approaches, such as lifestyle changes that reduce stress or modify situations that maintain smoking behavior (Elder et al., 1993; Windsor et al., 1993). There are group approaches, such as training programs to support resistance to peers and mass media (Evans & Raines, 1990). There are sociopolitical approaches, such as the legal advocacy of organizations such as Action on Smoking and Health (ASH) that have led to many of the victories of nonsmokers over smokers on airplanes, in public places, and in certain workplaces (Brigham, Gross, Stitzer, & Felch, 1994; Gomel et al., 1993; Jeffery et al., 1993; Mullooly, Schuman, Stevens, Glasgow, & Vogt, 1990; Schauffler, 1993), as well as contributing to the swing of the general attitude against smoking. In coming years, we will see new efforts against secondary smoke that puts nonsmoking spouses and children at mortal risk; against smokeless tobacco, which is now making its way into the children and youth markets (Glidden & Whigam, 1987); and against smoking while pregnant (Windson, Warner, & Cutter, 1988). We will likely see new social marketing approaches trying to deliver the health-promotive message as well (Altman, 1990; Crawford, 1978; "Hooked on Tobacco: The Teen Epidemic," 1995; Samuels, 1993).

The overall results show a reduction of smoking nationwide, but with certain sectors where smoking is increasing—adolescent and college-age women—and where smoking is stubbornly hanging on—blue-collar workers (Cummings et al., 1994; Elders et al., 1994). The message has not yet gotten to everyone, nor have the alternatives to the effects of smoking been promoted, although some approaches seem to work more effectively than others (see Bruvold, 1993).

Suicide Prevention

Suicide represents another major problem for primary prevention. It is probably the case that no one can prevent a person absolutely determined to commit suicide. Szasz (1986) argues that it is not the business of mental health professionals to act as psychological police, nor do they have the expertise. But we do know a good deal about suicidal behavior, and can publicize the signs that a person considering suicide often expresses (Kalafat et al., 1993; Rubenstein et al., 1989). These include

- being in a depressed mood, in combination with any four of the following that continue most days for a 2-week period:
- recent change of appetite, weight, sleeping patterns
- reduced interest or pleasure in usual activities or sexual behavior
- slowdown in clarity of thinking, concentration, or decisiveness
- thoughts or comments about death or suicide
- prior suicide attempts

By alerting schoolmates, family members, or others, it is possible to identify those at risk who might be able to receive preventive help.

The "hot line" approach to prevention is discussed in Chapter 4 (III.C.3); it represents a social response to the need for emergency confidential discussions about depressed feelings and thoughts of suicide.

II. The Second Dimension

Dew et al.'s (1987) analysis of the overall effectiveness of suicide prevention centers is not encouraging, even though these centers appear to be effective in attracting callers who are thinking about suicide. It is very difficult to prove that these centers do or do not prevent suicide. This means that we still need to consider innovative ways of reaching people and helping them appropriately (see Durkheim, 1951; Garland et al., 1989; Shaffer et al., 1988).

There are special settings where suicidal risk is unusually high, such as local jails during the initial 24 hours of incarceration, especially when the person is intoxicated and in isolation (Winkler, 1992). Likewise, certain groups, such as AIDS victims, have high rates of suicide. This situation raises a related but opposite situation that has recently been made public, the suicide-aiding professional. This situation has provoked the question of the place of a service to help terminally ill people commit voluntary suicide in a humane way (see Clark, 1993, and Crowther, 1993, on euthanasia). The ethical issues this question raises deeply challenge and disturb the public and helping professionals, including preventers (Bloom, 1993; Downing & Smoker, 1986).

3. Reducing Behaviors That Harm Others

Unfortunately, there is a long list of behaviors in which others are harmed to various degrees, but a much shorter list of successful preventive methods. The literature provides some very important beginning points that I will review here. First, consider the task of preventing behaviors that harm others. One person (or more) becomes an attacker of another, of either the other's property or person. Preventers have to be able to identify that would-be attacker and make such changes in the attacker, the object of the attack, or the situation so as to render the possible attack less likely or less virulent and the support for the would-be victim stronger and more effective. In those occasions when family or friends are the aggressors, we have a more complex preventive task on our hands.

Prevention of Juvenile Delinquency and Acting-Out Behaviors

The antisocial behaviors that youth perform can range from the normative-obnoxious (Fine, 1988), to the pathological (e.g., setting fires, destroying property, attacking innocent victims), to responses to aggression from others (such as some running away behavior). They can include verbal aggression and physical aggression; individual behaviors and collective actions; and problems at home and problems in school, work, and the community. Fortunately, these behaviors tend to diminish in most children over time, but for some, these severe and persistent antisocial actions—termed *conduct disorders*—represent significant problems that carry over into adulthood (Kazdin, 1990; Michelson, 1987; Reiss & Roth, 1993).

The problems for prevention of these conduct disorders are many and varied and the successes few. As Burchard and Burchard (1987) point out, the major successes are in the area of identification of risk factors (see Werner, 1987). A few studies provide some general guidelines for the prevention of juvenile delinquency and conduct disorders. As Berrueta-Clement, Schweinhart, Barnett, and Weikart (1987) note, only the broad outlines of a prevention understanding are present; to the future belongs the task of filling in the important details.

Major Models Regarding the Prevention of Antisocial Behavior

Hawkins and Weis (1985) offer a conceptual model that takes into account the complexity of personal, social, economic, and cultural factors. These authors offer a primary prevention approach that has proven useful in many contexts. Young people are socialized into society through three major institutions—the family, the school, and peers. There are three types of processes that each of these institutions must use if youths are to develop bonds of attachment and commitment to, and belief in, conventional society as organized by law and following a common moral code. These processes include opportunities for interacting with conventional or mainstream people, the level of social skills these young people have in obtaining reinforcement for their conventional behaviors, and consistent reinforcement for conventional social actions.

Hawkins and Weis (1985) propose a stepwise developmental sequence in which children obtain (or fail to obtain) a social bond with their family, which then helps to obtain (or fails to obtain) a social bond with the school. Then, the youths may obtain (or fail to obtain) a social bond with their peers. In each case, Hawkins and Weis are looking for opportunities for involvement in these three institutions, what skills may be developed, and what behaviors get rewarded. They propose a social development or sequence of likely events in which the three institutions have the opportunity to socialize the youths in prosocial ways. At each stage, they propose some guidelines to encourage young people to bond to the social order (in contrast with an antisocial order).

For example, bonding in the family may be facilitated by training parents to give children age-appropriate participatory roles as contributors to the family (and thus a stakeholder in it), to use good communication skills (active listening) with their children, and to provide clear and consistent expectations and sanctions for family members. These types of parent training ideas are believed to facilitate a child's bonding with the family. Similar suggestions are given for aiding the school system to enable children to form healthy social bonds with that institution and likewise to bond with prosocial peers. These three types of social bonds make it less likely that a youth will choose to get involved with delinquent behavior. Hawkins and his colleagues (Hawkins, Doueck, & Lishner, 1988; Hawkins & Lam, 1987; Hawkins, Von Cleve, & Catalano, 1991) have been engaged in community research documenting the usefulness of these ideas.

Michelson (1987) offers a cognitive-behavioral analysis that may be seen to fit within Hawkins and Weis's (1985) institutional model. Michelson asserts that antisocial youth fail to demonstrate needed social skills at various points in their life course and that the progressive nature of these (untreated) behaviors turns into serious social, legal, and clinical problems. Thus it is theoretically possible to construct various kinds of preventive programs at the many stages of the life course that attempt to reverse these cognitive-behavioral deficits.

Several major prevention projects have been conducted within these conceptual roadmaps. The Perry Preschool Project has provided very encouraging data on the effects of early intervention for later adolescent and early adult criminal (and other) behavior (Berrueta-Clement et al., 1987; Schweinhart & Weikart, 1988). Preschool-age children in a low-income black neighborhood, all whom were at high risk for educational failure, were randomly assigned to experimental and control groups in 1962. The experimental group was provided an enriched preschool education, following the hypothesis that if children could achieve success in their early schooling, this would be linked to success in schooling to the end of their secondary education. School success is conceptually linked to reduced rates of antisocial behavior. (This line of thinking follows the thrust of the Hawkins & Weis, 1985, model, although it employs a

Piagetian form of training. See Schweinhart & Weikart, 1988.) Longitudinal data support these predictions. Barnett (1993a) summarizes cost-benefit analyses from this early childhood education project for a 25-year period, including less delinquency for experimental participants as compared with controls.

The research of Spivak and Shure and their colleagues focuses on some of the specific mechanisms by which antisocial behaviors may be reduced (see Chapter 2, I.A.2). By providing training in the specific skills needed to resolve ordinary interpersonal challenges, experimental children performed more effectively than controls who did not receive this skill training in a formal manner. Some children receive problem-solving training in the course of their everyday lives; the problem is that not every child does. The programmatic studies by Spivak and Shure have shown that large numbers of children from diverse social and cultural backgrounds can all learn effective problem-solving skills.

Michelson (1987) presents information about parent management training (PMT), strategies that enable parents to interact more effectively with their children, especially around problems of aggression and acting-out behaviors. PMT follows the basic work of Patterson (1982) and his colleagues on how coercive interactions exacerbate aggressive behaviors and lead to full-blown acting-out disorders. Like Gordon's (1970) parent effectiveness training, PMT seeks to reduce coercive interchanges and promote prosocial behaviors. Research data support the efficacy of this approach.

Michelson's (1987) work on behavioral social skills training suggests some strategies related to those mentioned above but more focused on specific adaptive behaviors through enhanced communications in interpersonal skills. In general, these programs following the large-scale and small-scale road maps represent encouraging leads for dealing with the enormous problems of antisocial behaviors. It is difficult to list principles for the prevention of delinquency per se. It is becoming clearer that promoting interpersonal problem-solving skills, interpersonal conflict resolution skills, and generalized support of success in basic social settings of school, family, and among peers represents the best current plan for reducing the wide range of antisocial behaviors. (See also Boruch and other participants, 1991; Burchard & Burchard, 1987; Cairns et al., 1991; Davidson & Redner, 1988; Fagan, 1987; Huey & Rank, 1984.)

II. The Second Dimension

The Prevention of Rape

Rape presents another difficult problem for prevention. Rape is not viewed as a sexual invasion per se, but as a deliberate degradation of the victim physically, emotionally, and socially (Brownmiller, 1975). Rape is an act of violence and power perpetuated through the use of sexual and other means, toward females predominately but also toward males, with almost no age group exempted as objects of attack.

We are at the very beginning of our understanding of ways to prevent rape. I distinguish distal prevention from proximal prevention, referring to the distance from the ultimate untoward event that the preventive efforts involve. Furby, Fischhoff, and Morgan (1989) illustrate the more distant or distal approach to prevention, whereas Zoucha-Jensen and Coyne (1993) represent the more immediate or proximal study.

Furby et al. (1989) present a study of the perceived effectiveness of strategies for rape prevention and self-defense among a diverse group of women, a group of men, and a group of sexual assault experts. The 30 strategies, 16 on rape prevention and 14 on self-defense, were the most commonly mentioned among the more than 1,000 specifically mentioned ways (Fischhoff, Furby, & Morgan, 1987). The findings of the perceptions of these three groups—at the time there were few hard facts bearing on the efficacy of any of these strategies—suggest that each of the 16 rape prevention strategies, if used consistently, would reduce the risk of assault in half. Women were much more likely than men or sexual assault experts (mostly women) to rate these strategies as effective, despite national reports that many of these techniques were attempted—and still the incidence of rape remains extremely high.

Let's look at these distal strategies for rape prevention. One category includes methods

1. to reduce accessibility of women to potential assailants by locking doors to residences, to the car, and so on
2. to increase women's perceived ability to cope with an assailant by walking briskly and appearing confident
3. to increase perceived changes of outside intervention by going places with friends, parking in well-lighted places, and the like
4. to increase the perceived chances of punishment of rapists
5. to reduce men's propensity to rape by eliminating pornography in the media

6. to increase women's ability to implement preventive measures by staying vigilant and through frequent public awareness programs on rape

Each of these possible strategies requires that the potential victim know what resources are available to her (or him), what resources the assailant has (that might be used to counteract the potential victim's actions), and the circumstances of the situation. In most circumstances, however, all these facts are rarely known. This is why it is so difficult to provide empirical information about preventive strategies. For example, locking one's doors may be useful for strangers, but would not be effective in date-rape situations. Moreover, suggesting that women always go in groups in well-lighted places may reduce risk, but there is a price to be paid for this restriction of freedom.

Zoucha-Jensen and Coyne (1993) present some tentative information about the effects of proximal resistance strategies regarding actual rapes or attempted rapes. (Note: The difference between strategies in this study and the prior one is that Zoucha-Jensen and Coyne dealt with an immediate interactive situation between would-be rapist and victim, whereas Furby et al. dealt with strategies distant in time and place from any actual attempted rape.) The surveyed medical and legal records recorded outcomes (rape, nonrape, additional physical injury, if any). These data were connected with resistance strategies reported by the women. Five categories of resistance were used:

1. No resistance
2. Nonforceful verbal resistance (pleading, crying, or assertively refusing)
3. Forceful verbal resistance (screaming or yelling)
4. Physical resistance (wrestling or struggling, pushing, striking, biting, or using a weapon)
5. Fleeing (running, walking away, or fleeing in a car)

Multiple resistances were coded for their most forceful category.

The results, although limited in number (to 150 women) and time and place (1988-1989, Omaha, Nebraska), are very suggestive: No resistance and nonforceful verbal resistance were associated with being raped (chi square [$df = 4$, $N = 149$] $= 22.93$, $p < .001$). There was no significant relationship between resistance strategy and additional physical injury. The other strategies showed much higher avoidance of being raped:

II. The Second Dimension

- 45% avoided rape by running or fleeing
- 50% avoided rape by forceful verbal resistance
- 55% avoided rape by physical resistance

In contrast, 6.5% and 4.2% avoided rape by no resistance or by nonforceful verbal resistance, respectively (Zoucha-Jensen & Coyne, 1993, p. 1634). There were other limitations of this study, but as the best available information, persons threatened with rape would probably be well advised to use physical resistance, forceful verbal resistance, or fleeing—even though nothing can be predicted with any certainty about whether or not these strategies will avoid additional physical injury or not. See Pithers, Kashima, Cumming, Beal, and Buell (1988) on the prevention of relapse in sexual aggression and Gondolf (1987) on changing the behavior of men who are spousal abusers. Both of these are forms of treatment aimed at preventing new episodes of abuse; both may be suggestive of purely primary prevention ideas as well. (See discussion of relapse prevention in Chapter 3, II.C.5.)

Violence Against Others

Abuse against persons, from infants (including in utero) and children (Cappelleri et al., 1993; Conte et al., 1988; Kornberg & Caplan, 1980; Lutzker, Wesch, & Rice, 1984; Ramey, Bryant, Campbell, Sparling, & Wasik, 1988; Stiffman, 1992; Stilwell & Manley, 1990) to classmates and teachers (Huey & Rank, 1984; Sherif, Harvey, White, Hood, & Sherif, 1961) to dating partners (Levine & Kanin, 1987) to strangers (including helping professionals) (Novaco, 1977) to spouses (Schinke, Schilling, Barth, Gilchrist, & Maxwell, 1986) to elderly parents (Powell & Berg, 1987) or people in institutions (Matsushima, 1990), has come to mark our society as one of the most violent in history. The problem of violence toward others is very complicated because the aggressors may come from social units that ordinarily are sources of support against aggression and violence—such as family and friends. The same models of primary prevention are generally applicable, however. The configural equation directs attention to individual strengths and weaknesses, group supports and stresses, and physical environment resources and pressures. Preventive or promotive efforts are applied to both victim and aggressor in cases where they are part of the same social system. Moreover, these preventive or promotive efforts must be designed in tandem as far as possible.

II. The Second Dimension

Table 3.2 Representative Characteristics Associated With Violence Within the Family

Configural Dimensions	Would-Be Victims	Would-Be Aggressors
Individual	Female—infant, child, adolescent, adult, elderly	Male—adult, adolescent
	Differentiating features (premature, retarded, crying, etc., especially chronic condition) that seem to provoke the abuser	Anger, frustration
	Lack of good communication skills	Lack of good communication skills
	Use of alcohol (as in date rape to lower resistance)	Use of alcohol, drugs (especially as associated with unemployment)
	Low self-esteem	Low or lost self-esteem, anxiety, depression (often associated with loss of job)
Primary Group	Social isolation	Social isolation
	Onset of parenting	Onset of parenting
	Marital discord	Marital discord
		Stresses in family, such as financial difficulties, inadequate housing
	Disputes over disciplining, money, etc.	Disputes over disciplining, money, etc.
		Divorced, single-parent family
		Intergenerational experience with domestic violence

(continued)

Tandem Primary Prevention Strategies. Table 3.2 illustrates how tandem strategies might work. I will enumerate the classic list of factors associated with violence toward primary group members (children, dates, spouses, parents, siblings, other friends, and relatives) distinguished by would-be victim and would-be aggressor. Then I will discuss some strategies for prevention, in this and other sections of this book. The main point is to

Table 3.2 Representative Characteristics Associated With Violence Within the Family (Continued)

Configural Dimensions	Would-Be Victims	Would-Be Aggressors
Secondary Group	Low socioeconomic status	Low socioeconomic status (although abuse can occur at any socio-economic level)
	Not employed outside the home	Unemployed, lost job
	No membership in outside associations, club, union, church	No membership in outside associations such as club, union, church
Culture	Sexist victim: accepts dependent role, self-blaming, subculture supports victim role as "wife's duty" etc.	Sexist: power as prerogative of males
Society	Few laws protecting would-be victim, little prosecution of whatever protective laws available	Laws unclear about abuser in family context, police are loath to jail one family member because this puts more strain on whole family
	Courts appear to be unsympathetic to victim	Courts protective of the rights of the abuser
	Acceptance of violence in culture	Acceptance of violence in culture

SOURCE: Swift (1988) and Nietzel and Himelein (1987).

recognize that each strategy has to be modified because of the operation of the others within the same social system.

Given the intricate pattern of abuser to abused and the representative (but not exhaustive) list of factors shown in Table 3.2 associated with violence in the family, tandem preventive strategies are likely to be successful. The major recommendations on prevention of various aspects of violence in the family are familiar; what may not be emphasized enough is that tandem or dual preventive services may be needed.

For example, with regard to individual characteristics, efforts to help would-be abusers prevent uncontrolled anger should be paired with social skills training for the would-be victim to identify situations that generate anger so as to change them, as well as to learn assertive skills and what the law offers as protection and one's fair rights. Both kinds of training should take place in a context of improving communication skills so partners can share what has been problematic between them and what each has done to resolve the sources of the problems and hence the (violent) symptoms of the expression of these problems. Tandem services represent a kind of contingency planning by the prevention service worker, substituting a "no lose—win/win" situation for the problematic one (Gordon, 1989).

Moreover, as the configural equation directs one to consider, these tandem changes should take place within the context of other changes, such as reducing social isolation by connecting both partners with support groups, service networks, and friends. The stresses associated with unemployment should be addressed by helping people return to work (see Chapter 3, II.E.3); workers and family members should also be connected with various mutual aid and support groups so as to deal with the dual problems of social isolation and lack of resources within the family itself (see Chapter 4, III.B.1, III.B.2). Stresses associated with parenting can be reduced through various methods, from family planning to family life education (see Chapter 3, II.E.4).

At the same time, prevention workers should be participating in larger societal efforts to end sexism and racism, not only for the specific part they play in violence in the family but for their general sake as well (see Chapter 5, IV.D.2, IV.D.3). The basic principle is to remember that a whole configuration of causes is involved in any violent situation and preventive solutions require balancing the efforts for both parties and the sociocultural context. (See also Barth, Hacking, & Ash, 1988; Boruch et al., 1991; Budin & Johnson, 1989; Cairns et al., 1991; Ferre, 1987; Lutzker et al., 1984; Taylor & Beauchamp, 1988; Tzeng, Jackson, & Karlson, 1991; Violence Prevention Coalition of Greater Los Angeles, n.d.; Walther, 1986.)

4. Behavioral Rehearsal Through Role-Playing

One way to reduce individual limitations is to learn how to cope effectively and to practice this new behavior until one becomes able to perform it effectively. The sequence of events related to such practice is long and involved, from recognizing the problem and getting motivated to act, through the practice sessions themselves, to the reactivation of the skill when it is needed. This section addresses the rehearsal part.

Meichenbaum (1985) notes that two general modes of action are needed to get clients to put their coping strategies into action: imagery or cognitive rehearsal (discussed on p. 105) and behavioral rehearsal. Behavioral rehearsal, such as role-playing, requires the client to imagine the stressful situation very vividly, but in addition to thinking about (and feeling) the stress, the client now engages in physical actions that practice what might be done to reduce the tension. For example, when enabling youths to buy contraceptives in a public situation—a potentially embarrassing and inhibiting scenario—the practitioner and clients simulate a drugstore setting so as to practice how to accomplish this task effectively. Beyond simulation, there is also guided practice in real-world contexts.

In role-playing contexts, filmed simulations are sometimes used with discussions of what is happening. In this case, behavioral rehearsal is accomplished by vicarious modeling, that is, by observing holistically what a model does in a similarly stressful situation and noticing what happens to that model (Bandura, 1986). At other times, the client or the practitioner might take the role of the client in acting out the scene. Other variations include members of the group taking turns acting out one or another role and providing feedback and support for the other actors (Schinke et al., 1979).

Meichenbaum (1985) notes a variety of contexts in which behavioral rehearsal has been successfully used: with patients in pain (Turk, Meichenbaum, & Genest, 1983), in coping with anger control by police officers and adolescent offenders (Feindler & Fremous, 1983; Novaco, 1977; Sarason, Johnson, Berberich, & Siegel, 1979), in seeking help from others (Wasik, 1984), in being assertive with one's physician (Sobel & Worden, 1981), in resolving conflicts between adolescents and parents (Robin, 1981), and in handling job-related stress by nurses (West et al., 1984).

Bandura's (1977, 1989a) self-efficacy theory suggests that simulated coping will generalize to the real world most readily when clients believe they can do what is called for (efficacy expectation) and that an adequate response will lead to successful consequences (outcome expectation). (See a related discussion of the Health Belief Model [Rosenstock, 1990] and the theory of reasoned action [Carter, 1990; Fishbein & Ajzen, 1975] as well as other aspects of Bandura's social learning theory in Appendix B.)

5. Relapse Prevention and Booster Shots

This section examines two terms that are relatively new to the practice scene and need further discussion in connection with primary prevention (contrasted with treatment). The term *relapse prevention* has received careful definition by its originators, Marlatt and George (1984), who build on the concept of self-efficacy (Bandura, 1977). The notions of preventing attrition in one's research sample or preventing dropout from treatment have long been with us, but only recently have planned efforts been conceptualized and tested to achieve these goals in primary prevention.

Briefly stated within the primary prevention context rather than the treatment context of Marlatt and George (1984), the idea is to identify high-risk cues or situations for relapse from some newly attained healthful status, to bring this risk to the attention of the client, to discuss together the factors specific to this individual that might lead to relapse to being at high risk for a preventable problem, and to offer suggestions and practice to counteract these factors so as to resist these pressures toward relapse. This concept belongs to the general cognitive-behavioral framework, suggesting that factors of self-efficacy and reinforcement will play a large part in the prevention of relapse.

Many people relapse from treatment; most who do, do so shortly after their initial change attempt (Rimer, 1990). This is especially true in the addiction area, where the person may be "dried out" (as in alcohol treatment programs), but the sociocultural and physical environments have not been changed much as a result of this person's private treatment. When such ex-clients return to their ordinary environments or happen as if by chance to go to these areas, all the cues that set them off in the first place still exist (McCrady, 1989; Wallace, 1989).

Professionals do not know whether or not people will relapse to a high-risk status, but the dynamics seem so similar to those of treatment relapse that I will assume relapse is possible. Marlatt and George (1984) describe relapse prevention as a self-control program designed to help people who are trying to change their behavior to anticipate and cope with the possibility of relapse. Thus relapse prevention is a psychoeducational program combining both behavioral skill training and cognitive interventive techniques.

Meichenbaum (1985) brings this discussion closer to primary prevention in his consideration of relapse prevention in stress management (see

Chapter 3, II.B.2). Ordinarily healthy people facing ordinary stresses in society need ways to manage these stresses and can learn them. But slips, failures, or relapses of various degrees are bound to happen on occasion and, rather than assume that the client will rebound and continue with the preventive effort, the people involved may view these slips as evidence of inadequate personal efficacy and may give up the healthy behavior patterns previously learned. To reduce this possibility, Meichenbaum suggests ways of encouraging clients to anticipate some failure or setback experiences and then has them rehearse how they will respond effectively so as to recapture their feeling of self-efficacy. One must not push the probability of failure too strongly, however, or one will risk creating a self-fulfilling prophecy. Rather, relapse prevention should be included among a range of responses that the client learns about dealing with stress. The relapse concerns being subjected to new risk factors, not to threats to personal self-image. To emphasize this point, one might term this *risk relapse prevention*.

Meichenbaum (1985) also makes the important point that stress always exists, even after clients have learned successful training. The goal of stress inoculation training is to learn how to respond adaptively to changeable situations, to be resilient in the face of momentary failure, and to accept that which cannot be changed and go on with life as best as possible.

Most of the literature on relapse prevention concerns work with people who have just undergone treatment and have emerged at some desired level of functioning. A new set of learnings is engaged such that the participants will be able to maintain control over their formerly antisocial behavior over time and across varied situations. Sandahl and Rönnberg (1990) discuss relapse prevention in the context of brief group psychotherapy for alcohol-dependent patients. McCrady (1989) aids couples involved in addiction with relapse prevention. Stark et al. (1990) address the issues of relapse prevention at the time of the first phone contact with substance-abusing clients. The interview prompts to workers are instructive:

> Sometimes people [who] decide to get help never make it down here. Is there anything you can think of that might stand in your way? (Listen to obstacles generated. Prompt, when needed, as follows:) What about problems in transportation, child care, finances, other people who think it's a dumb idea, you changing your mind, perhaps because you think that you are really doing well,

or doing really badly? (Generate workable solutions with caller for each possibility.) (p. 71)

Primary prevention can learn some valuable lessons from work in relapse prevention, including from studies that did not show successful outcomes (such as Killen et al., 1990, in which smoking relapse prevention worked for men but not for women; Ito, Donovan, & Hall, 1988, in which there were no differences between a cognitive-behavioral relapse prevention group and an interpersonal process aftercare group, as related to drinking outcomes; or Stark et al., 1990). Successful relapse prevention studies also provide suggestions.

Pithers et al. (1988) make the point that a continuum of antecedents is likely with regard to the untoward behavior. Some antecedents are at a long distance from a specific antisocial behavior (such as a recovering alcoholic who is feeling vaguely upset and moody); others are events that are apparently irrelevant to the antisocial behavior but in fact move one closer to it (such as a recovering alcoholic who happens to walk into a bar to get change for a phone call and bumps into old drinking buddies); others are high-risk crises (such as that recovering alcoholic's friends calling for a round of drinks for old-times sake); and others involve having inadequate coping behaviors (such as not being able to say no to friends).

A risk relapse prevention program attempts to analyze each category and provide appropriate self-strategies for dealing with them. For example, if one is feeling moody (something that had been associated with drinking in the past), then one acts to change that mood by any number of methods such as relaxation techniques (see Chapter 3, II.D.3) or problem-solving methods (see Chapter 2, I.A.2) to oppose any condition that might lead to antisocial behavior. For antecedents that are apparently irrelevant, one must recognize the past stimuli associated with the problem (such as going into bars) and look for alternatives immediately (such as locating a drugstore or gas station to get change instead).

High-risk crises need planned escape strategies and interpersonal skill techniques (such as saying assertively that one must meet a friend elsewhere and leaving promptly). Antecedents involving inadequate coping behavior suggest that booster shots are needed for the appropriate coping skills, ones that presumably were learned in the initial service program.

In general, one or more of these categories may be relevant for a given primary preventive situation; individualized discussions should be held before the problem occurs. Let's take a direct prevention example. Suppose a person has learned to incorporate condoms in her view of what safer sex methods mean and that she has become committed to safer sex while continuing an active sex life. In the context of this preventive achievement, the prevention worker might raise a series of questions or, better, ask the client to anticipate possible situations that might reduce the likelihood of using condoms. The client should take each situation and work it through for a preventive risk relapse strategy—to avoid going back to a situation without safe sex:

Worker Suppose you meet a terrific person at a party and are immediately attracted to him. Matters between you are going very well and you both experience the desire for sex, but you discover that you left your condoms in your other jacket.

Client Something like that happened a while ago, so I know what you mean.

Worker OK, if this is a possible kind of situation, what can you think of to prevent your having sex without condoms? What can you do? What could the other person do? What alternatives are there to having sex without condoms?

Client I suppose I could bring up the topic of protection with that person to see if he has any on hand. Or maybe we could go some other place and, on the way, stop off and get some condoms.

Worker Those ideas sound reasonable. Are you sure you could in fact say those things to a new date?

Client I'm pretty sure I can talk frankly about safe sex, just like we learned to do in the group. Like the TV ad says, "Sex is wonderful, but I'm not willing to die for it."

Worker What if the other person is pressuring you to have sex right away? What could you do in this situation?

Client Well, if my date really wanted to get going, maybe I could ask a friend at the party if he or she could loan me a condom. I know one other thing that could be done—I could say, "Hey, no sex until we have a condom," but frankly, I'm not sure I could handle that.

Worker If you're sure this is the critical stage where you're going to have sex whether or not you have a condom, then knowing this, your plan should always be to do something to get that condom before things get to this stage. You mentioned various methods at earlier points in the relationship that would work quite well . . .

There are many situations that clients might dream up that could lead them to neglect preventive or protective actions just learned. It is a different kind of teaching to have the client think about strategies of maintaining safe sex and continuing communications with a desirable partner. These strategies can be quite challenging to suggest, but the very act of thinking about them clarifies the nature of safe sex and the stages of preparation required to be a "great lover" (Hatcher, 1990).

In general, prevention workers may have to be quite assertive in helping clients think about and overcome possible cues that would get them back into habits making them at risk once again. Showing that people have attained a desired preventive objective does not guarantee that they will stay at this desired level forever. Talking about possible situations and cues that could lead to relapse from a desired level of preventive or protective activity may be the ultimate in individualizing the prevention program; only the participant can identify for himself or herself factors likely to lead to that person's unique relapse.

Booster Shots

The phrase "booster shot" refers to a medical situation in which one set of immunization shots has been given and, at a later date, another set is given to complete the preventive effect. The term is used loosely in the prevention literature, but it has great potential if incorporated into the flow of events termed *primary prevention*.

Let me define some parameters of the situation that might involve booster shots. First, the booster shot comes after an initial prevention program has been presented and there is some evidence that desired movement to a criterion level has taken place. At this point, there are several choices: "Declare victory" and terminate (while the worker is ahead) or maintain contact with the clients on a planned or unplanned basis to support their progress (or to study successful programs or both).

Second, at some later date, the worker evaluates the situation again to determine whether there have been any changes. If there are improvements or the client remains at the same level of success as seen before, either terminate or maintain contact. If there is some deterioration, the worker must decide what to do next. This is the context of the booster shot.

The worker may decide to offer another full dose of the original program (if the deterioration is severe) or, more likely, offer a modified program (such as a brief review program or possibly a new program adapted for older, more mature clients). The worker must evaluate once again to ensure that the criterion level has again been met and either terminate or maintain contact, that is, initiate a new booster program after another period of time.

A fundamental issue regarding the booster shot is knowing when clients have attained and maintained a successful criterion level of preventive or promotive achievement. Workers cannot give booster shots forever; nor can they foresee every kind of temptation. Rough norms need to be established, such as if 50% to 75% of the sample succeeds in maintaining the successful criterion level over a reasonable period of time, then that program will be declared successful for the range of time including the booster period. These participants may face more extreme or different challenges later, for which new prevention programs will be needed. This moves out of the booster period into another consideration for primary prevention.

A typical study in the need for booster shots was conducted by Peterson and Mori (1985) regarding the prevention of child injury. These researchers used the problem-solving approach to aid children (aged 7 to 9) to produce their own plan of action regarding safety and the prevention of injury and to self-reinforce these actions. The children were trained to prevent injury to an acceptable level of competence. Five months later, they were retested and retrained on any module where they did not achieve the acceptable level of competence. There was some decline in safe behavior during this time, but the children did not return to baseline levels. Booster training quickly brought them back to their earlier achievements. Thus booster shots may be a cost-effective expenditure of money and effort.

I offer the following principles with regard to booster shots as part of an integrated primary prevention program:

1. Have clearly defined goals of the primary prevention project so that one knows baseline and intervention period levels of performance on the activity in question. Performance and learning involve cognitive as well as affective and behavioral components, and an assessment of outcome should include an examination to ensure that participants understand, are in favor of, and can perform the desired behavior to some criterion level.

2. At some appropriate time after the project has been terminated, retest former participants for the level of the targeted performance behav-

ior. The timing for retest is not clear. It would be reasonable to give the participants time to embed these new learned behaviors in their life situations and to let the natural supporting processes take over. It is also easier to correct minor deviations than major ones, which would argue for going in sooner than later. Balance going in too early with going in too late. The nature of the target behavior is relevant: Life-threatening behaviors should be monitored more closely and in shorter intervals than others.

3. If at the retesting it is determined that some slippage has occurred, then the worker and the participant must determine how serious the decrease is and whether or not it is worth the effort to reenter the situation formally. (Merely discussing the situation with a former client probably reactivates some of the preventive understanding and actions that may be helpful in itself.) Some participants, such as school children, may not be directly involved in discussion of their progress, although their parents should be, as should school officials and the researchers. For example, Flay et al. (1989) note that the desired effects of their social influence approach to smoking among 6th graders (in which they taught students how to resist social pressures from peers) had been essentially wiped out by the 12th grade. They raise the point about the need for booster shots in each succeeding grade, a decision teachers, parents, and administrators must ultimately make. As junior high and high school students become involved, it becomes increasingly important to have them participate in these discussions (Young, Elder, Green, de Moor, & Wildey, 1988).

4. The actual booster shot must be adapted to the level of performance and need of the target group. A brief reminder of previous training may be adequate for some participants, whereas a complete replay may be needed by others. It may be helpful to involve the participants in deciding on the booster shot, because this puts some of the responsibility for the renewed learning in their hands.

5. Conduct another monitoring or evaluation period to assess the level of performance after the booster shot had time to take effect. At some point, a program has to end. More research is required to examine the long-term effects of primary prevention programs as these become embedded in ordinary life events. Longitudinal studies, such as the Perry Preschool project (Schweinhart & Weikart, 1988), can demonstrate the costs and benefits of specific programs even as these become blended into, or diluted by, the ordinary flow of life events.

II. The Second Dimension

6. Reducing Prejudice and Discrimination

Dr. Seuss's (1961) book, *The Sneetches*, is quite instructive about the nature of prejudice (attitudinal prejudgment) and discrimination (harmful behavior, by acts of commission or omission, directed toward a person based on group characteristics, not on individual factors). Members of a group of creatures are exactly the same except some have "stars on thars" (on their belly buttons, to be precise), whereas others lack these stars. The ones with the stars lord over those without, who become very unhappy because of their lack and the attendant discriminatory behaviors directed toward them.

Somehow the situation gets reversed, and the reader comes to realize that creatures are all basically alike or, at least, having "stars on thars" is not a basis for superiority but merely a difference. In this way, the incomparable Dr. Seuss tells his story of prejudice. This section presents methods for preventing such prejudice and discrimination.

Smith (1990) makes the point that the context of prejudice and discrimination has changed over the past half century from explicit and open actions in segregated schools, public facilities, and the like to the situation at present, when the expression of racism has grown more subtle. It is even harder today for individuals to understand their own life training in prejudicial thinking and action. (The same training has probably been given in the other *isms*—for example, see Albee, 1981, on the prevention of sexism.) If one believes that one is not prejudiced, then there is little need to engage oneself in antiprejudice training; such self-deception is present among helping professionals as much as anywhere else.

This historic shift toward subtle racism occurred because of changes in the law that preceded public sentiment (especially in affected locations; see Chapter 5, IV.D.3). So, for example, President Dwight D. Eisenhower sent in federal troops to enforce the Supreme Court's decision on school desegregation. Only later did attitudes change toward segregation.

Attitudes, particularly those involving prejudice, are learned early in life, essentially at the parents' knees. Children simply accept family attitudes as the way of the world. They may find support in homogeneous communities or they may find opposition in heterogeneous ones. These attitudes are rarely thought-out points of view. As children grow, their education extends into schools and social settings where the prejudices of their families may be challenged. Such challenges may stimulate change or crystallize the views further—the full dynamics of each are not well understood. People may carry their prejudices, suitably disguised in adult forms, throughout their lives—perhaps supported by, perhaps in opposition to, the many social groups to which they belong.

In this section, I use the topic of racism to stand for all other forms of *isms* for simplicity of discussion, even though I recognize there are many differences among ways people dislike and oppress others. The distinction among personal, institutional, and cultural racism is important. *Institutional racism* refers to collective policies or standards of practice (such as criteria of admission, rewards for advancement, laying off workers) used by one group, intentionally or not, toward another group that serves to create or maintain advantages or opportunities for the first relative to the second. Institutional racism is built into the system through a cobweb of interconnections all serving the same function in different ways. Poll taxes and qualifying tests for voter registration, segregated schools, job discrimination patterns, and selective banking practices in providing housing loans all work together to weave a self-fulfilling prophecy that a minority group is less adequate than the majority group. No one knows exactly who put these laws, policies, and rules into effect, and so pervasive is it that institutional racism is as invisible as the air we breathe or the civil rights we hold dear (for ourselves).

Individual or personal racism involves the prejudicial attitudes and the discriminatory behaviors that one person holds toward members of some group. Both attitudes and behaviors are learned; presumably for them to continue to exist, there must be some pattern for their reinforcement. One can hold prejudicial attitudes but not act on them in performing discriminatory behaviors; or attitudes and behaviors may go in tandem. Likewise, it is possible for personal and institutional racism to exist together or independently.

Cultural racism reflects both individual and institutional expressions of the superiority of one race's cultural heritage, value system, and lifestyle over those of other races (Ponterotto & Pedersen, 1993, p. 11). Cultural racism proposes one's own culture as the standard of reference against which other cultures are in some ways deficient.

Much of current thinking on understanding and dealing with prejudice and discrimination is based on the watershed writings of Gordon Allport (1954a, 1989). The core ideas, emerging from theory, research, and practice, first defined prejudice and discrimination as being derived from false stereotypes. Allport (1954b) proposes seven general classes of ways to counter prejudice:

1. Legislation: This includes civil rights legislation, employment legislation, and group libel legislation. Allport (1954b) notes that legislation may increase prejudice, such as the laws that legally established second-class citizenship for African Americans in the South. No legislation aims at controlling prejudice per se, only the expression of prejudice. In the long run, thoughts and attitudes will fall in line with behaviors.

2. Formal educational programs: These include more than basic information about other groups because "information seldom sticks unless mixed with attitudinal glue" (Allport, 1954b, p. 373). Experience suggests that direct and experiential programs work best. It is also possible to teach positive tolerance for differences among peoples, as well as teaching to prevent prejudice.

3. Contact and acquaintance programs: On the basis of research knowledge, Allport (1954b, p. 376) proposes an action hypothesis that specifies planned contact between two peoples under conditions of equal status and power in pursuit of common objectives. Subsequently, a number of classic experiments were conducted to illustrate this hypothesis. One study involved a simulation in which two teams of campers were made competitive (by manipulating the rules of sporting and other camp activities), which rapidly led to intergroup fighting (Sherif et al., 1961). These conflicts were resolved when new camp activities required that the teams cooperate in achieving a common goal, suggesting how norms of competition or cooperation create conflicting or friendly relationships between groups.

4. Group retraining: This approach involves the use of group dynamics, an understanding of human relations in group settings. Blanchard and Cook (1976) conducted research that suggests that constructive interracial attitudes may be fostered by having small-group members engage in helping behaviors. (See Davis & Proctor, 1989, for guidelines for practice with individuals, families, and groups in contexts related to race, gender, and class conflicts.) Aronson and Bridgeman (1979) conducted a number of studies involving an interdependent learning situation in which children were given portions of a single class exercise. Each individual had to learn his or her own part and then communicate it to the others so that the whole team could achieve its common goal. Children had to learn how to communicate meaningfully with others (including minority people), how

to listen carefully, and how to ask good questions. Because of the structure of the project, a kind of social "jigsaw puzzle," each person was seen to be making an important contribution to the common cause (see also Rooney-Rebeck & Jason, 1986; Slavin, 1981).

5. Mass media: Research was just beginning when Allport (1965b) developed his strategies for reducing prejudice through the mass media, but he proposes several principles based on tentative information: One needs a campaign, not merely a single program, to influence attitudes through the mass media. The campaign should focus on specific effects and use prestigious symbols (such as the musician who organized the worldwide benefit on behalf of AIDS victims). Propaganda campaigns need to be sensitive to their intended audiences; for some people, prejudices are part of their underlying personality structure; for others, they may be due to a lack of accurate information. In general, Allport recommends allaying anxiety; otherwise, such propaganda will tend to be resisted. When attitudes cannot be changed, mass media can attempt to change the context so that the prejudices cannot be legally expressed.

6 and 7. Exhortation, catharsis, and therapy: Allport (1954b) does not see much accumulated effects of generations of exhortations through preaching or ethical pep talks or in catharsis as such, although an explosion of feelings may have a temporary effect. On the other hand, Allport sees a strong contribution from individual therapy (and, I would add, group therapy).

Ponterotto and Pedersen (1993) expand this perspective in their guide for counselors and educators. These authors suggest that professional helpers first must understand racial or ethnic identity development (see Cross, 1991; Phinney, 1989, 1990). Then they must assess their own racial or ethnic development and take steps to develop their own racial identity. Finally, they can employ a variety of methods of aiding others to achieve a high level of racial or ethnic identity development, which is associated with better mental health and lower levels of prejudice.

Ponterotto and Pedersen (1993) cite various authors in presenting a series of prejudice prevention methods. Walsh (1988) is cited with regard to building a climate of respect among students and teachers who are to engage in discussions on prejudice. Teachers promote critical thinking, the rights of all to be heard, and the self-esteem of the participants within a multicultural and nonsexist educational environment. (Walsh notes that high self-esteem is associated with lower levels of prejudice.)

II. The Second Dimension

Role reversals have been used to reduce prejudice, especially under conditions of "blaming the victim" (Smith, 1990). In these situations, one group is encouraged to imagine itself as the other group so as to become emotionally involved with the images, feelings, thoughts, and expectations of being born in some other racial group. These experiences can increase the self-awareness and self-control regarding making prejudgments that are based on stereotypes held about some group.

Stereotypes are, by definition, simplistic overstatements that either devalue or overglorify a group and thereby minimize individual differences that may be different: "Blacks are lazy, live on public welfare, and are good musicians and athletes." "Asian Americans are quiet, hard working, and good at math." Stereotypes may be logically inconsistent— lazy and good athletes. Yet they organize people's perceptions and actions toward the object of the stereotype, as when a storekeeper becomes extra observant when a minority teenager walks into the drugstore.

Stereotypical beliefs are very strongly held, probably because they are often based in part on individual experiences that reinforce the stereotypes. One minority youth may have swiped something from the drugstore when the shopkeeper happened to be looking; this may have been the only time she saw a theft in action and this piece of evidence is very central to how she organizes her attitudes. She may "know better" in the sense that she reads that the majority of criminals are white and the majority of people on welfare are white. The valedictorian at the local high school may be a recent émigré from Southeast Asia who did not know how to speak English when he arrived several years ago; now this person has a scholarship to go to MIT. A germ of truth makes stereotypes very resistant to change.

For primary prevention, the issues of prejudice and discrimination focus on to how to influence actions that unfairly and unequally (illegally and immorally) impose limits on members of one group in ways that are not imposed on all others. In addition to the suggestions presented above, I offer the following collective practice principles:

1. Obtain solid documentation of the discriminatory behavior. Prejudicial attitudes may be annoying, but these behaviors are most subject to action. Sometimes stating that one has such documentation may be the first step in getting the discriminator to make changes because of the implied threat of untoward publicity or legal action. The discriminator may also take strong actions to destroy that evidence, so be prepared for a variety of reactions.

2. Mobilize collective forces as far as possible in favor of the discriminated party (parties). A broad-based coalition of informed supporters makes it less likely that any one portion of that group would be singled out for attack because the information and activity are spread throughout the larger group. (Unfortunately, attacks may be physical as well as symbolic; many have lost their lives in the defense of civil rights.)

3. Organize that collective so that information and resources can be focused at the right place at the right time by the right people. Specialists in organizing or mobilizing evidence, such as community activists or lawyers, may be useful. Be prepared with all the facts arranged in persuasive ways; premature efforts frequently meet with failure.

4. Apply the responsive pressure to the discrimination through appropriate but friendly (or at least neutral) agents of the government. This may mean, at times, bypassing local agents in favor of state or federal ones, provided that the supporting laws permit their entrance into the problem. In general, ask what the law, statute, or ordinance provides with regard to the offending action and what redress can the discriminated person expect. In organizations, as contrasted with governments, there will be certain positions in the structure to whom one might turn for relief.

5. Agents of the discriminated group should approach agents of the discriminating group with legal, social, and other resources in hand, thus taking the status of an equal force and an equal power. In this contact or series of contacts, the steps are worked out whereby the offending group will cease its discriminatory behavior. Whether or not the victims receive any other redress is a complicated legal matter.

6. If there is any way that the two groups can be found to work toward a common goal, this might facilitate communication and cooperation. Attitude change may never occur, but the significant objective is behavior change. It is preferable, of course, to obtain both attitude and behavior change.

D. Physiological and Biological Aspects

1. Diagnostic Screening

In public health, the term *screening* has at least three different meanings: to count (as in actuarial statistics), to sort into categories for helping

Table 3.3 Seven Warning Signs of Cancer

Changes in bowel or bladder habits
A sore that does not heal
Unusual bleeding or discharge
Thickening or lump in breast or elsewhere
Indigestion or difficulty in swallowing
Obvious change in wart or mole
Nagging cough or hoarseness

SOURCE: American Cancer Society.
NOTE: If you have a warning sign, see your doctor.

purposes (as in triage), and to identify for purposes of possible intervention (as in periodic health exams). These meanings blur into one another depending on the situation. I focus here mainly on the last function, identification for possible intervention.

Screening may be done by other people (as in being given a mammogram by professionals at an office), by oneself (as in doing a breast self-examination; Mayer et al., 1987; Schechter, Vanchieri, & Crofton, 1990), or occasionally by machine (as in blood pressure machines). This section focuses mainly on screening done by others, but I want to note the importance of self-exams, both for the awareness of particular problems (such as the seven danger signs of cancer) and for the stimulus to think preventively about the problem itself ("I've got a smoker's cough, and I have to stop smoking to reduce my chances of getting lung cancer."). The seven warning signs of cancer presented in Table 3.3 are an important public health self-screening device.

A major use of screening occurs in medical contexts. For example, the risk in the general population of having a child with a major birth defect is between 3% and 5%; only a small fraction of these defects are detectable by means of diagnostic screening procedures such as amniocentesis (Grobstein, 1979). Some of the most important genetic disorders (in terms of numbers of people involved and the level of support victims require) can be discovered through existing screening procedures, however (Bolton, Charlton, Gai, Laner, & Shumway, 1985; Warheit, Auth, & Vega, 1985).

Methods of prenatal screening are of recent vintage. Amniocentesis, perhaps the most widely known, involves withdrawing a small amount of amniotic fluid from the sac that surrounds the fetus and contains cells shed from the fetus. Amniocentesis is best performed during the 15th to 17th week of pregnancy so that enough fluid is available to allow safe removal of a small portion. This puts the procedure in the second trimester, which raises some problems should abortion be called for. A more recently developed procedure, chorionic villous biopsy, is performed at the 8th to 11th week of pregnancy, in the first trimester, and thus reduces some of the problems associated with amniocentesis (Schild & Black, 1984, p. 47).

Schild and Black (1984) note that the major risk of amniocentesis is from miscarriage; data suggest that this risk is slightly elevated over the natural risk of miscarriage—1% to 2% (p. 46). It takes several weeks for the culture produced from these cells to grow and be analyzed. Part of the information obtained is a karyotype or picture of the 23 sets of chromosomes; the sex of the fetus can also be determined. This is very important in the transmission of some genetic disorders but it also has social and cultural meaning for the people involved.

A diagnostic procedure that is not invasive involves the use of sonography or ultrasound, in which sound vibrations are reflected off tissue of different densities, yielding measures of the size and shape of fetal structures (Schild & Black, 1984, p. 46). These and newer experimental methods are enabling people to learn about the fetus and its possible genetic defects in ample time to make an informed decision on what steps to take next, some of which are preventive in nature. (See Begab, 1974, on the potentials of such preventive actions.)

There are also many screening instruments for newborn infants (Magrab, Sostek, & Powell, 1984). The majority of infants with developmental disabilities were medically normal newborns, so it is important to screen all infants, such as with the Denver Developmental Screening Test (Frankenburg, Van Doorninck, Liddell, & Dick, 1976) or the Brazelton Neonatal Assessment Scale (Brazelton, 1973)—which has the additional psychological benefit of stimulating the parents' understanding of, and raised levels of interest in, their child (Brazelton, 1986).

There are also important screening tests used with young people and adults. Prevention-oriented health maintenance organizations use screening surveys to optimize good health while minimizing costly treatments for illness. Periodic health screening involves millions of persons in programs such as Kaiser Permanente in California (Fields, 1978).

II. The Second Dimension

Louria, Kidwell, Lavenhar, Thind, and Najem (1976) provide a useful review of the literature with regard to the types of health problems that adults are heir to and for which primary prevention is feasible. They recommend a 10-point program of selective screening that may be achievable, practical, and acceptable to consumers. This includes a Papanicolaou (PAP) smear for women over the age of 25 every 2 years; self-examination of breasts every 3 months for women over 30; a yearly test for blood in the stools for everyone over the age of 49; tests of blood pressure and blood cholesterol levels every 2 years (unless there is reason to suspect a problem); intraocular pressure tests every 3 to 5 years for everyone over age 35; hemoglobin test every 2 years; prostate exam for men every 2 to 3 years after the age of 49; screening for compliance of limitation or elimination of smoking; and the regular use of seat belts.

Starting at age 20, people should be tested every 5 years for both total cholesterol and high-density lipids (HDL), the "good" cholesterol. If either one is problematic, then one should be tested further for low-density lipids (LDL), the "bad" cholesterol. The goal is to have a total cholesterol measuring under 200 milligrams (per deciliter of blood; mg/dl), a level thought to reduce the risk of heart disease in most people. With a level above 240 mg/dl, one definitely needs testing of the LDL. An HDL above 60 mg/dl is considered enough to protect one against heart disease. An LDL level below 130 mg/dl is desirable; above 160 mg/dl, one needs to take action through diet, exercise, or medication (McCann et al., 1990).

Screening issues emerge in social research. Reinherz and her colleagues (Reinherz & Griffin, 1977; Reinherz et al., 1990) identifyed levels of risk among children scheduled to enter kindergarten. The screening battery included gathering family and health data and some psychological tests on learning efficiency known to predict special needs of kindergarten children. Some empirical findings emerged that have important preventive implications. By connecting levels of risk—high (immediate intervention), moderate (needing retesting and referral to specialists), or low—to the battery of tests, these authors discovered that "no child with speech problems emerged in any of the more positive ratings for social and emotional behavior, including temperament, attentiveness, social assertiveness, sleep habits, and bowel and bladder control" (Reinherz et al., 1990, p. 16). The implication is to watch out for children with speech problems as predictors of other untoward behaviors.

In general, screening possibilities offer specific tests of predictable problems, some of which can be prevented entirely (at various costs), whereas others enable family and other care providers time to plan for optimal support of a person with developmental disabilities.

Screening is a technical procedure; information derived from screening must be put into the larger equation of what we know about a situation and what goals people hold before options are presented to participants.

2. Genetic Counseling

Genetic counseling is the nonmedical aspect of genetic services. Magrab et al. (1984) define it as a communication process whereby a family is helped to understand

> 1) the medical facts including the diagnosis and treatment of any given genetic disorder, 2) the ways heredity contributes to the occurrence of the disorders (statistical probabilities) and the risk factors involved, such as mortality, developmental deficits, and recurrence, 3) the alternatives for dealing with the risks (abortion, adoption, acceptance), 4) selecting a course of action that is consistent with the family's goals and beliefs, and 5) making the best possible adjustment to the occurrence of a genetic disorder. (p. 52)

This section presents basic background information to enable the reader to recognize when a referral to a specialist in genetic counseling would be useful (Kessler, 1979; Rauch, 1988; Reisman & Matheny, 1969; Schild & Black, 1984)—although clients may not accept this information (Neal-Cooper & Scott, 1988; Nelkin & Tancredi, 1989).

The rapid developments in genetics dazzle the imagination while raising some awesome ethical issues (e.g., whether or not to inform people screened for Huntington's disease of their inevitably fatal status years before it is to occur; Meissen & Berchek, 1988). Yet basic genetic information may help people to make other behavioral choices that will prevent misery to themselves and to potential offspring. These choices have enormous social and financial costs, as the lifetime care costs of profoundly ill or retarded people are extremely high. In a time of scarcity, difficult decisions must be made as to where resources will be directed. For this purpose alone genetic counseling is of major value. Yet, in ways difficult to measure, having information related to reproduction expands human options and the value choices these entail. I propose putting genetic counseling in the context of the configural model, which involves looking at issues of reproduction from the perspective of individuals, small and large groups, society, culture, and history—all are directly or indirectly affected by personal decisions. All are shareholders, in both the burden of the decision and the costs of the outcomes. Recognizing these burdens may lighten the challenge facing the particular individuals involved.

A study of genetic counseling by Sorenson, Swazey, and Scotch (1981; as reported in Schild & Black, 1984, pp. 7-8) suggests that the basic reasons people come for genetic counseling are to learn more about the etiology of the medical problem and to learn about the risks for recurrence of the problem in future children. Clients also want to talk about "sociomedical" issues— their feelings about having a child with problems related to their genetic makeup, questions about schooling and other special programs, financial costs of raising such a child, what effects this would have on their relationships with their other children and between spouses. Ethical and moral questions abound and helping professionals must be comfortable among such issues, which means that they have to know their own values and be able to listen and respect the values of others. Books, such as that of Loewenberg and Dolgoff (1992), are helpful at points of departure.

Basic Genetic Information

This section represents a brief review of what readers are likely to have learned in undergraduate biology or human development classes. It is not intended to be an exhaustive coverage of the major concepts in the rapidly changing field of genetics but a presentation of the terms that specialists will use in case conferences.

Genes are the smallest unit of inheritance of specific characteristics. Most traits are produced by large numbers of genes. They are composed of pieces of deoxyribonucleic acid (DNA) located in the nucleus of each cell. Genes group together in paired strings called chromosomes, one strand coming from each parent (ovum and sperm cells). Humans possess 23 pairs of chromosomes in each cell, or 46 chromosomes. The first 22 are matched pairs (autosomes); the 23rd is the sex chromosome, in which the female is indicated by XX and the male by XY.

Human inheritance involves the combination of male and female chromosomes and the resulting division of cells into specialized groups.

One type of cell division (meiosis) involves the uniting of sperm and egg cells so that the fertilized egg contains only 46 chromosomes. The other type of cell division (mitosis) occurs as the fertilized cell reproduces itself.

For various reasons, errors occur in these divisions, leaving too few or too many chromosomes; sometimes errors occur in the structural arrangements among genes, which produces birth defects and abnormalities of various types. It is estimated that about 1 in every 200 live births involves a chromosomal disorder—this involves about 20,000 infants each year in the United States (Schild & Black, 1984, p. 24).

In the case where there is an extra chromosome present in the fertilization process, the resulting cell has 47 chromosomes and is called a trisomic cell. Where one chromosome is missing, resulting in a cell with 45 chromosomes, one speaks of a monosomic cell. The most common trisomic error occurs in the form of Down's syndrome, where the chromosome involved is number 21; this condition is also called trisomy 21. When there are structural defects in the chromosomes, other abnormalities are produced; this occurs about once in every 500 live births (Schild & Black, 1984, p. 26).

Genes may be dominant or recessive. Dominance means that the gene is manifested in a single copy (offspring) of itself; recessive means that a gene is not expressed in a single copy. There are three types of single-gene disorders—that is, those conditions associated with a specific abnormal gene (Rauch, 1988): autosomal dominant inheritance (such as Huningon's disease), autosomal recessive inheritance (with such major diseases as sickle-cell anemia, cystic fibrosis, and Tay-Sachs disease), and X-linked recessive inheritance (such as hemophilia and colorblindness). These illustrative diseases are only a few of the nearly 2,800 confirmed or suspected genetic disorders (see Schild & Black, 1984, p. 32). A fourth pattern, termed *multifactorial inheritance,* involves the interaction of genes and the environment. Among the common forms of this disorder are asthma, cleft palate, diabetes mellitus, some forms of mental retardation, and spina bifida (Rauch, 1988). Details of the transmission process are given by Schild and Black (1984). Assuming that there are appropriate indications for referral to a genetics clinic—such as known congenital abnormalities, acknowledged familial disorders, multiple miscarriages, incest, or if the mother is 35 years or older (see Schild & Black, 1984, pp. 40, 78-79)—then the exact nature of the problem needs to be determined by biochemical and physical analysis along with a study of the family

II. The Second Dimension

history (a genetic pedigree for the family tree). The resulting picture of the chromosomal patterns (the karyotype), in combination with the other information, provides the basis for counseling.

In part, this information involves transmitting technical genetic information to the involved persons, but more important for nonmedical personnel is the interpretation of these facts. People who seek counseling are looking for answers to questions such as, What does it mean that I am a carrier of sickle-cell anemia? What should we do now that we know we are a PKU family? Schild and Black (1984) emphasize that these genetic diagnoses are always a family diagnosis in the sense of an assessment of inheritance, future reproductive risks, and the personal implications of being "affected" by some genetic error. These kinds of information impose great stresses on the involved people and the relationships between and among them. Decisions reached in one generation will affect the succeeding generations, often magnifying the problem.

Schild (1977) has identified the psychological and situational tasks these facts generate; I am condensing and combining several of her points:

1. Reaffirm one's self-worth as one's self-concept is being reorganized in the face of this genetic information.
2. Accept this new genetic identity, including a changed body image, possibly a felt difference, probably more ambivalence regarding future procreation, and perhaps a perceived social stigma.
3. Grapple with the limitations of this genetic diagnosis, including the potential loss of a desired, healthy, normal child or the mastery of new social roles such as person with a genetic defect.
4. Accommodate the special needs of a child with a genetic disorder, including getting special treatment, special education, and respite services, all which require altering prior lifestyles for all parties involved.

Schild and Black (1984) consider the monumental ethical and value problems genetic counseling often entails, from those related to folk beliefs versus scientific understanding to those concerning the future birth of a developmentally delayed fetus to immature mothers in highly stressful contexts. Although knowledge of genetics is expanding rapidly, this arena of genetic services is still heavily embedded in a value context and strong controversy, as are studies about biological markers of risk (Searight & Handal, 1986; Shiloh, Waisbren, & Levy, 1989; Tabakoff & Hoffman, 1988; Tolan & Lorion, 1988). Another aspect of the future concerns drugs that are supposed to make people smarter (Cantebury & Lloyd, 1994) or affect their life course (as in the flurry of interest in the drug melatonin or Vitamin E or other miracle drugs).

3. Relaxation Training

Benson (1975, 1992) advocates the use of "the relaxation response" by healthy but harassed people as a way of counterbalancing the stresses of everyday life. He reports clinical studies of this approach, but large-scale objective studies are lacking. Benson notes that folk wisdom—from Zen Buddhism, yoga, and, more recently, transcendental meditation (TM)— has long prescribed similar methods. (It is not necessary to join any philosophy or cult to gain benefits related to relaxation.) He has extracted four basic components needed to bring about this response:

1. A quiet environment, with as few distractions as possible
2. A mental device to prevent the mind from shifting back to its usual logical, task-oriented functions (This mental device must be a constant stimulus, such as a word repeated over and over, silently or aloud. In TM, this word or sound is known as a *mantra;* see Clements, Krenner, & Mölk, 1988. A secret and private mantra is not necessary—any word that keeps the mind from its ordinary distractions will do; eyes are closed; breathing is normal; other distractions are minimized as far as possible. Another approach to prevent mental distractions is to gaze at one object continuously.)
3. A passive attitude and a receptivity or "let it happen" state of mind. (This is difficult for some people to achieve—distracting thoughts will occur and can be "turned off" in favor of returning to the mantra.)
4. A comfortable position as a way of reducing distractions (However, falling asleep is not the same as relaxation, so one must assume some position that is comfortable but not so much that one falls asleep.)

Benson (1975, 1992) proposes that one deeply relax all one's muscles. His method of relaxation is similar to many others (Jacobson, 1934; Wolpe, 1958) in consciously relaxing one set of muscles at a time by first tightening them up (enough to feel the tension and heat) and then releasing them (and thus to feel the sense of relief and pleasure). As Meichenbaum (1985) points out, instructing the client to tighten his or her fist and then relaxing it easily demonstrates some fundamental principles: that one cannot be both physically tense and physically relaxed at

II. The Second Dimension

the same time and that one can influence one's level of relaxation. (See also biofeedback as a preventive tool, making use of awareness of one's bodily states; Chen, 1995; Dunajcik, 1994.)

Meichenbaum (1985) suggests that the practitioner discuss with the client what it means to be relaxed, as some people think relaxation is just a mind game or even something detrimental to being alert. Clients have to learn to give themselves permission to relax; this is important in reducing their stress. Relaxation for Meichenbaum (in distinction to Benson, 1975) involves being both physically relaxed and mentally alert. For Meichenbaum, one uses one's state of relaxedness to challenge a low-intensity stressful cue, as is done in systematic desensitization.

Meichenbaum (1985) notes that relaxation is an active coping skill, one that requires practice. Relaxation will have a gradual effect. The object is to manage stress, not to remove it, because some stress is stimulating. In learning to relax in combination with other kinds of coping skills, the client should be reminded that he or she should attribute this success to his or her own actions as a basis for improving perceived self-efficacy.

Some people use relaxation as a way of turning off intense thinking and problem solving for the day—so as to be able to go to sleep.

E. Holistic or Multifactor Approaches

1. Trends in the Prevention of Substance Abuse

This section illustrates how one topic area has evolved over time from optimistic study of single causal factors to more realistic study of multiple factors. This story of developing sophistication in thinking about preventable problems probably is relevant to all the specific fields of interest and may be a kind of intellectual marker of the progress of their development. The point of including this discussion is to encourage readers to expand their own thinking about primary prevention, both conceptually and in terms of the configuration of practice.

Botvin and Dusenbury (1989) describe three stages or trends in research in the substance use field. The first generation of research in primary prevention practices tended to involve simple, linear thinking. For example, in prevention in substance abuse areas, the major conceptual guidelines suggested that information about the hazards of smoking or drinking or using drugs would be sufficient to change young people's behavior in these areas. Results commonly showed that these students did learn some of the information presented but went right ahead and smoked, drank, and experimented with marijuana. (These are the so-called gateway drugs that lead some to harder drugs.) Similar studies varied the information with fear-arousing messages or moral appeals—but with no better results (Weinstein, 1987; Chafetz et al., 1970; Natham, 1985).

Then followed what I term a transition phase away from simple, linear models to simple but diffuse programs, such as the many varieties of affective education (Chapter 2, I.E.3). For example, values clarification helped young people be aware of the different values they and others held, possible inconsistencies within any value set, and the process by which values are learned—all without making any judgment of which was to be preferred (in contrast to Kohlberg's, 1981, 1983, nonrelativistic view of moral development; see Chapter 2, I.B.2). The general goal of affective education involved helping school children "understand themselves and others better and to be able to apply this understanding in everyday situations" (Cooper et al., 1980, pp. 24-25). A large number of programs and curricula were developed independently. Some of these programs emphasized feelings and inner awareness; others focused on causal analyses of everyday events (Linkenbach, 1990). They differed also in the rigor with which they were constructed and tested in field settings. Research evidence summarized by Botvin and Dusenbury (1989) indicates that these methods were generally ineffective, probably because the teaching methods used were not focused on particular skills needed to deal with real-world events, such as substance use.

During this time, the rigorous and conceptually strong work of Evans and his colleagues (Evans, 1976; Evans et al., 1978; Evans & Raines, 1990) ushered in a second generation of research on the psychosocial factors involved in smoking—peer pressure and mass media instigations of smoking. A multifactor program was constructed that addressed these pressures directly. This involved teaching students how to say "no" to peers without losing a friend (Chapter 2, I.E.2). The program also provided techniques for dealing with advertising pressures to smoke. The successful results, as well as the elegant design and methods, encouraged many others to construct variations along the lines of Evans's work.

These variations led to another transition period, when the focus on teaching specific techniques spilled over into various kinds of targets,

II. The Second Dimension

employing various but specific resistance skills. These transition studies taught not only what to say but also how to say it (Englander-Golden, Elconin, & Satir, 1986). Various "teachers" were employed—older peers, regular classroom teachers, outside specialists. Generally successful results have been encouraging, as have follow-up studies (Botvin & Dusenbury, 1989).

The third generation of research on primary prevention practice may be here in the form of comprehensive, systematic projects that employ empirically grounded specific techniques. Botvin and Dusenbury (1989) are an exemplar of this third generation (see also Schinke & Gilchrist, 1984).

The hallmark of this third generation of research and practice in primary prevention is the organized delivery of a complex curriculum composed of specific but integrated units. These include factual information relevant to the topic and age group (e.g., the immediate adverse effects of smoking as contrasted with long-term effects), self-directed behavior change (i.e., the development of self-esteem and a sense of personal control), decision making (which involves critical thinking and independence of thought), coping with anxiety through use of anxiety reduction techniques, and social and interpersonal skills (in particular, ways of effective communication with the opposite sex). Each of these units is delivered with regard to smoking, drinking, and use of marijuana in 20 sessions in the 7th grade, a booster set of 10 sessions in the 8th grade, and another set of 5 sessions in the 9th grade (Botvin & Dusenbury, 1989).

There is a conceptual rationale for each of these units, although they appear somewhat independent as educational tasks. Each unit contains specific techniques focused on specific outcomes. Manuals facilitate precise dissemination of the content (although school contexts vary considerably). The overall project is being studied with careful attention to the research design and the measurement instruments. The intention is to present a well-conceptualized package that is rigorously studied so that the results may be used to advance primary prevention practices in this area.

These third generation primary prevention projects have set a challenging benchmark against which to compare the literature. This kind of systematic theorizing, practice, and research should continue the contributions to the advance of primary prevention that the first two generations made in their time.

The lessons to be learned from this example may be summarized as follows:

1. Consider what types of variables are assumed to be causing the major outcomes of a given area and how they are related. If simple descriptive linkages are being proposed, even well-operationalized ones, is it possible to raise the conceptual level of analysis of the project? Raising the conceptual level involves locating the whole ecology or configuration of interrelated systems and asking how each affects the others within some steady dynamic supersystem. As we raise our conceptual sights on the nature of the problem and possible resolutions, we find more factors that justifiably could be making significant differences in the situation.

2. With the growth of realistic complexity in a given problem area, one must make choices or set priorities regarding the targets chosen and how one set of targets is linked with other sets of targets. Such interrelating may eventuate in economies of shared resources among the different sets of targets. Interrelated service packages also bring the advantage of snowballing effects, each part reinforcing underlying skills in the others. (For instance, the same problem-solving skills may be applied to smoking or drinking or other specific situations. Also, the positive self-esteem emerging from mastery of one area may be useful with efforts in another area.)

Conceptual sophistication tends to run ahead of tactical sophistication. (See Milgram & Nathan, 1986, for a review of alcohol abuse prevention approaches—such as legislative penalties for drunk driving, price manipulation, and changes in drinking age—and programs—such as Boost Alcohol Consciousness Concerning the Health of University Students [BACCHUS]; Students Against Drunk Driving [SADD]; and Cambridge and Somerville Program for Alcoholism Rehabilitation [CASPAR], a teacher-training workshop for secondary school students). We are still at the beginning stages of developing effective prevention programs in abuse of substances and foreseeing what interrelated effects each portion of the service package will have on the others.

2. Stress Management

The "management" of stress has become big business in this age of anxiety. The stresses of modern life are everywhere, from the pressures for achievement in school to the demands for productivity on the job and for "success" in interpersonal relationships. Such stresses take their toll, as indicated by the 5 billion doses of tranquilizers Americans are said to take each year (Powell & Enright, 1990) and in the two out of three office visits to family doctors prompted by stress-related symptoms (Cotton, 1990).

Stresses or challenges are intrinsic aspects of modern life, however, and may be viewed positively as being useful and stimulating. I will use the more neutral term *stimuli* to refer to internal or external experiences that require a person to respond to avoid an undesired outcome or to achieve some desired one. When the person has the resources (his or her own or "borrowed" resources from others) to deal adequately with the stimuli, then the stimuli are viewed as a positive or growth experience, what Hollister (1967) intends by his term *strens* or what Cotton (1990) calls *eustress,* good or positive stress. If the person lacks resources and cannot obtain additional ones, then the stimuli are viewed as stress or distress, a negative or destructive experience. There are degrees of stress, or accumulative amounts of stress that lead to varying degrees of destructiveness, but challenging stimuli that are resolvable are essentially pleasant. Modern people spend much effort trying to avoid or reduce stress. We don't spend nearly as much conscious or systematic effort trying to engage strens.

These terms maintain the usual intended meaning of stressful stimuli as negative without closing off the possibility that the same stimuli may lead others to positive experiences or strens depending on how the person responds to these stimuli in the given context. One person may see a glass as half empty, another person may see it as half full, both looking at the same stimuli. Writers on stress management refer to seeking a balance between "the client's individual resistance to stress and the amount of stress in his or her environment" (Cotton, 1990, p. 5), but in fact it might be more accurate to suggest that we seek an imbalance in favor of strens. Certainly, one must resolve stress-causing problems by countering them with "resistance," but included in that resistance is a positive movement toward individual growth, fulfillment, and social contribution.

Let me define stress management (or stimuli management) broadly as the analysis of, and suitable adaptations to, internal and external stimuli and the correlative adaptive efforts (by oneself and others) so as to optimize growth-promoting stimuli (strens) while minimizing growth-inhibiting stimuli (stress). (See also Gullotta, 1982, on methods to ease the distress of grief; Schinke et al., 1986, regarding stress management in family situations; Solomon, Frederiksen, Arnold, & Brehony, 1984, on stress management delivered over public television; and Tableman, Marciniak, Johnson, & Rodgers, 1982, on stress management for women on public assistance.)

There are some important sequelae of experiencing either stress or strens. One comes to think of stress in terms of these negative sequelae, as the concrete manifestations of stress reactions are legendary: There may be physical signs, such as aches and pains, nausea, and frequent urination or defecation; there may be cognitive signs such as irrational thinking (hard to concentrate or make decisions, forgetful) or depressed affect; or there may be behavioral signs, such as excessive drinking or drug use to deaden the stress, accident proneness, loss of sexual interest, or avoiding anxiety-producing situations (Cotton, 1990; Powell & Enright, 1990).

Some theorists locate stress solely in the cognitive sphere, such as Ellis (1985), who constructs an A-B-C-D framework in which some Antecedent event appears to cause some unpleasant Consequence, but in fact it is the Belief about that event that determines the consequences. Irrational beliefs in particular—such as the ideas that one has to be loved or approved by everyone or that one must be perfectly competent and achieving to be considered worthwhile—produce the unpleasant feelings or stresses people experience. Therefore, one must Dispute these irrational ideas and change them into rational ones—it would be preferable if one were approved by everyone, but that isn't likely to happen, so stop worrying about the impossible goal and work toward fulfilling a more rational goal of having some friends who approve of one—to be released from paralyzing stresses. (Also see Seligman, 1991, on promoting learned optimism; Chapter 2, I.B.3.)

If one takes stress out of the purely individual context—where most commentators deal with it—and looks at its large-scale context, one finds important sociocultural or physical environmental indicators of differential affect, such as the disproportionately high rates of hypertension among blacks, depression among women, suicide among men, or anomie (normlessness, nonconnectedness) in urban versus rural areas. There are no direct measures of the effects of oppression; perhaps disproportionate rates of hypertension, depression, and suicide are the kinds of proxy measures we should be studying—and changing as part of a configural analysis of stress management (see Chapter 3, II.C.6).

II. The Second Dimension

The sequelae of strens are not so well understood, but they presumably include physical signs, such as experiences of fitness and good muscle tone; cognitive signs, such as experiences of sensitivity and acuity, being in control, and feeling that one is able to accomplish some action (self-efficacy); and behavioral signs, such as involvement in social situations, mastering tasks using new techniques, and greater interest in personal aspects of life, from food to sex. The holistic health movement may be an endeavor to counteract the emphasis on stress in an age of anxiety by trying to promote strens and recognize its sequelae just as we do the more familiar signs of stress. Whether or not emphasizing the positive (strens) will also reduce the negative (stress) remains to be studied. Likewise, reducing the social and cultural oppression that creates stress on minorities would free up great amounts of energies for productive contributions to society (Noble, 1987; Renzulli, 1973).

Powell and Enright (1990) employ a cognitive social learning perspective and thus incorporate the particular techniques of Meichenbaum, Beck, and Ellis, whose practice methods and concepts are well represented in this book—although I have arranged them in a different conceptual package. Powell and Enright offer the following ad hoc self-help techniques: relaxation training, including various instructions for progressive muscle relaxation training; methods to control hyperventilation (rapid breathing and feelings of faintness in periods of high anxiety or stress—this may be controlled by stopping one's activity, calming oneself, consciously breathing slowly, and rebreathing, i.e., making a tent of fingers over one's face and breathing in some trapped air that is rich in carbon dioxide); distraction methods, including thought stopping, meditation, and focusing on the environment or on some bridging object (i.e., some kind of security blanket); cognitive-behavioral techniques, such as Meichenbaum's self-instructional methods and stress inoculation training; Beck's techniques, such as developing awareness of one's thought processes (to cut anxiety feelings down to realistic size); restructuring; and Ellis's techniques related to the A-B-C-D approach of rational-emotive therapy. I discuss all these (except hyperventilation) in this book. To summarize briefly these points, I list the following statements:

1. One should view all life as stimuli to which one has to adapt both to survive and to prevail. Stimuli become stressful or positively enjoyable, as circumstances (including one's own efforts) make them so.

2. When stimuli impinge at rapid and intense rates, one can get overwhelmed, turning what may be pleasant stimuli into stresses (e.g., holidays with the in-laws). The primary suggestion is to organize the flow of stimuli and to prioritize one's responses to them. Which of all the things that have to get done is most important, requires special resources, is required for solution of later problems? (If the boss makes multiple demands, smile and ask what about the priority among these demands because you can't do them all at once or in the limited work time.) When one controls the flow of stimuli, one also gains a sense of inner control over one's life, which also imparts a sense of direction to one's life (Kobasa et al., 1982).

3. Included in organizing and prioritizing stimuli is the involvement of other people or physical environments. These others may share the burden and the enjoyment, so that time spent connecting with them in the stress/strens context is time well spent.

4. There will be times when undelayable deadlines all come due at the same time. One must be prepared but think about reorganizing affairs so as to avoid such overloads. Call out the troops for help, just as one should stand ready to help friends in like circumstances on occasion (Hersey, Klibanoff, Clyburn, & Pobst, 1981).

Stress management is, or can be, a natural activity—we do some of it automatically as part of living in the contemporary world. It might be helpful to be more self-conscious about it and to build some of these methods into our everyday lifestyle. On occasion, we may need a little help from our friends. Or we may need help from professionals when the traumas or the accumulation of assaults becomes too much for our ordinary means of resolving stress.

3. Prevention of Problems Associated With Job Loss

An important example of focusing on decreasing an individual limitation or problem within a configural context is given in the work of the Michigan Prevention Research Center, specifically the project on coping with job loss (Caplan, Vinokur, Price, & van Ryn, 1989; Vinokur, van Ryn, Gramlick, & Price, 1991). When an individual loses his or her job, along with the salary, fringe benefits, status, and social supports that a job entails, there are concomitant risks of depression, anxiety, and decreased self-esteem and life satisfaction (Vinokur, Caplan, & Williams, 1987). One kind of primary prevention program is directed toward reducing these untoward outcomes (i.e., reducing individual limitations), but in the context of increasing individual and social strengths, as will be seen in this exemplary project.

Many social networks surround the unemployed worker, from the primary group consisting of family, friends, and close work associates to the secondary group connections to union, community, and cultural groups. The Michigan team has conceptualized an experimental intervention in terms of the process involved in motivating continued job seeking (and the seeking of quality jobs), along with inoculation against setbacks in the job-seeking process. The process involves addressing personal factors: first developing a trusting relationship with the client and then addressing the motivation and skill needs of that person. In addition, social supports are directed to enhance an individual's self-esteem, to communicate belongingness, and to provide material aid. Prior research indicated that a worker's spouse plays a key role in developing attitudes and expectancies regarding the value of job seeking (Vinokur & Caplan, 1987).

Eight training sessions average between 16 and 20 participants who provided mutual peer support. In the course of the training sessions, small groups are formed to brainstorm or problem solve with regard to some case examples. In addition, a buddy system evolves where people who have become friendly in the training sessions are paired up to do some problem solving by phone between sessions. Training is given in using social networks to obtain job leads—friends of friends who may know about jobs in certain companies. The fact that the trainers make contact with participants at state employment compensation offices and that a prestigious university is conducting the training sessions also represents linkages between the individual and macrosocial components in society.

In short, the Michigan team of researchers has developed a conceptually formed and empirically grounded project dealing with an issue critical to our times—nearly 10 million people lose their jobs annually (Caplan et al., 1989, p. 759). The entire package of training takes into consideration the individual worker, the worker-trainer pair (or trio, because pairs of trainers are used), buddies within the group, small groups within the larger training group, the spouse of the participant, and ultimately institutions in the state. Research conducted with the participants in this project has showed that, as hypothesized, the experimental intervention produced higher rates of reemployment for participants than for controls. The researchers counted both the experimental participants who actually attended the sessions and those who did not as part of the total experimental group. Other research on the nonattenders discovered a self-selection process, that people who needed the job skills training and benefited from it were drawn into the project, whereas many of those who did not attend were able to find jobs on their own (Vinokur, Price, & Caplan, 1990). A follow-up study of these participants also suggests strong cost-benefit analyses: large net benefits to participants and to state and federal government programs that supported this project (Vinokur et al., 1991). See also health promotion strategies for unionized workers (Grozuczak, 1981) and other studies of primary prevention at the worksite (Vicary, 1994).

4. *Parent Effectiveness Training*

In this section, I illustrate a theory-guided practice program that has received wide attention. Thomas Gordon's humanistic methods—he was a student of Carl Rogers and draws much of his ideas and practices from the Rogerian philosophy—have been taught to over a million parents (Gordon, 1970) around the United States and abroad, as well as to more than 100,000 school personnel (Gordon, 1974) and to large numbers of business people (Gordon, 1977). At its core, these effectiveness training approaches seek to enable people to attain their goals without being overcontrolling or overpermissive, or without forcing people to one's way of doing something, or without bribing people to do it your way. Gordon's program is more than a technique for attaining some goal.

Effectiveness training represents a philosophy about a fundamental relationship between parent and child, teacher and student, employer and employee. That philosophy is essentially democratic, a participatory two-way interchange between people who each have something of value to share. Gordon suggests that this democratic method of problem solving fosters well-being and thus is a useful primary prevention strategy, albeit one that involves individual thoughts, feelings, and actions in interpersonal contexts. Many factors are involved, which is why I have chosen to place it here as a holistic approach.

Beginning in 1950, Gordon experimented with leadership training methods based on his experience as a counselor in the Rogerian tradition.

The communication skills needed by the therapist are based on exactly the same principles that parents (and teachers and employers) need in connection with their children (students, employees) to have a happy and productive situation for all people involved. Gordon eventually developed these ideas and packaged them in a clear accessible way. Several thousand instructors have been trained in these methods and are now licensed to teach in every state and many countries abroad. Nearly 40 years later, Gordon is still developing new applications for his core ideas (Gordon, 1989). Let's examine these ideas.

Gordon (1970) emphasizes several major dimensions of the parent-child situation for which interventive methods are proposed:

1. There exists naturally in every human relationship what can be called areas of acceptable and unacceptable behaviors from the given actor's point of view at a given time and context. What is acceptable may change as people, context, and time change.

2. People "own" their own behaviors—they are responsible for performing and for changing these behaviors. Other people may find a given behavior undesirable from their own point of view. For instance, a child may be noisy when the parent is on the phone and can't hear. Being noisy is not a problem to the child even though it is for the parent, whereas, for example, a child may be unhappy about not having a friend to play with. This is the problem that the child feels (and thus "owns"), of which the parent may not be aware.

3. Unacceptable behaviors may become points of conflict, especially if communications exchanged are not clear. Gordon identifies 12 typical ways in which parents communicate ineffectively (e.g., ordering, threatening, preaching, blaming, ridiculing, withdrawing), all which speak to the child (with destructive blaming—"You stop making so much noise!") rather than to the issue at hand (the level of noise at this time and place).

4. Gordon begins with *active listening,* in which the listener tries to understand what the sender is feeling and what the message means by putting that understanding in words and checking with the sender. (Parent to distraught child who has just come home from a day at school: "Sounds like you think your teacher is mean to you." Child: "Well, not mean, exactly, it's just that he doesn't ever ask what we think of all the homework he assigns.") Active listening is termed an *all-purpose people skill,* meaning that it is a fundamental way of relating to others in many contexts (Gordon, 1989).

5. The communication pattern in destructive blaming takes the form of "You-messages," ineffective confrontational statements (such as "You stop that! You should know better. You're acting like a baby.").

6. "I-messages" communicate to the child how the parent feels. These messages are less apt to provoke resistance and begin to place responsibility on the child, as well as modeling honest direct messages. (For instance, to a child who has pulled out pots and pans in the kitchen just as the parent is starting to prepare dinner, "I can't cook when I have to walk around the pots and pans on the floor." This assumes that the child has the ability to understand the message and can make decisions to change.)

7. Gordon proposes a "no-lose" communication method, as contrasted with a parent win-child lose (authoritarian situation) or parent lose-child win (permissive) situation. Essentially, this is an interactive problem-solving approach, a mutual search for a solution acceptable to both parties.

Step 1. Identify the problem.
Step 2. Generate possible alternative solutions.
Step 3. Weigh these alternative solutions.
Step 4. Decide on the best acceptable solution.
Step 5. Work out ways to implement this solution.
Step 6. Evaluate how it worked (and presumably make modifications as needed).

This method also involves some interpersonal negotiating for an acceptable compromise, assuming parties are granted about equal power. This is the revolutionary point in Gordon's work, the idea that parents, teachers, and bosses can literally work with their charges in a participatory way because in real life, children, students, and employees have power even if they cannot always overpower the other. As Gordon (1970) points out, "powerless" kids can be coerced to do something but can make life a hell in so doing. The point is to find out what mutually acceptable ways all parties might agree to that would constitute meeting everyone's needs without anyone's "losing."

Gordon (1989) recognizes that this crash course in counseling psychology may be misleading to some people who rush off and try I-messages inappropriately (e.g., "I like the way you finally are taking some responsibility for keeping your room cleaner"—which essentially gives a preachy and child-blaming message).

II. The Second Dimension

Gordon (1989) also points out that it may be more appropriate at times to make environmental changes, such as diverting a young child with appealing activities rather than discussing a given conflict or childproofing an environment so a greater range of permissible activities can occur. The focus of Parent Effectiveness Training (PET) is on communications and negotiation, assuming that children are basically good, cooperative, and problem solving if only given the opportunity to do so by their parents. Moreover, this teaches children self-discipline, which is exactly the skill they will need to become effective adults. These same principles can be applied in the school room and in the factory or office situation.

Gordon (1989) cites a variety of research in support of his general thesis. For example, the work of Johnson, Maruyama, Johnson, Nelson, and Skon (1981) shows that of 122 studies published from 1924 to 1980, 65 found that cooperation was related to higher levels of achievement than was competition; 8 were in the opposite direction; and 36 found no statistically significant differences. This same team of researchers also found that cooperative learning as compared with competitive educational arrangements facilitates closer ethnic relationships (Johnson, Johnson, Tiffany, & Zaidman, 1984).

A set of studies by Levant (1983) and his students reviewed comparative studies involving PET. Of 35 comparisons, 69% respondents favored PET, none favored the non-PET control group, and 31% showed no significant difference (see also Cedar, 1985). These and other studies provide some encouragement for the effectiveness training approach (Gordon, 1989). This also means that we should consider the approach by which Gordon disseminated his work to a large population, building a cadre of people who can be trained as teachers of this method, with the whole organization being put onto a paying basis. Helping professionals don't always think about fiscal issues, but someone has to pay the bills for the helping services provided in society and this free enterprise approach is one model to be considered. (See Broussard, 1989, and Lavigne, Reisinger, Bernard, & Stewart, 1983, for other systematic approaches to training parents of infants to preschool-aged children. Also see Forehand, Walley, & Furey, 1984, and Jason, Kurasaki, Neuson, & Garcia, 1993, on preventive efforts in teaching child-rearing skills.) Whether PET can be applied in high-risk situations remains to be studied (Huxley & Warner, 1990).

METHODS OF PRIMARY PREVENTION

Dimension III. Increasing Social Supports

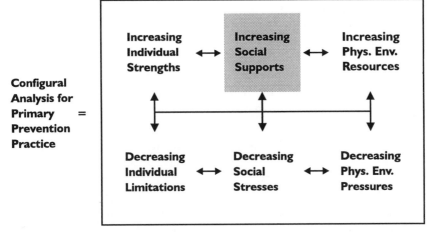

Figure 4.1. The Configural Equation

With this chapter, I enter the social context for problem-solving in primary prevention. Building on Chapter 2, Increasing Individual Strengths, and Chapter 3, Decreasing Individual Limitations, I now examine how social contexts influence individuals and groups and how they may be influenced to help people obtain desired goals and objectives. Four major types of social contexts are distinguished with regard to increasing social supports (and, in Chapter 5, decreasing social stresses): interpersonal supports, primary groups, secondary groups, and sociocultural contexts.

Dimension III. Increasing Social Supports
- A. Interpersonal Aspects
  1. Helper Therapy Principle, Peer Tutoring
  2. Attachment, Bonding
  3. Friendship
- B. Primary Group Aspects
  1. Social Support, Mutual Assistance, and Self-Help Groups
  2. Natural Helping Networks
- C. Secondary Group Aspects
  1. Social Empowerment, Advocacy
  2. Consultation
  3. Concrete Assistance From Social Groups
- D. Aspects Involving the Sociocultural Context
  1. Institutions as Vehicles of Primary Prevention
  2. Symbol Systems
  3. Mass Media

This chapter addresses the first social facet of the configural analysis, the various contexts having to do with social supports. As Albert Einstein wrote, "Many times a day I realize how much my own outer and inner life is built upon the labors of my fellow (human beings), both living and dead, and how earnestly I must exert myself in order to give in return as much as I have received" (quoted in Hersey et al., 1981, p. 32). We are always involved with other people, giving and receiving.

The main hypothesis of the configural analysis is that primary prevention goals are more likely to be achieved by increasing the strengths of the individual, sociocultural supports, and resources from the physical environment, in combination with reducing individual limitations, sociocultural stresses, and pressures from the physical environment. This general hypothesis is indicated by the configural equation at the beginning of Chapters 2 through 6.

People are so completely socialized and social that it is inconceivable to consider any helping modality without embedding it in the many social contexts that make up life as we know it. Social scientists have categorized portions of this social world for convenience of study, but ordinary citizens walk through the complex maze of social statuses, roles, organizations, norms, sanctions, and the like with little apparent difficulty. Even a young child knows how to behave at school, at home when the grandparents are visiting, or at the ballpark.

III. The Third Dimension

This knowledge of the social is only apparent, however, because many people experience great difficulties with the social sphere. Something is wrong in practice and in theory when divorces equal the number of marriages, when rational people permit huge federal deficits to build up ("on the backs" of future generations of our children), when violence occurs seemingly on a random or irrational basis.

First, some definitions: I use the term *social context* to refer to four persisting social relationships. The first type involves interpersonal relationships viewed as essentially two-person groups. Some type of ongoing communications between two parties takes place such that each has certain knowledge and expectations of the other, and his or her own part in that relationship. I will refer to several specific *interpersonal relationships*—peer tutors, parent-child bonding, and intimate friendships or confidants—that play a vital role in the life of the individual in social contexts.

A second aspect of the social context involves *primary groups,* those ubiquitous small groups where members hold diffuse role relationships to one another and meet frequently on a face-to-face basis. Included are families, peer groups, small work teams (such as a platoon of soldiers or a team of workers on a common project), and neighborhood enclaves (often with a cultural substratum). From such groups one receives various forms of assistance and through such groups one gives one's share of assistance to others. Thus the label of *mutual assistance groups* is commonly used to refer to these primary groups.

I distinguish two forms of mutual assistance groups, those that are *natural* in the sense that they are found in existence in the everyday life of a community (Collins & Pancoast, 1976) and those that are *constructed,* usually by outsiders working to obtain some planned goal by bringing people together who have some shared fate or goals. An example of the latter is Silverman's (1988) Widow-to-Widow program, which is described more fully in this chapter.

The third form of social context involves *secondary groups,* whose many manifestations include a school (not a specific class within the school), a union, a church (one of such size that members may not know everyone by name, in contrast to a small congregation of long-standing members), or a workplace (again, one of large scale). In addition, I include political parties, professional groups, and special interest groups (such as people with special hobbies) whose participants extend far beyond the local area and who probably do not know most of the other members. A most

III. The Third Dimension

important type of secondary group is the voluntary organization, which is dedicated to a social cause. For example, Action on Smoking and Health (ASH) represents a volunteer-supported organization to reduce or eliminate the use of tobacco as a dangerous health hazard.

In short, secondary groups involve relatively large collectives organized to achieve some common end, whose members may not know many, perhaps most, of the participants and may never see them directly. Secondary groups are highly diverse and yet share common functions of coordinated actions toward some common end where each party has a specific role vis-à-vis the others in the group.

The fourth type of social context involves society and culture. By *society,* I refer to the composite of all groups tied together by a civic bond, all being members of one political system that assumes control over collective defense and social welfare functions. Society is divided into various units, each related hierarchically to the whole, such as cities and towns, counties, states, and the federal government. Formal obligations (such as taxes and defense of country) and benefits (such as protection from aggression and laws determining fair play) are connected to membership in society and its constituent parts. The relevance of society, as I define it, to primary prevention emerges as laws are enacted, policies are administered and critiqued (as through an ombudsman role), social change is undertaken, and social integration is achieved—all these specific aspects of the societal structure are relevant to the focus of this book. The working units of society are broken down into various institutions; I will examine how these units may be employed in primary prevention.

Culture refers to shared lifestyles, values, language, and history that characterize a particular group of people at a particular time and place (Ponterotto & Pedersen, 1993). Culture plays a part in primary prevention by supplying meaning and zest to (civic) life, empowering individually weak people to be collectively strong, and integrating large numbers of people on the basis of a lifestyle and a collective history (including a shared language and religion) rather than formal legal relationships.

Multinational corporations may be considered a part of culture because they have great influence on many aspects of our lives, albeit without fanfare. The "home" of a multinational group may not be in any one place—unless it is cyberspace. It is a network of organizational units situated in different nations, which acts in concert on its collective behalf, rather than for the benefit of any one nation.

These four types of social contexts are overlapping and interrelated. National organizations such as the Sierra Club or the Audubon Society may have state and local organizations that operate as kinds of primary groups for the individuals involved. Two minority group members working together on a continuing project for a large labor union of governmental workers may be conceptually placed in all four of the above categories. More important than categorization is the fact that people fit together in the social system by various bonds of connectedness; this is the underlying meaning of the term *social*. Sometimes connectedness generates conflicting loyalties, however. A tight-knit family may not permit its younger members to leave the area even though better jobs may exist in another state. Voters may continue to elect a cultural compatriot to office even when a better-qualified person of a different ethnicity is running. Fans may "root, root, root for the home team" even when they know it is a bunch of greedy, self-aggrandizing, spoilsports.

Thus the social context becomes a critical feature of any plan for primary prevention, both to promote social supports and to reduce social stresses that stem from the very same sets of relationships. With this as background, I will focus on particular types of social supports identified in the literature.

A. Interpersonal Aspects

1. Helper Therapy Principle, Peer Tutoring

Friends have always helped friends achieve goals that the one person could not achieve on his or her own. A special form of this common experience has been singled out by a distinctive label—*the helper therapy principle* (Riessman, 1965, 1976)—that has many potential applications in primary prevention. Riessman focuses on the helping person who has a characteristic similar to the person being helped. When such persons are induced to help others less well functioning than themselves, a special effect may occur: Helping may help the helper as much or more than the person being helped.

This outcome is particularly likely when (a) the helper is only slightly more advanced on the content of the help than the person being helped (e.g., an older student who is not strong in reading may benefit as he or she helps a younger child with basic reading skills), (b) the helper has a slightly less serious condition than the person being helped (e.g., a widow who has dealt reasonably well with her own personal situation may volunteer to help a newly widowed person work through the stresses of transition), or (c) ordinary people with no particular problems may benefit from the help they give others. The principle may even be applied to professionals and paraprofessionals, who all may benefit from the help or teaching they provide for others. Likewise, this principle may be related to the situation when ordinarily inactive group members are propelled into leadership roles.

How can a person who gives help be transformed by giving help? Riessman (1965, 1976) suggests several reasons. As the helper teaches or guides the helpee to think about some topic or to perform some skilled activity, so the helper has to think about it in an organized way or practice the skill to be able to help the other. This effort of thinking or practice seems to help the helper, perhaps through overlearning or self-persuasion.

In addition, the helper observes his or her own behavior through the helpee's responses to the educational content and makes suitable improvements in his or her own performance: "I must be pretty good if I can help others." (This adds to the perceived self-efficacy of the helper, in Bandura's, 1986, terms.) Helpers may be distracted from other pursuits that may be problematic while engaged in helping others.

Riessman (1965, 1976) also notes that the positive feeling of usefulness adds to the beneficial effect. There may be social approval and various kinds of recognition and reinforcement both of the helping act and through the helper's own improved performance of that skill. Helpers may come to realize that they are part of the helping community, thereby giving them a stake in that community. This positive self-feeling probably accounts for the enormous amount of volunteer work that undergirds the entire health and welfare system in the United States.

I must comment on the term itself, *helper therapy principle,* in the context of this book. The important point of Riessman's (1965, 1976) contribution is on the educational effects for both helper and helpee. There is no "therapy" as such, and this idea is a "principle" only in the sense of representing an apparent common pattern of experiences. It is not used in the technological sense. I will continue to use the term only because it has an established meaning, but it merely points to a fruitful idea of a peer helper.

One important application of the helper therapy principle is in the area of peer tutors, when one older or educationally stronger person instructs another younger or less educationally strong person in a school context.

In an important critical review of the early literature, Devin-Sheehan, Feldman, and Allen (1976) summarize the major trends in the then-existing research: Although there is a large body of anecdotal evidence supporting peer tutors, there is a substantial group of well-designed research reports as well, involving a variety of participants, goals, and procedures. The tutors include students at the elementary, junior high, and high school level, as well as adults and college students. They may be volunteers or paid (or given school credits). The tutees are usually grade school students. The goals of tutoring are mainly academic, but there are some social behavioral goals as well.

The overall trend of results is fairly consistent: Tutoring can be beneficial to both tutees and tutors. Looking at some of the specifics, Devin-Sheehan et al. (1976) report the following: A broad range of students may benefit from acting as tutors—there is evidence that students characterized as having behavior problems or being low achievers and even being institutionalized may benefit from acting as a tutor to another person. Whether the tutor or the tutee benefits more is an open question—the evidence is mixed. Studies report not only improvement in reading and other academic content but also improved attitudes toward teachers and school as well as increased self-concept.

There is no evidence favoring same-sex or opposite-sex dyads as resulting in more favorable outcomes (Devin-Sheehan et al., 1976). A greater age difference between tutor and tutee yields somewhat better academic results for the tutee, but some benefits may be derived at the social level if the age difference is not too great. There is not enough information to consider race or socioeconomic status on peer tutoring. It is an open question as to what training—if any at all—is associated with more positive tutoring outcomes. Devin-Sheehan et al. (1976) close with a lamentation on the quality of the research, even though they praise a number of studies as being of adequate rigor.

Later research has continued to pursue the analytic question of what kinds of tutors and tutoring with what types of tutees in what contexts produce what results (see Telch, Miller, Killen, Cooke, & Maccoby, 1990). One study in a programmatic series by Joseph Allen and his colleagues provides an example. Allen, Philliber, and Hoggson (1990) report on the national replication study of their Teen Outreach Program, a school-based prevention of teenage pregnancy, school failure, and school dropout. The Teen Outreach Program, identified by the National Research Council (1987) as one of three approaches with documented effectiveness in reducing teenage pregnancies, was replicated in 35 sites across the United States. On the basis of 4 consecutive years of data, there was evidence showing that this program reduced teen pregnancy, school failure, and dropout rates by 30% to 50% relative to matched comparison groups of students (p. 506; see also Philliber, Allen, Hoggson, & McNeil, 1989). What works? With whom? Under what conditions?

Allen and his colleagues pose these questions to two alternative theoretical frames of reference with regard to the volunteer activity involved in this outreach program. Students from the 7th to the 11th grades volunteered at least ½ hour a week at school or in the community (e.g., hospitals, nursing homes). The focal question in this research study was the effects of volunteer service on these students. Note that some of the services they performed were in school (as tutors), but other services were performed in the community. Measures were taken by anonymous self-reports of problems these volunteers were experiencing in their own lives—course failures, school suspensions in prior year, and pregnancy-related problems. These items were repeated at the end of the school year and were correlated with the intensity of the volunteering, how it was structured (e.g., in or out of school, with or without credit), and how much of the outreach curriculum materials were used in the training.

Findings reveal that Teen Outreach Program participants have "significantly lower levels of suspension, school dropout, and pregnancy, and insignificantly lower levels of failure in courses than comparison students, even after controlling for levels of problem behavior at entry and significant demographic factors" (Allen et al., 1990, p. 515). Teen Outreach Program students went from having significantly more problems at entry to significantly fewer problems at the end of the project than did comparison students.

The authors examine the details of these positive findings. They report that the greater the intensity of volunteer work students contributed, the fewer problems they demonstrated at the end of the project (controlling for entry level problems). They also note that the effect of volunteering was more strongly observed for older students than for younger ones— which they interpret to mean that the usual preventive axiom of intervening early should be qualified: Make the preventive experience age appropriate, not merely early in a person's developmental history.

The helper therapy principle provides one explanation for these results, but these results also help expand some conceptual and empirical boundaries of the principle. A variety of kinds of volunteer services appear to serve the helper—Allen et al. (1990) do not distinguish academic tutoring results from other community services. It appears important that adolescents have responsible activities, including those outside the conventional student role. These authors note that these results provide "important lessons for other preventive interventions targeted at adolescents" (Allen et al., 1990, p. 522), including letting youths with various degrees of personal or social problems get into helper roles that may enable them to help themselves. How this self-help occurs as volunteer helping goes on still needs study, but a sufficient empirical base exists to begin exploration in earnest. (For other studies in peer tutoring, see Haven & Stolz, 1989; Jason & Rhodes, 1989; Wallston, McMinn, Katahn, & Pleas, 1983. See Jason, Johnson, Danner, Taylor, & Kurasaki, 1993, and Jason, Kurasaki, Neuson, & Garcia, 1993, for a comparison of peer and parent tutors. For adult-level peer helpers, see Halpern & Covey, 1983; see Oster, 1983, for negative results.)

I offer the following statements reflecting this literature on peer helpers:

1. Young people of almost any type—except those with serious interpersonal problems from which the helpee might possibly be injured—should be considered for the peer helper role. One must not stigmatize the "problem children" by making them peer tutors; rather, a range of children should be selected, including those with their own deficits in the tutored topics (e.g., reading or math).

2. The type of tutoring should depend on both the needs of helpees and the skills of helpers. Obviously, the helper has to have enough skill to provide constructive help, but helpers do not have to be scholars on the topic in question as long as they are more advanced than the helpees.

3. The research literature is not clear about the age, race, sex, or social class of the helper-helpee dyad or about what training, if any, the helper needs. "Training" to be helper may be an acceptable avenue for students who tend to resist ordinary academic procedures. As a general rule, the more clear and well structured an assignment is, the more likely the student will be able to master it—even when that student is the peer tutor.

III. The Third Dimension

4. The research literature appears to be clear about other features of the peer tutor situation: The helping may be volunteered or paid (in money, credits, or whatever unit is relevant). There should be some reasonable reward structure for peer tutoring, whose concrete expression will depend on the developmental age of the helper (Piaget). Included in this reward situation should be social approval by authority figures (such as teachers and parents).

5. Tutoring should be done in relatively short periods of time so as not to tire either helper or helpee, but the amount of time depends on the ages of the children involved. The lessons to be covered should be selected by the teacher of the helpee in consultation with the teacher of the helper so as to be real to the helpee and manageable by the helper.

2. Attachment, Bonding

There is no question that infants form strong and persistent relationships with their parents and other caretakers, just as these adults unquestionably form strong and persistent relationships with their children. However the path to forming these relationships is neither necessary nor smooth, and so developmentalists have studied many facets of this vital period in the lives of children and parents (Ainsworth, 1991; Bond & Joffe, 1982; Kent & Rolf, 1979; Osofsky, 1986; Roberts & Peterson, 1984).

Bowlby (1988) postulates in his quintessential contributions to these studies that attachment behavior characterizes human beings from the cradle to the grave. Many strong relationships exist between friends and lovers, between foxhole buddies, between colleagues at the workplace or church or in the gym—just their opposites exist in the same places. And so one finds publications with titles such as *Attachment Across the Life Cycle* (Parkes et al., 1991) and *Attachment in Adults* (Sperling & Berman, 1994), despite the critical attacks on the entire enterprise (Belsky & Benn, 1982; Eyer, 1992).

These complicated and contentious discussions are important for primary prevention practices, as well as many other areas of concern, and so I will attempt to sort out aspects of the story that bear directly on the topics relevant to this book, guided by Michael Rutter (1981), a model of a scientific and humane explorer of human development.

The crux of the issue is whether attachment, bonding, or any human relationship has as its fundamental beginning something that is built into the human species, something innate or instinctual, or whether it might start operating at certain critical periods in a person's life (not before or after these critical periods). This is, of course, a current version of the ancient nature versus nurture debate, but depending on what one believes "the answer" to be—or more likely, what complex sets of answers emerge that correspond to the complexity of human beings interacting in social environments—one will generate very different kinds of primary prevention programs.

The 20th-century version of the story begins with the work of Sigmund Freud and his instinct-based theory of human development, where unconscious strivings meet the resistance of societal demands; the developing person is formed in response to these conflicting forces, as are all the human-relationships that build on these personality characteristics. Freud's followers (and dissenters) added variations to what is built into the human being, with a common theme being the importance of early mothering. If early life events are not smooth, the resulting individual will likely have rough sailing throughout life.

At the same time, professions emerged to deal with the resulting problems—from disturbed children to neurotic or addicted adults. These professionals gained status and power from working with problems they defined to be present and for which they were the primary experts in resolving. Organizations such as mental hospitals and child guidance clinics emerged, through which these activities were delivered.

Eyer (1992) and feminist writers (Chafetz, 1988; Tavris, 1992) point out that these cultural structures and forces were dominated by a male-oriented ideology about many things, including the "proper role" of women—to stay at home with the baby, not to get a paid job, and to manage home and hearth.

Thus the view of human nature that emerges at any given period of time appears to be the confluence of ideology that established what is good and not good, professional organization that defined the problem and its solution, and the emergence of a rationalizing theory about instinctual forces that led to a number of related ideas about human relationships and to foster them in the most appropriate ways.

After the horror of World War II, which left many orphaned children and separated families, the World Health Organization asked psychiatrist John Bowlby to report on the situation. Bowlby's studies and resulting publication on maternal deprivation sent shock waves around the world:

Children who were institutionalized for their own health and safety were in fact being harmed by these placements because they were deprived of maternal attention to their instinctual needs. Damaged children were being seen in clinics as well as in the juvenile justice system. Major psychosocial problems were emerging from tiny instinctual beginnings. The results were major institutional changes and great efforts by psychiatrists and social workers (among others) to encourage mothers to stay at home with infants and young children.

Bowlby (1951) developed his ideas into a theory of attachment, which says, in brief, that infants have innate or built-in emotional and behavioral patterns that impel them to attach themselves physically and psychologically to their parents or caretakers. How these caretakers respond to the child's innate needs determine that child's mental health and personality.

Mary Ainsworth, a colleague of Bowlby, later developed a standardized test in which 1-year-old infants come to a "strange situation"—a laboratory room with toys and such—where they are exposed to some mild disturbing experiences, including a brief departure of the parent from the room (Ainsworth et al., 1978). Observations on what happens constitute the basis of categorizing attachment styles:

1. The securely attached child shows signs of distress when the parent leaves the room, but seeks out the parent after the parent's return, holds the parent for a while, and then returns to exploring and playing.
2. The avoidant child also shows distress at the parent's leaving but avoids or rejects the parent after the parent's return.
3. The anxious or ambivalent child shows high levels of distress and a mix of approaching and rejecting during the return period.

Ainsworth and others project that these personality styles, which emerge in infancy, may hold for long periods of the individual's life (Parkes et al., 1991).

All of these theories and research studies have been resoundingly and increasingly criticized and yet they continued to grow and take different forms. Eyer (1992) claims that the bonding studies are an extension of the attachment paradigm. But bonding has an important place in preventive theory and practice and thus needs special attention here.

Klaus and Kennell (1976) introduced the term *mother-infant bonding* to describe the emotional attachment that seems to form at a critical

III. The Third Dimension

period soon after the birth of the baby when there is skin-to-skin contact between mother and child. They studied a group of 28 lower-class black women having their first child. A randomly selected group was given 1 hour extra contact with their newborn within the first 3 hours after birth, plus an additional 15 hours of contact within the first 3 days. The control group received the traditional hospital routine—a glimpse of the infant at birth, a brief contact (for purposes of identification) 6 to 8 hours later, and a regular feeding schedule of 20 to 30 minutes every 4 hours. All other experiences were the same for both groups.

Certain differences between the two groups appeared soon and remained over a period of years (Ringler, Trause, Klaus, & Kennell, 1978). After 1 month (Klaus et al., 1972) and after 1 year (Kennell et al., 1974), mothers who had the extra contact with their newborn infants were more attentive and involved with their children, according to a small number of significant findings out of a large number of studied interactions between mother and child. By the second year, linguistic differences appeared (Ringler, Kennell, Jarvella, Novojosky, & Klaus, 1975). Mothers in the experimental group used significantly more words per statement addressed to their children and used twice as many questions as did mothers in the control group.

By the 5th year, the differences between children in the experimental and control groups persisted (Ringler et al., 1978). Of 19 mother-child pairs continuing participation in this longitudinal study, the 5-year-olds in the experimental group expressed themselves significantly better than did the control children. The more mothers used language rich in adjectives, the higher the child's IQ score was at age 5. These findings cannot be explained by differences in the mothers' IQ scores.

Other research supports these initial findings. Cross-cultural research using methods similar to Klaus and Kennell's (1976) original study finds that early mother-infant contact is associated with better infant health and growth and increased duration of breast-feedings (Lozoff, Brittenham, Trause, Kennell, & Klaus, 1977; Sosa, Kennell, Klaus, Robertson, & Urrutia, 1980). Another intriguing development associated with bonding is the finding that infants with extra contact with mothers are less likely to experience abuse, neglect, or failure to thrive (Lozoff et al., 1977).

One can understand the excitement that this simple procedure caused—merely placing the naked infant on the body of his or her mother soon after birth apparently leads to all types of very important psychological

III. The Third Dimension

and social outcomes. These positive results of a low-cost preventive action seemed like a dream come true: Simply reorganize the hospital routine to encourage this mother-infant contact.

Critical reconsideration of every aspect of these studies began to clarify the active ingredients of the bonding experience, however (Belsky & Benn, 1982; Eyer, 1992). In looking beyond the bonding process, Belsky and Benn (1982) discovered that "opportunity for early contact with the newborn may initiate a process of parental familiarization or orientation which heightens awareness of the distinctive features of the newborn" (p. 287). Heightened awareness encourages maternal sensitivity in caring for the newborn, which then leads to the positive outcomes previously mentioned. Thus Belsky and Benn argue, rather than skin-to-skin contact stimulating an innate response system, the active ingredient that appears to produce the positive effects is parent-neonate interaction, a set of learned—not innate—events that is easily activated, such as by going through the Brazelton Neonatal Behavior Assessment Scale (Brazelton, 1973, 1986) with the new parents to acquaint them with the reflexes, orienting, and interactive responses of their baby (see also Farran & Haskins, 1980; Trad, 1993).

Belsky and Benn (1982) caution that these and other positive results they review are only tentative hints about the causal factors related to early infant development. We have much to learn about the dynamic transactions between infants and parents (and other caretakers) that aid or hamper the children's development (see Jason, 1992; Sameroff & Chandler, 1975). Belsky and Benn note that fathers (mainly ignored in early research) have an important part to play in infant development. In addition, they call attention to the other social system components, from rooming-in facilities at a hospital (or giving birth at home) to the large number of other social supports that new parents depend on.

Eyer (1992) is not so gentle. The full title of her book is *Mother-Infant Bonding: A Scientific Fiction.* She questions how we could have been so taken in by (a) a series of flawed experimental designs: "Do the behaviors that are designated dependent variables, such as holding the infant en face, actually represent better mothering?" (p. 19); (b) vaguely undefined key terms—the definition of *successful bonding* is never consistent and shifts from study to study; (c) invalid measurement methodology used as the basis of success—only 5 of about 75 measures showed statistical significance; (d) unexamined basic assumptions about innate or instinctual systems presumed to underlie bonding; and (e) the organizational and ideological props supporting this work. Eyer presents evidence for her case and some of the refutations by supporters of bonding and attachment. It makes interesting reading for primary preventers as a cautionary tale about believing too strongly whatever it is one hopes is the case. Whether or not Eyer proves her point only the future will reveal, but the tides of science will move back and forth over the years, to find evidence for nature (innate, instinctual forces), and then again to find evidence for nurture (learning by planned and unplanned experiences), and then again to find evidence for synthesis (wonderful social learning experiments that push the boundaries of biological limitations, and biological limitations that hold down the exuberance of social learning experiments).

We are at an awkward moment in translating research in primary prevention into practice strategies: Later research will clarify, correct, and perhaps reverse previous information. Yet we must act on the basis of the best available information. So, the caution that Belsky and Benn (1982) recommend is well justified—not to go beyond the evidence in translating research into action strategies—as long as the other half of their caution is noted—make use of all information available within a family and community context so that any one recommendation is placed within that context. In the case of bonding, they suggest that we transform every evaluation of infants and children—in medical, educational, or psychological settings—into learning experiences for parents that heighten their awareness of the skills and limits of children within family and community contexts. This would include the Klaus and Kennell (1976) approach and any other contact among parents, child, and professional helper. Belsky and Benn also note some ethical issues related to bonding, that some parents who cannot perform that postbirth contact (due to premature birth or illness) feel as if they have let their child down on some essential experience in life.

Kennell and Klaus (1976) attempt to correct this by saying that bonding does occur later in the lives of parents and children, even as they reiterate their original notion that there is a sensitive period in the postbirth time, thus trying to have their cake and eat it too. Trying to have an argument come out every way one wants it is a failing that all preventers are potentially err to (Tizard & Hodges, 1978; see also Hawkins et al., 1988, on social bonding in the societal sense).

III. The Third Dimension

Yet it is the preventer's lot to seek happy and effective attachments over the life course. Perhaps I can offer some tentative principles of what we have learned, good or bad, from this experience with attachment and bonding:

1. Communicate well in age-appropriate ways throughout the life course. For parents and newborns, these communications largely involve physical interactions in which parents give sustenance, warmth, and safety attention to their newborn, who in exchange presents exciting curiosity as well as demanding and continuous attention, particularly as he or she matures into a thinking and feeling individual. Parents and children need to learn effective communications in both directions (Gordon, 1989). School mates must learn how to communicate effectively so as to get their point of view across without losing friends in the process (Englander-Golden, Elconin, Miller, & Schwarzkopf, 1986; Englander-Golden, Elconin, & Satir, 1986). Marital partners need to learn effective communication to help promote happy and stable marriages (Markman, Floyd, Stanley, & Storaasli, 1988). Employees and employers need to learn better ways to communicate for the sake of productivity and satisfaction (*Journal of Primary Prevention,* 1994). Dying people need to learn to communicate with loved ones (and not-so-loved-ones) so as to integrate the pieces of their lives as they are bound up with the lives of those who survive them (Erikson, Erikson, & Kivnick, 1986). At each life point there is a way of communicating that one can learn so as to promote quality of life; if it involves using some biological aspect of our species, that is well and good.

2. Foreknowledge leaves one forewarned. Parents must really want a baby to endure all the continuous demands infants inevitably make. Preventers need to do a much better job informing sexually active people about what is potentially involved—there is life after sex. Even when unplanned and unwanted babies emerge, preventers can do a better job informing parents about human growth and development—the simple and basic things such as when most children learn to walk and talk and become emotionally secure and independent and how to effectively and constructively discipline children—by consistent yet loving communication. Social supports (health, education, and welfare) are needed for those who lack them, as the future of society (and support in our old age) will depend to a great extent on how well these infants become capable workers in the future (Ozawa, 1986).

3. Problem solving and potential achieving are continuous life tasks. They are amenable to improved methods for their accomplishment at each juncture over the life course. The very reason for forming close relationships with others is to learn how to problem solve and to be assisted in problem solving. Whether this reason is determined by gigantic evolutionary reasons—to give the fittest of the species a better chance for their gene pool to survive—or whether one can convey these ideas and skills to children through intentional or unintentional lessons following some learning model is a moot point. Parents have to act as if they know what they want to achieve and how they can flexibly work to achieve it and help their children learn these same lessons (Shure & Spivak, 1988).

4. In short, all must work at establishing and maintaining good quality attachments and social bonds between parents and children, among family members and friends, among students and teachers, among participants in the workplace, everywhere in the social world. We have to use the "best available information" of our day, not uncritically—we have to think about the underlying assumptions and what social structures and forces benefit or are harmed by these procedures—but actively. We must put the ideas to work and to the test and we must be willing to listen to the full results and adapt accordingly. Let me conclude with this quotation from Rutter (1981) in which he updates his 1972 study of maternal deprivation and related issues:

> [There has been a] continuing accumulation of evidence showing the importance of deprivation and disadvantage as influences on children's psychological development. Bowlby's (1951) original arguments on that score have been amply confirmed. However, . . . it is now very clear that deprivation involves a most heterogeneous group of adversities which operate through several quite different psychological mechanisms. Thus, insofar as deprivation is a causal factor, the acute distress syndrome sometimes shown during admission to hospital or to a residential nursery is probably due in part to an interference with attachment behavior and in part to the effects of a strange and frightening environment, with the disturbances after return home probably due in part to the adverse effects of separation on parent-child relationships; intellectual retardation is likely to be a function of a lack of adequate meaningful experiences; conduct disorders are in part a response to family discord and disturbed interpersonal relationships; and affectionless psychopathy may be a consequence of abnormal early bonding. . . .
>
> The old issue of critical periods of development and the crucial importance of the early years has been reopened and re-examined. The evidence is unequivocal

that experiences at all ages have an impact. However, it may be that the first few years do have a special importance for bond formation and social development. (p. 217)

3. Friendship

Readers may recall from their introductory psychology class the classic experiment by Solomon Asch (1952) in which a group of eight college students were sitting in a semicircle looking at two sets of cards with lines on them.

One card had three lines of different heights; the other had only one line. The task was to decide which of the three lines was the same height as the one line. It should have been an easy task—all one had to do is to look at the lines on the cards. But it was a difficult task for the only true subject in the group, the person sitting at position seven. Seven confederates of the experimenter gave their planned (mis-) judgment as to which of the three the test line was most nearly like. Pictures taken of this experiment show seven relaxed confederates, whereas the one true subject is straining forward looking at the lines and trying to figure out what is reality—how can it be that these other college students like himself say that the very short test line looks the same as the long line on the three-line card? This famous study on group pressure and conformity produced troubling findings: About one true subject in three went along with the confederates' patently incorrect answer and thus conformed to the group's definition of reality. A less well-known finding from this study is that if at least one other confederate selected the true line while the previous six confederates selected a false line, then the true subject always gave the correct answer and never bowed to the pressure of the group. One friend makes reality.

So it appears to be in real life. The importance of at least one good friend or confidant appears, in the gerontology literature, to be the basis for maintaining high morale among elderly persons (Lowenthal & Havens, 1968; see also Pearson, Cowan, Cowan, & Cohn, 1993, on the consistency of attachments of adult children and their aged parents). In a discussion of depression in women, Nicol and Erlenmeyer-Kimling (1986) note that "the most powerful protection from depression in the face of severe environmental circumstances was the presence of an intimate relationship" (p. 36). Bolton et al. (1985) conducted a preventive screening of adolescent mothers viewed as being at risk for child maltreatment. These authors discovered certain patterns of stressors relevant to the present discussion. These stressors include personal, environmental, and educational isolation from information on successful child rearing. The recommendation for preventive action is the presence of an "official" friend, who helps the pregnant teenager through the medical, welfare, and educational systems, and an "unofficial" friend, who shares the stresses and excitement of pregnancy and provides realistic support and reality testing. They see this unofficial friend as one who helps the adolescent's self-esteem and problem solving, not just for the immediate situation, but for life in general.

Most people have both formal and informal friends of this kind, but certain people at high risk lack one or the other or both. Bolton et al. (1985) are suggesting that primary prevention can identify groups of people at risk and supply, in one way or another, these friends. This can be done in individual lives as Sosa et al. (1980) did, or preventers can organize to generate friends on a large scale.

California established a mental health promotion bureau in 1978 with the mandate to develop a statewide mental health prevention program (Roppel & Jacobs, 1988). After a period of time to survey state needs and study preventive programs, the bureau established a statewide educational initiative that has come to be known as "Friends Can Be Good Medicine" (Hersey et al., 1982). The major program objectives were to inform the public about the health-promoting effects of supportive personal relationships, both for physical and mental health; to encourage individuals to invest more time and energy in their personal relationships; and to create opportunities for individuals and communities to come together to strengthen relationships.

A variety of materials were developed for mass distribution, such as television and radio public service announcements and a 64-page booklet containing poems, exercises, photographs, and passages dealing with the interplay of health and supportive personal relationships. Research by Hersey et al. (1982) suggests that the friendship message successfully reached a large proportion of the California audience. Later studies by Taylor, Lam, Roppel, and Barter (1984) suggest that initial gains in positive attitudes and knowledge about health were maintained a year later. Various groups and local organizations adopted the project at the conclusion of the state program, suggesting that there was some institutionalization of a program perceived to be successful. No research has been reported that specifically links this mass media approach with created friendships and health, however. (The notion of institutionalizing a successful program may appear too obvious to be mentioned, but in fact a whole different set of skills and activities is needed to disseminate and embed a good preventive program in the ongoing workings of society. The topic is beyond the scope of this book, but good material exists on this subject; see Dearing, Meyer, & Rogers, 1994; Rogers, 1973, 1983.)

Life is more complex than simply generating a friend and thereby guaranteeing health. For example, marriage is a highly intimate and persistent relationship between a man and a woman. Many researchers have noted, however, as Gordon and Ledray (1985) express it, that marriage appears to have a protective effect for men and a detrimental effect for women. Bernard (1972) compiled sets of observations on the advantages and costs of marriage to males and females: Married males exhibit superiority over never-married males on measures of mental health (fewer signs of mental disorders), physical health (at least starting at middle age), suicide rates (married men have half the rate of unmarried men), survival (married men live longer), and reported happiness.

Married women report a different story: More married women than married men report unhappy marriages, marital frustrations, considerations of divorce, and seeking of marital counseling. There are reports of higher rates of depression in married women as compared with married men or unmarried women (Field & Weishaus, 1992). Thus we are only at the beginning of understanding the protective value of having a friend. Many years ago, George Herbert Mead (1934) spoke about the dynamics by which a person becomes who he or she is, through interactions with significant others. Harry Stack Sullivan (1953) theorizes that it is developmentally crucial that youngsters form chum relationships to begin the process of self-discovery and self-formation. Novelists and artists have long portrayed the bittersweet attraction and repulsion of intimacy. The helping professions have been described in terms of the purchase of friendship, a professional friend when no private individual takes a friendship role with the client. (The professional brings other characteristics than just being a friend.)

The field of primary prevention as a whole has yet to incorporate this potentially powerful tool of friendship in a systematic way for various populations at risk (e.g., for child abuse or neglect, spousal abuse, lonely individuals [Perlman & Peplau, 1984; Rook, 1984]—especially the elderly or AIDS victims), although telephone assurance systems do provide some friendly contact and increase the awareness of possible problems.

Another example of telephone contact involves youths who have come to the attention of the authorities for various conduct problems. These youths stay at home until their cases are heard—so they will not be stigmatized or criminalized for being placed in jail—on condition that a volunteer telephone caller finds them at home whenever a random call is made (except when the youths are supposed to be at school or at work, for which another security check is made). The telephone caller is not a "friend" as such, but an aide in diverting the youth from being sucked into the criminal justice system. The cost to society is very low; the benefits are probably high, with these youths being given another chance to exhibit lawful social behavior without too much stigmatization.

Friendships can be formed through natural contacts, that is, in ordinary living contexts where individuals share common experiences—such as parents pushing the children on park swings or students standing in line to sign up for classes or picnickers sharing foods. But the several studies discussed above also suggest that friendships can be constructed—that is, they can be purposively nurtured by helping professionals. People can be employed to be friends to those without friends (or without constructive friendships). College students can be given class credits; poor people can be given exchange credits (see Chapter 6, V.A.3); retired people can be given money or awards or simply the pleasure of helping (see Gillmore et al., 1992). Such constructed friendships may or may not involve training.

Teaching people to be friends of the constructive type involves the presentation of *active listening skills:*

1. Regardless of who initiates a conversation, it is the role of the "active listener" to listen to what the other person is saying. This may involve being silent and waiting for the other person to speak or to continue speaking. Interest may be indicated by a warm tone of voice, friendly eye contact, and a posture of leaning slightly forward toward the other person.

2. Active listening may involve brief probes to get further information or expression of feelings from the other person: "Tell me more about that" or "What do you mean?" Sometimes a nonverbal message, such as nodding the head, may encourage the other person to continue speaking.

3. Active listening may involve repeating a phrase of what the other person has just said, but spoken as a question, indicating that the active listener wants more information: "You felt exhausted after people left?"

4. All of the above ploys encourage the other person to continue expressing ideas and feelings when this is appropriate to do so. Sometimes, when a topic has reached some closure, it is appropriate to ask a question that starts a new topic of conversation. But it is also possible to remain silent and let the other person continue the lead as to what topics to talk about.

5. The active listener should let the other person know that what he or she has said is fully understood. One can reflect the ideas and the feeling tone of the comments to indicate this: "I sense that you were feeling very lonely, even when some of your neighbors were still at the house." At other times, sharing one's own experiences at this point is helpful too: "I felt that way, even when my sister-in-law was staying with me; it is just somehow different when your husband isn't there."

Friends don't have to solve the other person's problems, although if they can provide moral support, information, or modeling, all well and good. But friends are frequently "people who are there" with the person at the right time and place, with no special agenda. Friends become problematic when they attempt to take on a professional helping role without adequate training.

The following statements attempt to summarize the action principles from the preceding discussion:

1. Connecting people with people for the purpose of generating friendships can have multiple constructive implications, although not including professional problem solving. Friendship has immediate validity to participants and rapid payoff—a kind of reciprocity, of feeling that one is part of this friendship group and one is contributing to it in one's own way and receiving from it in the ways friends are able to contribute. Simply bringing people together will not guarantee friendship, however. There must be some basis of shared interests and values sufficient to overcome whatever inertia or resistance the parties have for making the new contact and exerting energy. Preventers must find people with some commonalities as the beginning point of the contact.

2. Initial relationships should be supported with appropriate resources (such as an accessible place to meet in pleasant surroundings) but should be allowed to form on their own—one cannot force friendship.

3. People need help in identifying their growing positive feelings for their friends so that the connection will be more likely to grow and flourish. This identification may take the form of reflecting on the pleasant activities the friends have engaged in over time and how each connects the other with that pleasant association. This is not to label people as "friends" as much as to raise the consciousness of this point among the people involved.

4. Opportunities to help the friend may increase the friendly feelings regarding the association (the helper therapy principle).

5. Open communication ground rules facilitate the ongoing relationship. Indeed, active listening (Bloom, 1990) may be the essence of the friendship as well as its perpetuation.

B. Primary Group Aspects

1. Social Support, Mutual Assistance, and Self-Help Groups

By sheer number, groups offering social support are probably one of the major modes of providing preventive, protective, or promotive help (Barrera, 1986; Gottlieb, 1981, 1983; Maguire, 1991; Whittaker & Garbarino, 1983). A concept of many names, *social support* involves a relatively small number of persons coming together on a face-to-face basis regarding some concern that all share directly or indirectly by virtue of past or present events. Out of this small group interaction comes tangible or intangible assistance to one or more members, and the feelings or perceptions of being helped. The satisfaction of helping is also present, although this is less often discussed.

Constructed groups such as self-help groups, mutual assistance groups, and support groups may be said to seek some objective; in the technical language of social psychology, this would be termed a *task function* of the group.

Equally important is the *integrative function,* which involves members of the group getting along with fellow members. The kinds of activities devoted to achieving some objective often are different from those needed to keep good relationships among members, so that the group has to alternate task or integrative efforts in some fashion.

For purposes of this discussion, I distinguish natural support groups (such as a family helping its members) from constructed support groups of various types (such as those that are artificially but purposively brought together for an identifiable purpose). I discuss constructed support groups below and natural support groups in the next section. Both have their place in offering primary prevention practices.

To begin this discussion of constructed social supports, let me examine the Widow-to-Widow program developed by Phyllis Silverman (1970, 1988). Typically, there is a period immediately after the death of a loved one where many family members and friends help out a widow. Eventually, these people return to their own life situations, leaving the widow to start coping on her own. This can be a very stressful transition period, and it is to this situation that the Widow-to-Widow program is directed. Previously widowed persons, who are known to have successfully worked through their own experiences, are guided to reach out to a new widow with an offer of neighborly service—listening to the new widow, sharing experiences about how she herself dealt with these same stresses, and making suggestions as to where other aid may be located. These one-to-one contacts are typically awkward for both widows at first, but soon become quite natural. About twice a month the widows make contact, often initiated by the newly widowed person after the process has begun.

Over time, the widows may feel the need to share their problems and successes in larger groups and so group discussions and social activities are arranged. Sometimes several widows work together with a newly widowed person. There is no exclusiveness in the arrangements. Telephone hot lines and storefront programs have also been set up, showing considerable ingenuity in reaching out to the newly widowed.

Beyond the expression of profound and disruptive feelings stemming from the death of a loved one, there is also the need to redefine and reaffirm a new independent role in life for which many people have had little experience (Lieberman & Videka-Sherman, 1986).

Role models may make a greater effect than "academic" discussions by people who have not actually had this experience. One test of the success of the program is that many newly widowed persons later volunteer to be the next generation of helpers.

Widowhood is a challenge in a life transition for which the experiences of others who have gone through the same challenge may be particularly helpful to the newly widowed. Research on the program by various investigators is generally supportive, even though it is difficult to test whether or not emotional illness was prevented by means of this program (Silverman, 1988; see also Zambelli & DeRosa, 1992, on a bereavement support group for school-age children, and Jason, LaPointe, & Billinghom, 1986, on presenting self-help groups through the mass media).

Bogat, Sullivan, and Grober (1993) make an important point with regard to various social support services directed toward preventive interventions, namely, that most of these programs are directed toward women or attract predominantly female participants. Because research shows that women receive more emotional support in general, "support interventions seem to attract and target the very people who are most capable of forming supportive relationships on their own" (Bogat et al., 1993, p. 219). The main point is that primary prevention programs should ensure that all who are at risk are served, as long as resources are available.

To give a perspective on the prevalence of support groups of all types, I present the following listing found in the free local newspaper in rural central Connecticut: an adoption support group for Latin American parents, an AIDS support group, a group for people who have had a family member die, a parents' support group for "the toughest job in the world," a support group for adults and children with attention deficit disorders, a codependence anonymous group, a support group for divorced or separated persons, a debtors anonymous group, a depression anonymous group, a support group for parents of gifted and talented children, a group for substance abusers, a cancer support group, a group for parents of multihandicapped children, a support group for former foster children (over 18 years old), a group for people with mental health problems, a support group for persons with Huntington's disease, a gamblers' anonymous group, a panic management support group, a support group for women living with situations of domestic violence, a support group for family and friends of gay and lesbian people, a take off pounds sensibly (TOPS) support group, and a widows and widowers group. All for one average week, a breath-taking assortment of human problems and neighborly support.

The principles of this kind of lightly constructed support group system can be summarized as follows:

1. Enable people who have experienced the same kind of problem to meet together. One person in this meeting must have coped (or be coping) successfully with that experience, whereas the other person may be in the beginning stages of coping or problem solving.

2. Provide minimal training to the helper. The worker who brings the helper into gentle contact with the helpee has to have considerable trust in the power of the relationship that is to evolve naturally between helper and helpee. The worker sets the general goals—to address personal needs and necessary tasks (such as paying bills)—within the unique social context, but does not get involved in a direct helping role. (In the Widow-to-Widow program, the helper's efforts are a labor of love because they brings back vivid experiences and feelings of her own. This is the very point, that both widows can cry together as well as laugh together, while the helper models for the helpee some of the independence that can emerge in widowhood.)

3. Supply resources, as needed, over the course of the contact. These resources may involve information about community services, procedures to get through bureaucracies, and the like.

4. The rewards are intrinsic to the situation and are probably mutually contingent, that is, each party to the support group gets some kind of pleasure from the interaction even though these rewards are likely to be different for each party. (In the Widow-to-Widow program, the helper probably gets satisfaction from helping another through difficult times and indirectly gains by vicariously reliving her own struggle against the pain of widowhood. The newly widowed person is aided to express her emotions that others may not understand or care to hear; in expressing these feelings, she may gain control over them so as to move to another task of the widowed person, that of establishing an independent role in life.)

Let's consider another type of constructed support group where there is heavily constructed involvement by the helping professionals. Constructed social support groups at the macro level may be illustrated by the application of Paulo Freire's (1990; Shor, 1987) work on politicized education, that is, helping nonliterate people learn to read as a personal and political act, a part of the process of self- and social-empowerment. Freire, a Brazilian educator who was exiled by a military coup in 1964 for seeking to empower the poor people of his country, evolved a philosophy and method of "pedagogy of the oppressed." This is a way to interact with nonliterate people to teach them to speak about things they know, to link a handful of written words to this speaking and thinking, and thus to move to a basic education in the use of the written language that leads to self-respect and, potentially, political action. Education becomes a mutual process, not one where the all-knowing teacher bestows pieces of knowledge from the "bank" onto the student. This banking concept of education has many structural implications: The teacher is the authority, the one who controls, selects, punishes; the students know nothing, memorize—not think—and comply (Freire, 1990, p. 59).

Brown (1987) presents a highly accessible introduction to Freire's methods: Facing groups of Brazilian nonliterates who were fatalistic about their poor circumstances, Freire and his colleagues created small discussion groups that involved talking about a set of simple line drawings of people and nature. The nonliterate people could quickly identify the objects—a farming man, a pig, a well, a house—and distinguish things of nature from things of culture. The nonliterate people knew this distinction but the discussion gave them words to name and clarify it: They live in nature, but they make culture and pass it on to their children. In pictures of men using a bow and arrow and others of men using a gun, Freire and the nonliterates discussed how culture transforms people, perhaps to liberate them (from drudgery). The nonliterates recognized the part that education plays—only those who can read can earn enough money to buy things for technological development. Education involves the use of words and writing—and the effort to analyze one's own reality for its constraints and the actions needed to transform it. Freire (1990) calls this process *conscientization*. Now the stage is set for moving to the teaching of reading.

Freire and his colleagues would go to a community and meet with coinvestigators, the local volunteers with whom the educators would check their methods. They would select a short list of familiar words that contain in their syllables all the phonetics of the language (Portuguese, Spanish). These are called *generative* words because other words can be formed (and recognized in writing) from their syllables. First, a picture of a brick was displayed and the nonliterates would say the word *tijolo,* which means brick. Then a picture of the brick and the three-syllable word was displayed. The syllables contain consonants and vowels that can be combined with other words so that the sounds and letters can be formed into new combinations that Spanish-speaking people will recognize:

ta te ti to tu
la le li lo lu
ja je ji jo ju, etc.

By using these now-understood combinations of sounds and letters, the nonliterates came up with new words, such as *luta* (struggle), *lata* (tin can), and *loja* (store). With these words, they formed sentences and ideas: *O voto e'do povo* ("The vote belongs to the people"). Thus people were taught not only to read but to think about their social reality as well, a revolutionary idea that is understandably uncongenial to military dictatorships.

What types of practice principles regarding these strongly constructed social support groups can be suggested?

1. People who have had the same kind of problems should be connected with one another under the condition that one party in the group is further ahead than other parties in successfully coping. Freire and his colleagues approached villagers as coinvestigators and colearners, sharing the condition of oppression but with the understanding that they were able to teach the villagers how to talk and read about this situation—and how to change it.

2. With considerable sensitivity and planning, helpers arrange with helpees to talk together and to learn together and thereby evolve a social support system that takes them into political as well as social contexts. (Now educated villagers can participate in the larger social movements that the helpers have presented to them.)

3. Resources must be supplied as needed. (In the case of Freire's groups, these resources might be information on coming elections or other political actions villagers can take on their own behalf.)

4. The rewards must be intrinsic to the situation and are probably mutually contingent, even though they will likely be different for each party. (The villagers learn basic reading skills and develop self-confidence in being able to affect their own destiny to some degree. The teachers feel the satisfaction of the immediate success as well as anticipation of the possible successes as villagers exert their new skills.)

III. The Third Dimension

The practice principles on constructed social support systems are similar for lightly or heavily constructed groups.

Why do some people want to help other people in the first place? It is the task of the person who helps construct the support group to identify the reward structure for helpers and helpees. This is not an easy task—why, for example, should a widow wish to relive the difficult times after her spouse died for the sake of helping another recent widow? Why should a recent widow want to talk to a stranger about the stresses of widowhood? Indeed, why would a worker go into rural backwaters to teach people to read, especially when there may be government opposition and possible legal (or illegal) action against these teachers and villagers?

The helping professional must be clear about the rewards and costs of such constructed relationships and be able to get the contact started. There is an idealism involved, a belief in the goodness and worth of people and the goodness and worth of attempting to help them help themselves. These are the ideals that bring people into the helping professions; these are also the values that motivate the millions of volunteers around the world. The professional helper may be called on to give advice at points where the parties' commonsense and goodwill does not suggest a ready solution. It may not be easy to provide social support.

2. Natural Helping Networks

The natural helping network is a concept recently identified by social scientists (Collins & Pancoast, 1976) after millennia of experiences with this phenomenon. Better late than never. Collins and Pancoast (1976) recognize that natural helping networks are widely pervasive in the tissue of social relationships but that they are delicate and should not be crudely handled by well-meaning helping professionals. Citizen helpers perform their natural helping functions more or less well and might benefit from added resources, information, or moral support, but they should not be co-opted into becoming pseudo-psychiatrists or semi-social workers.

Natural helping networks represent naturally occurring groups, usually based in a neighborhood (Unger & Wandersman, 1983) or a particular physical setting, such as a bar, or a barber shop or beauty parlor, in which informal support occurs. Typically, natural leaders emerge in these contexts to facilitate the exchanges of services, material goods, or emotional support. (Note that these involve both task and integrative functions.)

III. The Third Dimension

These leaders are ordinarily not paid, are not necessarily schooled in the helping arts, and may not even be aware of their talents or reputation. They are simply doing what comes naturally to them, which others come to appreciate and value. Such leaders may receive assistance from others with regard to other concerns; they are not necessarily all-around "super-people" (Biegel, Magaziner, & Baum, 1991).

Collins and Pancoast (1976) describe some instances of natural helping networks. An anthropological study of homeless men (Dumont, 1967) identified a tavern bartender who aided the men who went to his bar by handling their welfare checks, loaning them money, and regulating their drinking behavior. He also was the proprietor of a boarding house for single men and served as a focal point around which the men interacted—thus providing them with a sense of belonging. Another example is the leading person in a single-room occupancy (SRO) building who built close relationships with the tenants, caring for them when they were ill, sharing money and material things, and providing companionship for drinking and card playing. Of these types of leaders, Shapiro (1969) writes, "They mitigate potential disorganization in response to stress and reduce disturbed behavior and neighborhood blight. They are, in fact, the unpaid and invisible staff of nameless and unendowed halfway houses" (pp. 649-650; see also Cochran, 1990).

Reissman (1976) compared professional and self-help groups and found many strengths in self-help groups, including the nearly equal status of helper and helpee (and presumably the feelings that this equality generates), the directness and immediacy of the help given, and the low costs. There is little rigorous research on the effectiveness of self-help groups, however, although anecdotal evidence of the intergroup satisfactions should stimulate such studies (Katz, 1993).

Gottlieb (1983) and others have warned about the overprofessionalization of support groups, particularly natural helping networks. Natural helpers possess important qualities of local acceptance, acknowledged skills and ideas that fit within the local culture, and a track record of success. Research has indicated that nonprofessional helpers can be quite effective (Durlack, 1979; cf. Berman & Norton, 1985).

It is easy to co-opt natural leaders by providing them with training, resources, and new directions, which of course mirror what the professional (who lacks local acceptance, acknowledged skills and ideas, and a track record of success in the neighborhood) would like the natural leader to do. The great challenge, Gottlieb (1983) points out, is to facilitate or support healthy primary group attachments among citizens without imposing the values and methods of professionals on leaders of these groups. There is another value conflict here because some natural leaders might wish to get a better-paying job or whatever and see the social service agency as an avenue for self-development. Is it co-opting to help these people change even at the cost of breaking up a natural helping network? A difficult choice.

What are the steps in identifying and supporting natural helping networks without damaging them? I suggest the following:

1. Identify natural helping networks in a given locale by finding a collaborator who lives in that area and is willing and able to share information. The kinds of information needed are on the kinds of problems and potentials the people of this locale have and what they are doing about them. Informants may include local clergy, police, social workers, and also people well informed about local people and happenings, such as bartenders, grocery store clerks, and mail delivery people.

2. Identify tactfully what the natural helper is doing. Because the natural helper may be performing roles that only intimate family members perform (such as handling a person's money), one must be cautious in learning about these activities as they might be helpful or exploitative—or even a bit of both. (In the homeless men example, there may have been a legal issue, such as receiving or signing another person's Social Security checks. Strictly speaking, this may not have been legal, but given the whole picture, if a man himself could not sign for his own checks, then he may have been institutionalized for his own protection, which may not have been what he desired. This informal maneuver permitted him to function in the community, even though it may have stretched the strict letter of the law. This kind of ethical dilemma is common to all professional helping.)

3. Form a comfortable relationship with the natural helper, learning about the help given and eventually offering some kind of services to the natural helper if needed. The professional can offer social approval and recognition of the services the natural helper is providing—if such recognition is wanted. The professional may also be able to offer further information or supplies to make the work of the natural helper easier. Note that the emphasis is on supporting the strengths of the natural

III. The Third Dimension

helping network rather than considering its weaknesses. Moreover, it is support of the existing network, rather than trying to make it over into something else the professional dreams of, that may or may not fit that specific situation.

4. Attach no strings for receiving this aid unless there are strong problems in how the natural helper is delivering the help. Obviously, not all natural helping networks are constructive and some may exact more cost than they provide effective services, as when a natural group extends protections to a person who really needs institutional services. If there is a serious problem, then the natural group itself may become a target of intervention to change it into a constructive force in that locale.

5. Remove oneself from the natural helping network when one is no longer needed. The natural helper should be given the professional's name and phone number in case the helper has specific questions or needs (see also Barth, Derezotes, & Danforth, 1991; De La Rosa, 1988; Des Jarlais & Friedman, 1988; Kenkel, 1986).

The family structure is perhaps an ideal type of a natural helping network—although as illustrated above, the term generally refers to nonrelated persons. The family as a unit of service and an object of service is discussed throughout this book, so I will not present any specific material here (Whittaker & Tracy, 1990).

C. Secondary Group Aspects

1. Social Empowerment, Advocacy

Empowerment is a complex term involving at its core the idea that power-deficient people gain some power over their own lives. How they gain that power—whether it is given to them by powerful others, or whether they are enabled to obtain it through the guidance by wise if not powerful others, or whether the power deficient get it all by themselves— is not clear by definition. Likewise, it is not clear that if the power-deficient people gain power, is it at the expense of the formerly powerful people (as in a zero-sum arrangement that what one side gains, the other side loses), or can the empowerment of the deficient group not affect the powerful group (a non-zero-sum arrangement)? Swift and Levin (1987) illustrate the latter point with the notion of parenting, that is, empowering a child to develop into an adult over a sequence of age-graded challenges that do not diminish the power of the parent.

Empowerment can refer to individuals, such as enabling a person to take advantage of some opportunity, but the term has focused on collective or social empowerment, as when a minority group or an oppressed group experiences empowerment (Albee, Joffe, & Dusenbury, 1988; Clark, 1981; Ferre, 1987; Freire, 1990; Rappaport, 1981; Simon, 1994; Solomon, 1976; Swift, 1992; Zimmerman & Rappaport, 1988). People may make mistakes when they have power over their own lives; no one has a monopoly on making such miscalculations. The philosophy of empowerment has to allow for everyone involved to make mistakes as being on the path toward experience leading to better decisions. In this sense, the expression of empowerment is like the expression of democracy in action.

Empowerment involves a configuration of persons in social contexts and physical environments at a historic time. The concept of power deficit involves the relation of power between one group and another in a given time and place. The content involved in that power relationship may range from economic resources to political or social statuses and has a concomitant of psychological effects (e.g., pride, inferiority) as well (Alinsky, 1969, 1972; Joffe & Albee, 1981).

The United States has experimented with versions of social empowerment, as in the Economic Opportunity Act of 1964, which established community action programs that were to engage the "maximum feasible participation" of the people involved in these programs. The intention appeared to be to empower the poor by helping them control portions of their own environment—and thus take away power from the established power brokers. The actuality was much more diverse. In some cases, bureaucrats or professionals attempted to represent the poor, whereas in other cases, the poor took control of aspects of their own environments. In many cases, this shift of power was problematic to the established forces; ultimately the War on Poverty ended without maximum feasible participation ever taking full hold. The germ of the idea, however, which is as old as the idea of democracy itself, has flowered into many different forms. (For a history of social empowerment in America, see Simon, 1994.)

For primary prevention, the core ingredients of empowerment may be described as follows:

III. The Third Dimension

1. A group of persons with some deficit of power, resources, or status comes to be aware of its relative position, not merely that members "live on the other side of the tracks," but come to an understanding in depth of the specific problems, illnesses, limitations to advancement, deprivations, and inhumanities they bear because of this deficit (Alinsky, 1969, 1972; Freire, 1990).

2. This group comes to recognize that, although individually weak, members may be collectively strong. It also comes to recognize that the difficulty is not due to individual deficits, but more likely to sociocultural forces that create collective deficits that all share regardless of individual differences. Members also recognize the philosophical value in exerting control over their own lives; if one has never done this, it takes a major shift in one's cognitive perspective to do so.

3. The group with the power deficit, either by itself or in conjunction with internal (indigenous) or external leaders, conducts a systemic campaign to make changes. For example, some groups gain empowerment by campaigns to register voters who then "vote the rascals out." Other groups gain empowerment by getting into the establishment and bringing pressure to bear on public bureaus to operate in ways more in line with the needs of the power-deficient people. Or more revolutionary paths are taken to "expropriate the expropriators" (Marx). All of these actions have as their aim the bringing to power of those who were inappropriately or unjustly deficient.

4. The social change that has been brought about is formalized in persisting social structures and norms—both to protect the recently empowered and to enable others to obtain their fair share of social goods. It is, of course, possible that those newly empowered may misuse their newly won rights by reducing access to others who may follow them, in which case the cycle of empowerment repeats itself (see George Orwell's *Animal Farm*).

What part do helping professionals play in these events? It is difficult to propose strategic steps in empowerment because helping professionals often represent the established interests that are, intentionally or not, the very forces maintaining the power deficit. Professionals have to be judicious and self-honest in their roles. Certainly, they can play a part in raising the consciousness of the power-deficient groups by clarifying the nature and depth of the effects of this deficiency. They can arouse feelings and motivate those in power to begin to explore ways to resolve deficiencies. They may take active roles in these changes, especially as they merge their identities with those they serve (Rothman, 1979).

What helping professionals should not do, as part of the democratic empowerment ideology, is legislate what the power deficient should do. Rather, empowerment involves degrees of facilitation to enable the involved people to discover for themselves what problems they are experiencing and what goals they would like to attain. At this critical point, professional helpers must supply accurate information on ideas, alternative goals, possible resources, options, difficulties, and the like—all without taking over the group's self-empowerment. Professional helpers may have to train the natural leaders in the power-deficient group—without co-opting them to be junior helping professionals—to be competent in leadership activities on a broader social stage. (See Eng & Hatch, 1991, on how a lay health adviser networked between black churches and social agencies. Likewise, Rappaport & Simkin, 1991, discuss healing and empowering through religious and mental health organizations.) Helping professionals also can affect the social environment in which natural leaders from the power-deficient groups may work effectively. These types of changes are important because they don't inhibit the natural leaders but merely open to them and others the options that they will later decide to accept or not.

Tadmor (1988) provides an example of empowerment involving a Caesarean birth (CB) population. CB is often a crisis to the involved persons, increasing the likelihood of postnatal depression and some lack of contact with the newborn in addition to the stressful medical aspects of the procedure. Tadmor points out that traditional hospitals treat the CB mother as a surgical patient, not a new mother, and that the whole arrangement of the procedure and aftermath reinforces this surgical patient role rather than one as a new parent. The CB mother's self-esteem is lowered because of these various assaults and the rooming arrangements (with mothers who delivered their infants ordinarily).

In formulating her model of perceived personal control to counteract the various untoward features of a CB in a traditional hospital context, Tadmor (1988) combined a number of features discussed previously: There is an anticipatory guidance session acquainting the CB couple with personnel and physical setting where the CB will take place, as well as an audiovisual presentation of CB and a realistic discussion of the pain and the recovery period. (See discussion of anticipatory instruction, Chapter 2, I.A.4.) Natural supportive networks are mobilized, as well as organized supports (in the form of a veteran CB couple who share their own experiences and ultimate success).

In the Tadmor (1988) study, the professional change agents were most involved in making changes in the hospital arrangements, but presumably former CB couples could have participated in these activities. The birth process itself was reorganized to permit the father to be present at the birth, holding his wife's hand and providing reassurance and confidence in the birth of their child (in contrast to the loneliness CB mothers ordinarily faced without their husbands present).

The anesthesiologist lowered the anesthesia level permitting the mother (and father) to make initial contact with the baby to promote bonding and then the anesthesia was raised to complete the surgical procedure. Postpartum events include the CB mother having early contact for breast-feeding while the pain level is still being controlled by regional anesthesia. Later, a veteran CB mother visits to initiate contact with a local CB support group. The new mother is encouraged to be a veteran CB mother for others (Chapter 4, III.A.1).

All of these changes required both social and physical rearrangements on the part of the obstetrics department at the hospital. The medical staff gave up some of its traditional prerogatives by empowering the CB patients, but in the end lost no real power and gained in healthier, happier mothers and infants. Effort was required to convince the establishment about these changes, but in a professional context that is presumably dedicated to client betterment, the changes were accepted on an experimental basis and then institutionalized when the success was documented—reductions in financial costs by shortening hospitalization and reducing the use of analgesia, as well as the advantages to the CB mothers and families (Tadmor, 1988). Other examples of empowerment include job training (Azrin & Besalel, 1980; Prestby, Wandersman, Florin, Rich, & Chavis, 1990; Vinokur et al., 1991) and breast-feeding policies in maternity wards (Perez-Escamilla et al., 1994).

2. Consultation

Consultation involves one party (the consultant) with special knowledge and skills communicating with another party (the consultee—another individual professional, a group of professionals, or an organization, usually through contact with representatives or leaders) so as to enhance knowledge, improve skills, and shape attitudes for the purpose of helping the consultees help themselves in their own professional tasks. The consultant offers suggestions; the consultee is free to accept or reject the ideas (Caplan, 1970; Kadushin, 1977; Mannino & Shore, 1986; Rieman, 1992; Tolan, Perry, & Jones, 1987).

Caplan (1970) categorizes consultation into four types that may be useful distinctions (see also Ketterer, Bader, & Levy, 1980, and critics Wynne, McDaniel, & Weber, 1986):

1. Client-centered case consultation: The consultant helps the consultee (such as a mental health professional) assess and plan strategies for a difficult case situation.
2. Consultee-centered case consultation: The consultant focuses on helping the consultee perform his or her work across all cases more effectively.
3. Program-centered administrative consultation: The consultant helps the consultee (e.g., administrators of a mental health agency) design, administer, or evaluate a program or policy.
4. Consultee-centered administrative consultation: The consultant focuses on helping the consultee (administrators, staff) perform planning and administering functions across the entire agency.

Consultation and education were part of a set of mandated services in the Community Mental Health Act of 1963 to encourage primary prevention activities in the local area, just as the move to deinstitutionalize began to reach full speed. Large numbers of disturbed and disturbing people were taken out of the mental institutions, were prescribed tranquilizers, and were told to check in at their local community mental health center for ongoing services. Unfortunately, two thirds of the original number of community mental health centers were never built and those that were often overwhelmed with heavy demands from very sick people; the primary preventive services became an impossible dream.

Drolen (1990) reports one recent survey of 69 mental health centers located in 27 states that shows substantial cutbacks in consultation, education, and other preventive services. In their place have emerged revenue-producing programs and time-efficient treatment methods. Priority is being given to the chronic mentally ill, but ability to pay has become a determining factor on who gets service. As ever, reality holds the sword over the heads of agencies that have to bring in revenues to cover expenses—or go out of business.

Many societal trends and cross-currents have woven together to produce swings in support for consultation and education within the community mental health center context. Mannino and Shore (1986) describe the history of mental health consultation, including the visiting teacher role that emerged from the settlement house movement initially to effect environmental systems changes. It was only later that visiting teachers became clinicians dealing with individuals. Clifford Beers's National Committee for Mental Hygiene consulted with local communities to develop child guidance clinics in the 1920s, another major step in consultation. Soon the need to prepare people for consultation service emerged, only to face the rising tide of psychoanalytically oriented individual services, which became popular in the 1930s to the 1960s with the consequent decline of interest in environmental and system approaches.

As Collins and Pancoast (1976) note, since the early days of Social Security legislation in the 1930s, trained personnel were required to help dispersing agencies meet standards and deliver services. There were other advances of consultation in the military during World War II, a need that arose from shortages of trained personnel. The National Mental Health Act of 1946 began the incorporation of the public health perspective in American mental health. Mannino and Shore (1986) point out the many contributions that Gerald Caplan made in defining and developing consultation in its contemporary outlines.

Crisis theory (Roberts, 1991) posits that people are particularly vulnerable at times of crisis, so that their immediate professional helpers should take advantage of the fluid situation to aid clients' progress. Because there are not enough immediate helpers, such as teachers, ministers, police personnel, and so forth, trained in mental health methods, social workers and others provide relevant consultation to those who were available (Schelkun, 1990). Kenney (1986) summarizes the research trends from a large consultation literature and finds generally positive results, with many methodological limitations. Zins (1995) is more cautious in interpreting the available results: "Although there is increasing evidence that consultation can have preventive benefits, this review suggests that the actual empirical support is not as strong as most of the literature suggests or that many consultants would like" (p. 295).

Ross (1980) presents an example of a crisis counseling service that led to a preventive program following the suicide of several students. The focus of survivor counseling and consultation services was on helping everyone in the school recognize the signs of suicidal depression (see Chapter 3, II.C.2) and respond appropriately. (See Park, 1982, for another example of combining treatment and prevention services.)

Roberts and Thorsheim (1986) used an ecological approach in a study of personal distress and alcohol abuse in members of 24 church congregations. Experimental congregations received consultation in providing social support and mutual empowerment (i.e., giving and receiving reciprocal support on a personal basis). Results favoring the experimental groups appeared in lower levels of distress and alcohol abuse (see also Forti & Hyg, 1983).

Consultation is a complex process and it does not always produce successful results. Cherniss (1977) describes one such failure, a consultation program directed to public school teachers that never became fully operational. Many possible weak points in the process were identified: An external group (a community mental health center staff) initiated the project without adequate involvement of the recipients of the program; there was insufficient institutional support; and the project leader was marginal to the organization. (For other examples of consultation, see Rieman, 1992; Wynne, McDaniel, & Weber, 1986.)

Wynne et al. (1986) present a checklist of questions to guide consultants. This checklist is divided into seven topics. I offer a brief summary below of a complex area of study and practice:

1. Explore the possibilities of consultation: Who is the consultee and what is the initial presenting problem? How did the consultee (and colleagues) decide to seek consultation at this time?

2. Contract: What are the initial target problems and goals that consultee and consultant agree to work on? Who is to provide what, where, and how? What are fee arrangements?

3. Connect consultant to the organization and staff: Who are the key players in the organization and how will the consultant link up with them, formally and informally? Who is in favor and who is against change in the organization? How can the consultant remain neutral among opposing groups?

4. Assess the situation: How will the consultant gather information about the structure of the organization, its history (stages of the organizational life cycle), current events that prompted the need, and relevant belief systems of the consultee(s)?

5. Implement the recommendations: How will the consultant make recommendations that fit within the belief system of the consultee and the organizational norms? How will change (e.g., new goals) be incorporated into the recommendations?

6. Evaluate the effects of the consultation: How will the consultant and consultee know whether or not the goals of the consultation have been met? Who is to judge? What are the plans for follow-through?

7. Leave the situation: How can the consultant best conclude the relationship with the consultee and the consultation system? Under what circumstances should further consultation be negotiated?

3. Concrete Assistance From Social Groups

We get by in life with a little help from our friends, as the Beatles' song goes. Indeed, the range of concrete assistance people receive from friends and family, as well as impersonal organizations and governments, is as enormous as it is vital. Caplan's (1964) Supply Model theorizes that to avoid mental disorder, people need three types of supplies: physical supplies, such as health, safety, food, and shelter; psychosocial supplies, including family and interpersonal relationships and interpersonal activities; and sociocultural supplies, such as access to work and education, social services, and social recognition. These are all obvious and basic factors in life but they tend to get overlooked in favor of sophisticated psychological therapies. Handal and Moore (1987) confirm Caplan's hypothesis that the greater the access to these supplies, the less mental distress and discontent people exhibit.

There are a number of examples of specific concrete assistance (and the effects measured), such as giving away free toothbrushes to young children and free condoms to bigger ones (Arnold & Cogswell, 1971; Hjorther, Nielsen, & Segest, 1990), providing respite for families in crises that might otherwise result in placing a child out of the home (Valentine & Andreas, 1984), helping homeless people establish living places (Rivlin & Imbimbo, 1989), and providing fluoridated public drinking water (Easley, 1990).

Concrete assistance has a checkered history in the helping professions. It was thought of as a form of charity and brotherly love and thus divinely sanctioned (Boswell, 1988). But it was also viewed as a danger that would create dependency on gifts rather than on working to support oneself and family. Even in current times, there is a dilemma about the source of support, from funds to which workers contribute over their career—a kind of social insurance—or general tax funds for people for whatever cause—a kind of general welfare relief. The United States has chosen a split-level system of social welfare, including both insurance and welfare, but this has been applied unevenly throughout the 50 states, each of which has the right to determine its level of, and eligibility criteria for, welfare benefits. (See Simon, 1988, for a critical analysis of this approach.)

There is also a fundamental dilemma between those who see the welfare system as residual, merely a backup for temporary problems when ordinary market forces and family systems are disrupted, and those who see it as a social utility. As such, it is seen as an intrinsic part of a complex society that cooperatively provides public education, universal health insurance, and the like as a basic right, without stigma, enabling all members of society to a fair start in becoming productive contributors to that society (Dryfoos, 1988, 1994; Wilensky & Lebeaux, 1965).

As people in primary prevention consider providing concrete assistance, it is necessary to be mindful of these public debates. Some concrete assistance to people with identified needs (such as emergency food and shelter) is readily supported, but usually on a temporary basis. Even able-bodied persons are provided assistance during periods when they are unable to work or work is unavailable to them, but these, too, are limited on the grounds that people should be able to get well and find new jobs. Current efforts to provide job skills training, day care, transportation, and the like reflect advanced thinking on the provision of welfare that addresses reality factors if people are to be enabled to help themselves. These reality factors are best seen within a configural perspective that considers the various pushes and pulls regarding any one action.

The tentative principles regarding concrete assistance can be summed up in this fashion:

1. Supply needed basic resources that people cannot obtain through their own efforts because of their stage of development (i.e., young children or elderly nonworkers) or social context factors (such as industrywide unemployment or personal disability). This is a humanitarian action that also serves future needs of society (Ozawa, 1986, argues that providing health, education, and welfare aids to poor minority children now will be more than paid back when they become productive workers).

2. Embed this action with as much dignity and respect for the strengths of the persons and groups involved as possible by providing paths by which they (or members of their extended family or group) can become

self-sufficient. This may require some very broad changes—see the discussion of prevention of prejudice and discrimination (Chapter 3, II.C.6)—as well as some very specific ones.

3. Recognize that the individual has to contribute to the extent possible to his or her own welfare so as to maintain dignity and self-esteem, but the "extent possible" requires careful analysis and possibly training. (Consider the communal barter system described in Chapter 6, V.A.3.) The individual's unique limitations likewise must be considered with regard to the "extent possible."

4. Recognize that a range of social support systems may be activated in providing natural aid (from primary groups) or constructed aid (from secondary groups). The cultural meaning of aid from either sector is important and should be weighed in terms of planning preventive or promotive programs (see Aoki, Ngin, Mo, & Ja, 1989; Cochran, 1989; Mays, 1989; Tafoya, 1989). Likewise, recognize the limitations of social supports and the various social pressures that may be placed in opposition to attaining client goals.

The welfare debate of the mid-1990s revolves around the issue of federal versus state or local selection of services to be funded within the larger context of an enormous national debt and growing world competition. Because primary prevention tends to be long term and indirect, it is particularly vulnerable in legislative assemblies focusing on immediate and direct services. Yet its philosophy of encouraging "teaching a person how to fish" rather than simply giving him or her a fish fits in well with the changing zeitgeist, if prevention professionals can only communicate their views clearly and strongly.

5. Recognize the range of effects the physical environment and historic time frame have on the current situation. Some may favor one or disfavor another type of preventive or promotive action. For example, women who killed abusive spouses years ago languish in prisons for murder, whereas recent changes in public understanding of spousal abuse make a defensive plea more acceptable. Physical access to services is a prerequisite to preventive or promotive services and has to be factored into the helping equation.

These last few principles are a rewording of the configural equation as applied to concrete assistance.

D. Aspects Involving the Sociocultural Context

1. Institutions as Vehicles of Primary Prevention

With this section, I begin exploration of the macrosocial dimensions of primary prevention. In particular, I consider institutions and organizations within the state and the community through which primary prevention is expressed. First, some distinctions. The term *institution* refers to a system of social practices that represents a societal solution to an enduring and common social concern. Five major societal institutions are commonly described: economic institutions to produce and distribute goods and services; political institutions to regulate the use of power and resources within the society; kinship institutions related to marriage and the family; social institutions that serve health, education, and welfare functions; and cultural institutions dealing with scientific, artistic, and religious concerns. All of these societal institutions have preventive or promotive implications.

Within any of these societal institutions are a number of specific organizations (which, unfortunately, may use the word *institution* but really mean a particular instance of that societal form). For example, schools are one instance of social educational institution, whereas adult education classes at a social agency are another.

Because institutions and their particular organizational forms are so pervasive, one tends to forget their persistent tasks until called on to deal with a preventive or promotive concern. Most primary prevention activities are predicated on adequate economic, political (as in equal opportunities and civil rights), kinship, social, and cultural arrangements (Bower, 1972). Unless people have some reasonable source of an adequate income; political rights and civil liberties; a stable and satisfying family relationship; adequate health, education, and welfare as needed; and access to cultural expression and enjoyment, any special service that preventers propose to offer has little meaning.

Yet in many instances in the United States, the assumption of adequacy in these basic institutional forms is not valid. Americans still exhibit many forms of discrimination; unequal access to health, education, and economic opportunities; and maldistribution of power. What is the proportion of women or minorities in the country at large and in the United

III. The Third Dimension

States Senate? Who serves on the boards (let alone in the factories) of the *Fortune* 500 businesses?

Primary prevention programs have to consider both specific service plans and basic institutional coverage (Caplan, 1993; Masterpasqua, & Swift, 1984; Pearson, 1981). Although it is usually impossible for a particular program to supply core health, educational, and economic opportunities, it may be possible to advocate for the adequate delivery of these services at large, which would also benefit the particular group affected by the prevention project (Wilensky & Lebeaux, 1965).

Davidson and Redner (1988) offer an example of institutional (organizational) change on behalf of a primary prevention objective. Preventing juvenile delinquency has proved to be a difficult and illusive goal (Burchard & Burchard, 1987). Diversion programs appear to offer some encouragement as a way of dealing with this complex problem. In the Davidson and Redner project, adolescents were identified between the time when they were apprehended by a police officer and their formal adjudication by the courts. This decision was made for conceptual reasons—to minimize the effects of negative labeling, which is thought to increase self-perception as a delinquent, while at the same time addressing high-risk individuals rather than assuming some broad category of predelinquent.

In the first of a series of projects, Davidson and Redner (1988) used college students to work with these adolescents for reasons of cost (nonprofessionals are far cheaper than professionals) and effectiveness of nonprofessionals (Berman & Norton, 1985; Durlak, 1979). The students received 6 weeks of training and ongoing supervision. They met with their charges, formed behavioral contracts with these youngsters, and served as child advocates to find community resources to facilitate their normal (and legal) development. Finding the first project successful in terms of recidivism rates over a 2-year period, these investigators conducted another phase of studies in which several organizational factors were varied to identify the active ingredients of the successful outcomes. I will take liberties in interpreting their study for purposes of emphasizing institutional factors.

One preventive condition involved use of a family model dealing with a family-focused behavioral program; another involved a helping relationship with a paraprofessional (the trained college student)—I term this a *social agency approach*; a third involved a legal model wherein services were delivered directly through a juvenile court setting; and the fourth condition involved a "nonspecific attention group" that the authors describe as like a natural helping network—student workers were trained briefly and only to use their natural helping skills—I call this a *friendship approach* because no professional skills are involved.

Davidson and Redner (1988) varied the organizational structure in dealing with youths diverted from legal jeopardy. The results from the second study showed that overall, in the 2-year follow-up, recidivism in the experimental groups was lower than recidivism in the control group (which received regular handling by the juvenile court). There were important internal variations, however: There was no difference in outcome among the group receiving the first study intervention (termed *action approach*) and the family or the social agency approaches. These three were superior to the friendship approach, the treatment approach delivered in the court setting, and the traditional juvenile court approach. Thus unstructured attention was not as effective as systematic efforts to reduce delinquency rates.

Davidson and Redner (1988) continued with new studies of the type of service agent and later with replication in a larger urban area. For our purposes, it is sufficient to focus on their contributions in the first two studies. The authors were able to vary organizational structures and relationships to discover which ones were more effective in achieving the goals of the project. These organizational manipulations required a great deal of effort and cooperation on the part of all system players, but given the common goal of discovering a better way to prevent juvenile delinquency, Davidson and Redner were able to make these changes. That several organizational forms produced similar results should not surprise us; there are many ways of arriving at any goal. One can ask further questions about the relative costs and effectiveness of these approaches to make future decisions in a cost-conscious but concerned society.

What practice principles can be extracted from this exemplary project? I suggest the following:

1. Select any predictable problem or promotable goal and one is likely to find it embedded in one or a combination of institutions (organizations) that currently are assigned to serve these concerns. If current service is not as adequate as one would wish, then consider a primary prevention program in which organizational changes are proposed in an orderly way.

III. The Third Dimension

2. Any changes proposed in the established way of doing things will likely meet with stiff resistance—after all, today's bureaucracies were yesterday's creative solutions and staff see little reason to eliminate their jobs. Organizational change might best be couched in terms of developments of existing structures, not replacements for them. Davidson and Redner (1988) speak of walking a tightrope between successful innovation and threats to existing organizational structures. There were problems with referrals to the experimental program and other problems in cooperation, but with skill and perseverance, the research project succeeded.

3. Consider program development in terms of how any of the organizational services might be delivered in a more effective and humane manner to prevent a predictable problem or to promote a desired goal. Assuming that every enduring human concern has economic, political, familial, social, and cultural aspects, consider specific programs within each of these for their probability of success.

4. Keep the cost-effectiveness consideration in mind always. This requires having control groups against which to compare experimental groups, with sufficient details of both the effectiveness issue (such as rates of recidivism) and cost considerations. In effect this means asking how much social gain can be purchased for a unit of cost. This provides powerful information for decision makers on future service programs.

5. Programmatic studies provide the opportunity to use results in redesigning the new project. Each phase should advance a specific question or questions, clarifying the limits of one organizational change and then applying this new knowledge to the next organizational change. Research and program development go hand in hand.

Other examples of institutional change include Allen (1986) on migrant workers' situations, Berlin (1990) on the role of the community mental health center in preventing disorders in children, Davidson et al. (1994) on a neighborhood injury prevention program in Harlem, Dryfoos (1994) on schools that serve health and welfare functions along with education, Fox et al. (1987) on promotion of safety in open-pit mines, Pransky (1986) on making changes in state laws, Warner and Murt (1985) on direct and indirect economic incentives promoting health, and Williams (1986) on improving care in nursing homes using community advocacy, to mention a few.

2. Symbol Systems

The phrase "symbol system" can be used to represent any system of ideas and beliefs, including cultures and subcultures, religions, and philosophical orientations. In each case, people generate a set of symbols, usually over a long period of time, that helps provide shared meaning to members of the group. Individuals are born into that group (or move into that group) and learn these shared meanings in terms of preferred goals and acceptable means of action regarding the world as it is understood in that culture.

Symbol systems are relevant to primary prevention for several reasons. Helping professionals must be sensitive to the culture, religion, or other belief systems of participants in projects. Table 4.1 summarizes some points about cultural sensitivity.

Symbol systems may set limits on primary prevention programs. For example, the Catholic Church and other religious groups have taken a stand against the use of artificial birth control methods. Any primary prevention project involving contraceptive planning will have to take into consideration this opposition to change the point of view, to neutralize it (in a political and social sense) so that it won't have any harmful affect on the preventive program, or to live with the opposition.

A classic way to address such value conflicts is to seek a higher order value that is shared, when this is possible. For example, regarding the tactics of pro-life supporters in connection with abortion clinics, it may not be possible to change their value position, but it is possible to encourage them to obey the laws of the land rather than risk fines or imprisonment for unlawful actions toward clinic patients and staff. Another example is when the Catholic Church supported universal health coverage legislation but did not support the provision of abortion services. A dilemma emerged in having to choose whether to support the whole legislative act (including the elective abortion provision) or risk losing the battle to get universal health care coverage. (For a discussion of the constructive role of religion in primary prevention, see Levin & Vanderpool, 1991; Payne, Bergin, Bielema, & Jenkins, 1991.)

Mays and Cochran (1987) describe the special concerns that black Americans infected with AIDS have because of cultural and psychosocial factors. They point out that the black community generally views AIDS as a "gay disease" (or a "gay white disease"), although in fact blacks are

Table 4.1 Culturally Sensitive Primary Prevention Practice

Steps in the Problem-Solving Sequence	Sensitivity Considerations
Step 1: Identify the problems and strengths of client and situation.	1. Begin where the client is in his or her personal, social, and cultural context, as this may affect the client's problems and strengths. 2. Use bilingual or bicultural workers or others experienced with the cultures involved. 3. Use accessible locations and appropriate methods of communication, maintaining client dignity at all times. Use surnames and other culturally appropriate forms of address. 4. Admit one's own cultural limitations, when necessary, in asking for help in knowing how to help the client.
Step 2: Identify alternative theories of behavior, and empirical and practice options.	1. Recognize that any theory must be modified by cultural considerations, as when young female workers may not be accepted as authorities by older male clients. Be prepared to adapt (e.g., having an indigenous older male as aid to the professional). 2. Clients may have folk theories about their problems and roles that have to be integrated with modern scientific methods as far as possible.
Step 3: Identify short- and long-term goals as part of decision making	1. Help clients formulate goals in terms of the multiple cultures in which they live. Accept client goals, unless laws and good practice dictate otherwise. Be careful of one's own biases. 2. Work to empower the powerless by developing personal skills needed to perform valued social roles. Also facilitate others in similar circumstances to join together in seeking their rights.
Step 4: Implement and concurrently evaluate the process and outcome of the preventive action.	1. Work with client's strengths, available social support groups, and physical environmental resources, rather than trying to remediate deficits and limitations only. 2. Show respect for clients at all times and do not use techniques that blame the victim. However, do not ignore clients' contributions to the problems. Understand them through a historical, social, and cultural analysis of the present situation. 3. Treat all clients with strict equality; have high standards of service for all.
Step 5: Maintain cost-effective elements after termination.	1. Compare client's current state with goals that include cultural contexts. No new problems should emerge when the initial problem has been handled. 2. Compare the overall costs to agency, client, and society, with overall benefits to same. Leave the client with a sense of self-competence and sociocultural supports to deal with new issues.

NOTE: See also Brown (1981), Devore and Schlesinger (1987), Green (1982), and Lum (1986).

disproportionately represented among AIDS victims. The largest percentage of AIDS cases among blacks does involve homosexual or bisexual males (about 39%), whereas heterosexual IV drug users are a close second (about 35%; Mays & Cochran, 1987, p. 381). The black community in general holds strong homophobic attitudes and strong ties of family solidarity. When black AIDS victims experience rejection by their families, they may be more severely affected than white AIDS victims, because whites tend to have access to a greater variety of other supporting groups. Furthermore, because of their negative experiences with the health care system in general, black AIDS victims tend to seek care later, when they are more seriously ill; they also may be misdiagnosed for cultural and communication reasons unrelated to their medical condition. However, black AIDS patients may demonstrate a strong fighting spirit, honed after years of surviving in a racist society, that may help them survive physically and psychologically. Mays and Cochran seek a fuller cultural understanding of black AIDS victims as a path toward better service for this group. Similar propositions may well be offered for every subcultural group (see Beiser, 1982; Coates, 1990; Cohen & Adler, 1986; De La Rosa, 1988; Fuentes & LeCapitaine, 1990; Mays, Albee, & Schneider, 1989).

Beyond setting boundaries, symbol systems may also provide positive opportunities for primary prevention projects. By bringing in culture to support the thrust of a preventive or promotive program, one draws on collective strengths, group pride, and the weight of tradition to underwrite a healthful action. One embeds the program in a context of accepted meaning (Keeler & Swift, 1982).

Johnson (1988) and his colleagues combined all these points in an exemplary program, the Houston Parent-Child Development Center, designed to be sensitive to Mexican-American culture. The center developed methods of preventing behavior problems in young children living in poverty and minority contexts. During the first year, the program was conducted in the homes of participants and included fathers as well as mothers and children. (The reason for this home-based phase is that Mexican-Americans are culturally unlikely to participate in a public program with people who are not immediate relatives.) Home visitors were women from the barrios who were trained to deliver lessons. Verbal instruction was conducted in Spanish over long periods of contact (about 550 hours over a 2-year period). Mothers were instructed in infant development and how caretaking influences that development. Some family workshops were held on weekends (to optimize attendance by fathers and other family members). After a year, activities took place at the center 4 mornings a week, with sessions conducted in a bilingual format. Mexican materials were used whenever possible to encourage ethnic pride and to promote positive self-esteem among participants.

Results from studies of this program are encouraging, both at the program conclusion and 5 to 8 years later. Parents, both mothers and fathers, became involved with the program and have fought for funding every year for the past 17 years (see also Fuentes & LeCapitaine, 1990; May & Hymbaugh, 1989; Zimmerman & Rappaport, 1988).

These examples suggest that symbol systems can be sensitively and effectively used in primary prevention projects. One must understand intimately the cultural group itself, both its strengths and its limitations, vis-à-vis the target of the prevention program. One must recognize the dual existence of members of subcultural groups within their own culture as well as within the dominant culture. This creates pressures and opportunities for primary prevention that careful planning might use to good advantage.

Allen (1986) provides some cultural practice principles in services to migrant farm workers. Stemming from a long history of setting up alternative cultures when a given situation placed people in high risk of psychological or social problems, Allen's project addressed the ecological system of stresses that followed Albee's formula (reproduced in Chapter 1 of this book). My summary of this work will emphasize the practice principles involving culture change (Allen, 1986, pp. 94-96) and a systematic strategy for implementing cultural change (Allen, 1986, pp. 94-101).

1. Culture change principles include the following:
   a. Involve all the people in decisions affecting them.
   b. Adopt non-blame-placing approaches and mutually beneficial solutions for both parties involved.
   c. Clarify both the immediate objectives and the long-term goals so that every change effort can have a clear focus.
   d. Show the connection between individual enhancement and organizational success; one cannot attain one without the other.
   e. Custom tailor any changes to all the local cultures involved.
   f. Focus on multilevel change strategies (i.e., consider all aspects of the configuration as used in this book), because changes at one point will

affect all the other configural components. Changes have to be personally fulfilling as well as organizationally desirable.

g. Develop a positive outlook and create a sense of community, that is, a shared fate in which the positive efforts of each party contribute to the well-being of all others.

2. Organizational change may be facilitated by a four-step process:

a. Analyze the existing culture and set objectives. If we use the migrant farm workers as an example, the wages for these workers were very low, turnover was very high, there were no toilet facilities in the fields, and workers were suffering from chronic health problems. The immediate objectives included doubling income and productivity in 18 months and upgrading substandard housing, among others.

b. Enter the cultural systems and gain commitment of all parties to seek alternative ways of attaining mutually related goals (e.g., income and productivity). What norms need to be changed to facilitate these goals?

c. Modify the existing cultural system, from the work of individuals to teams, levels of organization, and ultimately the whole system. In the migrant worker project, year-round employment opportunities were constructed, sanitation was improved, and fringe benefits were initiated (the first in the history of this industry; Allen, 1986, p. 103). Worker productivity increased at the same time.

d. Sustain the desired culture: I call this *institutionalizing* a successful project. In the migrant workers example, sustaining of the desired objective was initiated by weekly work team meetings to monitor the changes in productivity and income, as well as changes in housing and sanitation. These information and evaluation sessions were refined and continued over 5 years, reflecting major changes: "Annual worker income had quadrupled and turnover had reduced drastically. Instead of migrant camps, an 85-home model community had been developed" (Allen, 1986, p. 104) with social service programs, a library, and a homeowners association.

This example illustrates the not-well-understood point that preventive or promotive changes in cultural forces and social structures may be attained, resulting in important social benefits (see also Albee et al., 1988; Orlandi, 1986).

3. Mass Media

Mass media as a tool for primary prevention is coming of age. It has passed through the dark night of being ignored and left to antiprevention forces (see Davis, 1987, and Erickson et al., 1990, on trends in cigarette advertising and marketing). It has passed through the early days of excessive enthusiasm and naivete when it was thought that a short burst of scientific fact would be enough to get any right-thinking person to make fundamental changes in his or her behavior toward more healthful actions, the results of which would likely appear in a distant future. When early promotive campaigns failed to produce results, a cloud of pessimism arose in its wake (DeJong & Winsten, 1990) along with calls for more expertise in combining public health education and mass media. This collaboration has produced a number of successful health promotion campaigns (Abbott, 1992; Arkin, 1990; Flay, 1987; Freimuth, Hammond, & Stein, 1988; Katcher, 1987; Jason et al., 1989; Maccoby & Altman, 1988; Van Parijs, 1986).

In this section, I highlight the main principles emerging from successful public health campaigns as described by DeJong and Winsten (1990, 1992). These authors note that commercial advertising is largely intended to give direction to existing interests, whereas public health campaigns generally seek fundamental changes in lifestyles that affect health and healthy functioning. Of course, public health campaigns also reinforce the people who are already performing healthy behaviors and may help fine-tune the behaviors as well.

Fundamental change generally requires a long, often slow process of education, although some "crisis conversions" do occur—as when a peer dies of a disease caused by a behavior we, too, perform. However, this educational process is best conveyed as an issue of ongoing public concern that incorporates the "consumer" orientation of commercial marketing and the scientific knowledge regarding behavior change. DeJong and Winsten (1990, p. 32; 1992, p. 257) report six key elements in successful mass media campaigns:

1. Specify a well-defined target audience, differentiated according to geographic, demographic, psychological, and other relevant characteristics. This involves qualitative research to analyze various subgroups by demographic, psychological, or problem-relevant characteristics (Sherman & Reid, 1994).

2. Use formative research to understand the target audience and retest campaign materials. For example, a substance use campaign aimed at preteens would focus on delaying or postponing experimentation with

substances, whereas a campaign directed toward adolescents would address age-relevant tasks such as prevention of impaired driving. With regard to AIDS prevention through effective condom use, the mass media messages must counter the condom's negative image—such as reducing physical sensation and spontaneity—and replace it with a positive one—prolonging sexual contact and adding variety to foreplay.

3. Use mass media messages that build from the audience's current knowledge and satisfy its preexisting needs and motives. For instance, with preteens and adolescents it probably is more effective to convey the immediate effects of tobacco use—discoloration of teeth, body and mouth odor, and deterioration of physical performance—than long-term effects. Likewise, recent studies showing an association between smoking and impotence may influence the behavior of men who are unmoved by more distant risks such as death from heart attacks (*ASH Smoking and Health Review,* 1995). (See Jason et al., 1986, on self-help groups.)

4. Use messages that satisfy the audience's preexisting needs and motives, especially those not related to health per se and that can be gratified within a short time (DeJong & Winsten, 1992; cf. May & Hymbaugh's, 1989, campaign to promote Native American pride in health as part of a campaign to help pregnant women avoid alcohol and to educate them about its effect on the fetus).

5. Use a media plan to guarantee exposure of target-appropriate materials to the campaign. DeJong and Winsten (1992) remind us of the complexity of attitude change (discussed in Chapter 2, I.B.1); each step of the campaign needs to be checked for the appropriateness and effectiveness of the materials and methods of presentation. Each media has its own strengths and limitations (such as costs, contact time with audience, and types of audiences).

6. Use procedures for evaluating progress. This is a challenging task for any primary prevention program, but especially one that is delivered to a mass audience over public channels (see Maccoby & Altman, 1988, and the description of their projects given later in this section; Jason et al., 1986.)

7. Make a long-term commitment. The age of primary prevention in the mass media has just begun. Van Parijs (1986) presents an international perspective on public education in cancer prevention and notes four basic types of ongoing education programs:

a. Increasing the public's awareness of the problem, particularly as related to lifestyle behaviors causally related to the problem

b. Changing specific risk behaviors, such as education on the reasons for stopping smoking

c. Educating with regard to self-examination skills, such as breast self-examinations and testicular self-examinations

d. Promoting early detection of the problem so as to have an increased chance of effective treatment

These programs will take a lot of time, and prevention professionals have to be there over the long haul to sustain them. Because mental health professionals may be unfamiliar with these details of using the mass media, there is need for collaboration between the professions. DeJong and Winsten (1992) add other suggestions to enhance the effectiveness of these campaigns.

8. Recruit volunteers and program participants through the media and cement contact with local advocacy groups.

9. Produce self-help materials and make them available through media information. For example, liquid crystal thermometers for testing the tap water temperature at one's home were made available over mass media, and people could either call a number to receive a free thermometer or send in a request when mailing a check for the water bill (Katcher, 1987); the availability of support groups can also be announced through the media (Jason, Crawford, & Gruder, 1989), including the information superhighway.

10. Promote hot lines through mass media to permit person-to-person contacts, wherein general information may be individualized to some degree. With regard to sensitive content, such as direct discussion of condoms in a society where mass media is loath to offend sizable minorities who believe promoting condoms will lead to promiscuity, mass media often speak in vague terminology—"protection" and "bodily fluids." This makes the offer of a hot line and personal contact all the more valuable.

11. Help create and then inform the public of changes in public policy and social norms (see Coates, 1990, on notifying the gay community in San Francisco about the AIDS epidemic and ways to protect themselves and partners from it).

12. Become increasingly sophisticated in the use of effective commercial public relations strategies such as high-visibility news coverage,

securing "product placement" (or removal—such as not showing actors drinking and driving) in films and on TV, sponsoring sports and cultural events, and publishing targeted "lifestyle" magazines. (See Cherry & Redmond, 1994, on a social marketing approach conducted with recent immigrants from Afghan, an ordinarily abstemious Muslim group, in the face of an alcohol-saturated culture.)

As an example of these principles, DeJong and Winsten (1992) describe the Harvard Alcohol Project, a research-based mass media (advertising and public relations) campaign conducted in collaboration with the television industry. The goal of this project was to encourage the use of designated drivers (such as are legally required in Scandinavian countries) and to promote a fundamental shift in American social norms regarding driving after drinking. The three major television networks (ABC, CBS, and NBC), 15 Hollywood studios, and leading advertising agencies participated in the project to introduce dialogue into scripts to reinforce the emerging social norm that the driver does not drink. Research showed that high percentages of adults had seen public service messages and that there was a sharp increase in the reported use of designated drivers.

A benchmark of studies in using mass media for primary prevention is the Stanford Heart Disease Prevention Program, which involved the work of many researchers, including Nathan Maccoby and John Farquhar and their colleagues (Altman, Flora, Fortmann, & Farquhar, 1987; Farquhar, 1978; Farquhar et al., 1985; Fortmann, Williams, Haskell, Hulley, & Farquhar, 1981; Killen et al., 1988; Maccoby & Altman, 1988; Maccoby, Farquhar, Wood, & Alexander, 1977). This influential series of studies has reshaped the way we conceptualize primary prevention, and thus requires careful study.

Cardiovascular diseases (CVDs) have long been the major cause of death in America, even though predictors involving lifestyle and personal characteristics have been long known. The question has been how to convey this information to the public in a way they will accept and use. Given the scale of the problem, mass education through the mass media was an obvious consideration, but at the time (early 1970s), there was uncertainty on how to deliver the messages. With the use of social learning theory and models of attitude change, social marketing of "the right product backed by the right promotion in the right place at the right price," and diffusion of information, the Stanford Heart Disease Prevention Program (SHDPP) was undertaken. This project hypothesized that community health

III. The Third Dimension

education would be the most effective way to change health-related behaviors and the environmental contexts influencing those behaviors (see also the health education approach by Pless & Arsenault, 1987).

The first study was the Stanford Three Community Study, implemented from 1972 to 1975. Three comparable small towns in Northern California were selected and randomly assigned to one of three experimental conditions:

1. Health education through mass media
2. The same health education through mass media, augmented by face-to-face instruction for two thirds of a high-risk group
3. A control (receiving only national media exposure, as did the other two experimental towns)

These towns were relatively isolated from each other as far as common mass media were concerned (Maccoby & Altman, 1988).

Over the course of the 2-year project, surveys and some medical examinations were conducted among the 35- to 59-year-old residents of these three towns. A media campaign showered the experimental communities with specific behavioral information on how to reduce risk of CVD in English and Spanish, using television, bus cards, newspaper advertisements, billboards, pamphlets, booklets, and radio. The campaign ran for 9 months in 1 year, stopped for a follow-up survey, and then ran for another 9 months in the next year.

Results suggest that the health status in a community could be improved by an educational program delivered through mass media, especially when augmented with interpersonal contacts in natural settings (Maccoby & Altman, 1988). These findings led to the development of the Stanford Five City Project, beginning in 1978 and continuing into the 1990s. These five communities are much larger than the initial three towns; the health education programs are aimed at benefiting the entire population of these cities (while monitoring the 12- to 74-year-old range), and the educational program is more extensive, running 6 to 8 years rather than 3. There are also three comparison cities rather than one.

The hypotheses of the Five City Project include seeking a lasting reduction in the prevalence of CVD risk factors in the general population and a corresponding decline in CVD morbidity and mortality in the two education cities compared with the three comparison cities.

Maccoby and Altman (1988) describe three goals of the educational program:

1. To increase knowledge and skills of relevant parties so that CVD morbidity and mortality are reduced
2. To help generate a self-sustaining health promotion structure embedded within the existing organizational network: "The point is that community interventionists should plan carefully for their eventual departure from communities by promoting empowerment of community organizations and leaders and by relinquishing control over program design and implementation" (Maccoby & Altman, 1988, p. 171)
3. To derive a model for cost-effective community health promotion from these community studies.

Interim results suggest that the first goal is being attained; the other goals require more time for completion.

The SHDPP group is already considering the next generation of studies as part of the newly formed Stanford Center for Research in Disease Prevention. The initial project, funded by the Kaiser Family Foundation, is to establish a Health Promotion Resource Center for the 13 western states and, later, for the entire country. Maccoby and Altman (1988) describe the goals of this project:

> To encourage the development of innovative health promotion programs and materials, encourage the use of existing and effective materials and programs (e.g., promote replication), and tailor existing programs and materials that are effective or hold promise to the unique needs of individuals, organizations, and communities. Through processes of innovation, replication, and adaptation, the technology of community-based health promotion and disease prevention can reach its full potential. (p. 172)

See also successful programs by Freudenberg and Golub (1987), Hawkins et al. (1991), Pentz et al. (1989), Pless and Arsenault (1987), Puska et al. (1987), and Stunkard et al. (1985).

Mass media have been used in a number of primary prevention programs with less than successful results. Richardson, Reinhard, Rosenthal, Hayes, and Silver (1987) report that a large proportion of smokers are still unaware of the risks of smoking after 11 years of health warning messages on cigarette packages. Weiner, Morse, and Garrido (1989) note that mass media campaigns directed toward pregnant women drinkers have appeared to reduce drinking among moderate drinkers but not among heavy drinkers. Phillips and Carstenson (1986) note the increase in teenage suicides following television news reports about suicides. Gerbert and Maguire (1989) report on the public acceptance of the surgeon general's brochure on AIDS that was sent to every household in the United States in the summer of 1988. Only 59% of the nationwide telephone sample of 2,000 adults remembered receiving it; of these, 68% read most of it, whereas 20% read half or less. The most disturbing finding was that young people and blacks, two groups disproportionately represented among AIDS victims, were less likely to remember receiving the brochure. Enthusiasms about mass media must be tempered with caution and careful planning.

III. The Third Dimension

5

METHODS OF PRIMARY PREVENTION

Dimension IV. Decreasing Social Stresses

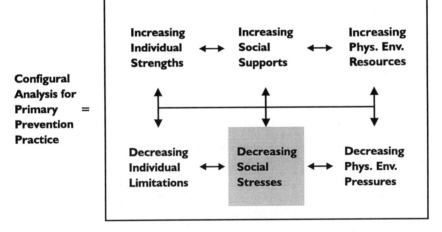

Figure 5.1. The Configural Equation

This chapter continues to address the social context of primary prevention practices concentrating on decreasing the omnipresent social stresses of everyday life. As in Chapter 4, four major types of social contexts are considered—the interpersonal, primary groups, secondary groups, and sociocultural contexts.

Dimension IV. Decreasing Social Stresses
    A. Interpersonal Aspects
        1. Aid From Peers

A. Interpersonal Aspects

1. *Aid From Peers*

The interpersonal approach to decreasing social stresses may involve two-person groups of peers, such as same-age chums, friends, or partners (including spouses and close work buddies). As Simmel (1950) points out, dyads are the simplest of groups but also the most fragile. They may be a source of great support against stress, but they may also cause great stress because of the intense feelings and intimacy that may emerge between peers in a context of shared values, secrets, and common ventures.

Natural dyads formed in the course of human events, such as chums, friends, or marital partners, are generally characterized by diffuse relationships; in principle, either party could take a leading or following position or both can share in all roles. This means that the stress-reducing function may go in either or both directions.

Constructed dyads are formed by third parties for specific purposes and usually involve identified ranges of interpersonal activities. Generally, the stress-reducing function goes in one direction (from helper to helpee), even though there may be some benefits for the helper as well. I will discuss the natural and constructed groups separately.

IV. The Fourth Dimension

Natural Peer Dyads

Natural dyads abound. They are one of the great sources of human pleasure—and pain. Leaving the painful side to novelists and pop song writers, I will focus on the pleasurable function of dyads related to reducing social stresses. Although "sticks and stones" (hand guns and the like) do break bones, "names" (name calling, insults, prejudices, denigration, and many other subtle forms) also hurt and may lead to sticks and stones being used. One must be concerned with the social, interpersonal, institutional, or symbolic forms of hurt as one inquires about ways that other social forms may reduce or prevent their harm.

Many of the topics discussed previously in ways social groups increase social supports are repeated here because of the close connection that exists between social help and social harm. I will also point out some unique social forms for reducing social stress.

Sibling relationships, confidants, and special friends constitute the largest sources of peer support for decreasing social stresses, as discussed in Chapter 4 (III.A.2 & 3). The particular issue for this chapter is how to promote this stress-reducing function of these relationships because these social supports do not inevitably emerge. I will not directly address how a family should promote positive sibling relationships or how individuals should locate best friends. Rather, I will assume that cooperative living in an atmosphere of kindness, reciprocity, and well-deserved trust enable such personal relationships to emerge (Bahr, 1988; Gordon, 1970; Guerney, 1988). The specific issue is how to make these social bonds that are assumed to exist work to reduce stress.

The distinctive nature of social stress is that the recipient has to be aware of the existence of the social-symbolic events and be acculturated into accepting them as a force that requires psychological and physical action to change. If one is not aware that some acquaintances are calling one names, or if one does not care about being called these names by these people, then there is no effect of the name calling.

Sometimes social stress is combined with physical problems, as in the case of victims of AIDS. Because of the often social nature of the disease, I predict a new social role will emerge, that of designated friend who attempts to initiate and maintain safe contexts and safety procedures during times of high-risk activity (such as anal intercourse or sharing needles among groups of drug users). The very fact that people are learning how to communicate with partners about sexual history and the immediate sexual experience means that a peer role is being formulated. Labeling such a role would make introducing sensitive discussions around safer sex and cleaner needles more readily performed: "Hey, who's going to be the designated friend in this relationship?" (Bandura, 1989b, 1994; DiClemente & Peterson, 1994; Kirby & DiClemente, 1994, p. 131; see also Padian, van de Wijgert, & O'Brien, 1994, on their couples counseling where one partner was HIV-infected, and Mata & Jorques, 1989, on needle sharing among Mexican Americans).

Natural peer relationships may be used to decrease social stresses through the following principles:

1. Because intimate peer support has been strongly associated with positive mental and physical health, the general directive is to cultivate these friendships (Gordon, 1970; Guerney, 1988; Roppel & Jacobs, 1988).

2. Friends, confidants, siblings, and other close personal peers may psychologically (as well as physically) help an at-risk person respond so as to reduce social stresses. Active listening (Chapter 3, II.E.4) informs the stressed party that another trusted and supportive person understands his or her problem and feelings. Sharing may make the burden more bearable but it may also introduce new ideas from the other on how to resolve the challenge or handle the feelings. Friends may refer the at-risk person to helping professionals if and when the need arises.

3. Active friendliness may be useful to inform the victim that he or she has support in this portion of his or her social world even if stress exists in another portion. To engage in active friendship, one should think about one's friendship and talk about it with friends, as appropriate: directly—"I love you," "This (the present mutual activity) has been great," "Thanks, you're a great friend,"—or indirectly—by means of a handshake, a hug, a smile.

4. Not only should one think and talk about active friendliness, one should engage in any appropriate activities that increase the at-risk individual's strengths (Chapter 2), reduce that individual's limitations (Chapter 3), increase other social supports for that person (Chapter 4), and make such changes in the physical environment as might be helpful (Chapter 6).

Constructed Peer Dyads

It is possible to construct peer relationships, even for limited periods of time, so as to promote healthy outcomes. Sosa et al. (1980), working in Central America, created a peer situation involving a doula, or untrained midwife, previously unknown to an expectant mother (presumably one who lacks other natural support systems). The doula stays in constant attendance to the mother-to-be from admission to the hospital through delivery, providing comfort, conversation, and friendly companionship during this crisis time. Results from this experimental-control group design showed favorable outcomes when the doula was employed compared with when she was not. The implications for a constructed role of this type are many—in children's hospitals when youngsters are undergoing routine operations, in schools with transfer students who get a buddy to show them the ropes, or in institutions with new or transferred persons who benefit from learning the informal culture (Felner & Adan, 1988; Felner et al., 1994).

Another role of ancient origins, the home aide, involves one person who provides certain types of help to another individual who requires that help so as to be able to maintain ordinary living conditions. Nielsen et al. (1972) describe a project in which home aides were assigned to frail elderly persons leaving a hospital after receiving needed medical treatment. The home-aide service enabled these discharged patients to remain in their own homes, rather than go to nursing homes. Even though they often required assistance in the activities of daily living, the elderly people were still in command of their lives by giving directions or involving family members to act on their behalf.

Widow-to-widow programs (Silverman, 1988) are discussed in Chapter 4; they represent another constructed dyad seeking to reduce stress and promote healthy roles for the recently widowed. The notion of constructed dyads serving to model stress reduction and growth promotion has many implications, particularly with life transitions, from the newly married, new parents, relocated neighbors to recently divorced persons and their children. Even international pen pals may be viewed as constructed dyads that seek to promote a richer understanding of different cultures and societies through personal contacts. Constructed dyadic relationships as strategies for primary prevention need further exploration in new social domains.

2. Aid From Nonpeers

Another aspect of interpersonal helping to reduce social stress comes from the variety of across-age friendship systems, such as parent and child, teacher and pupil, or master and apprentice. Although these relationships may have many other features, they clearly involve a dyadic relationship within various contexts. Sometimes people have natural and socioculturally sanctioned responsibilities to one another, such as parents to children and, later, children to parents. I refer to these as *natural nonpeer ties*. In contrast, other nonpeer relationships may be *constructed* in a contractual sense, regarding what behaviors each will perform vis-à-vis the other, such as in Big Brother or Big Sister relationships. The closeness of both types of relationships provides great opportunities for development but, unfortunately, also possibilities of exploitation and inappropriate behavior.

Natural Nonpeer Dyads

There are many examples of naturally emerging nonpeer dyads that reduce social stress for one (or both) parties. Parents are forever seeking to smooth life's way for their children, not so much as to eliminate stress as to introduce it gradually over the years so that children learn the necessary arts of resolving ordinary life challenges. Clearly, the methods parents naturally use (or are trained to use in family-life education programs, such as Parent Effectiveness Training; Gordon, 1970) to teach their children problem-solving and coping skills (Clabby & Elias, 1986; Shure & Spivak, 1988) are relevant here, particularly when minority children, who will have to face oppression in the larger society, are involved (Alvy, 1988).

A great deal of learning goes on without much public awareness when older siblings teach or model behaviors for younger siblings. Ample data suggest the untoward transfer of attitudes and actions, such as when younger siblings copy substance-using behaviors from older brothers and sisters. But there is also the likelihood of positive transfers that are largely unexploited by primary prevention. Like peer tutoring, nonpeer modeling conveys both information and values. The possibilities of what college-age youth could tell (model for) their younger siblings (and other youngsters) about life and love, truth and consequences, and great expectations and realistic opportunities are intriguing possibilities for primary prevention. Just as with peer tutors, certain incentives could be arranged for conveying information between people sharing natural relationships.

Constructed Nonpeer Dyads

It is also possible to construct meaningful relationships between persons of different ages. Some community programs have enlisted "heroes" to present preventive or promotive messages to their "fans." Enlisting local athletes or pop musicians and scientists or successful business people to promote a cause could provide effective role-modeling as well as open up possible futures for younger children. Off-season volunteer services for national athletes is another unexplored avenue for promoting health causes.

Another example of nonpeer dyadic relationships that can be used in primary prevention is the Big Brother/Big Sister approach, which matches a same-sex adult with a child in need; the adult provides guidance, resources, and encouragement that the child might not get in other ways. Edmondson, Holman, and Morrell (1984) report a research study of such a relationship between "surrogate parental role models" and 50 boys age 9 through 12. These authors found that high percentages of youths and their mothers felt the need for frequent individual interactions between the boys and adult men, even though most of the youngsters belonged to organizations where they had group contact with men. On the basis of these data, a Big Brother/Big Sister program was initiated; a second study was performed on the 116 active matches. Positive changes were noted in the children by both parents and volunteer Big Brothers or Big Sisters. Frequency of contacts was positively related to perceived behavior changes—measures included the child's self-worth, behavior at home, and relationships with friends. School attendance or behavior did not show significant changes. (The authors recommend contact at least once a week as the minimal frequency.) There were no differences reported in effectiveness in age, student status, or marital status of the volunteers. This was an exploratory study; long-term data are lacking. The Cambridge-Somerville study conducted at the beginning of World War II provided longitudinal data that suggest that experimental youths having Big Brother/Big Sister-like contacts did not do better as citizens than the controls in terms of police records and the like (McCord, 1978), so the status of this form of stress reduction (and the corresponding support promotion) is not clear.

Rosenberg et al. (1992) present information about a street outreach project on drug abuse and sequelae that has documented success in reducing risk behavior of drug users and their sex partners. Street outreach workers (whom I am assuming are somewhat older than the drug users) live in the area where their would-be clients live; through repeated face-to-face contacts, they establish some degree of trust. They counsel drug users to deal with their drug problems (which is treatment), but also to use condoms and to clean needles with bleach (which represents primary prevention for predictable problems for these drug users).

Culturally sensitive practice raises questions about how helpful adults can be with adolescents if these adults differ in various ways from their students. Jemmott and Jemmott (1994) conducted a study in HIV-risk reduction with African American youths and concluded that the same levels of reductions were reached regardless of the race and gender of the adult, the gender of the youth, and whether or not mixed groups were used to convey this information.

I offer the following principles derived from this literature:

1. The critical factor in providing preventive or promotive services in nonpeer relationships is the high level of sustained goodwill and energy on the part of the helper toward the helpee. Few other characteristics of the helper appear to be significant.

2. The provision of these kinds of services require time, both a concentrated time of getting together on one occasion and the continuity of contacts over a long period of time. This is relatively easy for family members living together, but it is a challenge for nonrelated adults. Time allocation can be facilitated by creating a routine: "Saturday, 8:30 a.m. Meet 'little brother' at the playground as usual. Lunch at the salad bar at 11:30."

3. Nonpeer relationships require the nurturing of communication skills so as to transmit information, both factual and socioemotional. Much of the learning will be by modeling, but the helper must develop active listening skills (Bloom, 1990) as well. Communication of significant information requires a level of trust that is earned over time and place.

B. Primary Group Aspects

1. The Buffering Function

Primary groups may be very important in primary prevention as mechanisms to decrease social stress, even though these same groups may generate some stresses as well. Buffering implies that a person or group—or sometimes the caretaker of such a person or group—is under stress and that the help of the primary group is directed toward reducing that stress. For example, a couple of neighbors may bring over a lunch to a family moving onto the block. This welcoming party recognizes the common phenomenon of moving-day stress and attempts to offer informational aid—the names of good plumbers and electricians and the like—and emotional support—"I remember how difficult it was when I moved in 10 years ago, but it will soon be over"—as well as food. In general, when a primary group seeks to help a party currently under stress, this is called the *stress-buffering effects of the group* (Bogat et al., 1993; Cohen & Wills, 1985).

In contrast, let's say that a person is going about her ordinary life routines without any particular problems or stresses when a group of friends invites her to join them at a community center that is having a demonstration of square dancing. A primary group (the friends) seeks to enhance a person's state of healthy functioning by a new experience (the dance demonstration); it is not a correction of a weakness or illness. In general, when a primary group seeks to help a healthy, well-functioning party, this is called a *main effect of social support* (Bogat et al., 1993; Cohen & Wills, 1985). This main or direct effect may also involve information, emotional support, or concrete assistance.

There is a technical controversy about whether personal well-being is related to social support whenever that support is provided or only when the party is under stress. The evidence is mixed and is compromised by methodological problems (Bogat et al., 1993; Cohen & Wills, 1985). Until the many factors in this discussion can be resolved, it seems most useful to primary prevention to assume that social support facilitates well-being in both contexts, but especially when the receiving party is well functioning (Maton, 1989a; Okun et al., 1988).

Cohen and Wills (1985) review the well-established positive correlation between social support and well-being, such as the 9- to 12-year prospective studies in the Alameda County samples by Berkman and Syme (1979), which showed that social support is related to mortality. (See also Cassel, 1976, who was one of the first to point to the buffering effects of strong social support, and an early review of the literature on social support by Heller & Swindle, 1983; Auslander, 1988; and Clinton & Larner, 1988.) The helping support may enter a person's life any place (or in several places) from when a stress is recognized—and the person is still healthy—to the onset of the effects of that stress—when the problem emerges full-blown and the time for primary prevention has passed. The support itself may be informational, emotional, or concrete (as in provision of physical assistance, money, gifts, and the like).

Let's look at some instances of the buffering functions of primary groups. A stressed worker comes home to his family and is received with love and attention—and diversions. The worker may be fed, entertained with news of the family, and informed about events of interest to the family. None of these, per se, removes the work-related stresses, but the stresses may be put aside or put into perspective by feeling a part of another social system (the family). The family is not organized specifically to be a buffer to the world of work, but it naturally functions this way—although the worker could as well come home to no meal, conflict in the family, and a pile of bills, which would add to the stresses of the work day. (See the entire issue of the *Journal of Primary Prevention*, 1994, on prevention in the workplace, and especially Felner et al., 1994. See also Vinokur & Caplan, 1987.)

The coaching staff of a college athletic team may be a primary group to the team members and yet may be organized to act as buffers to the pressures the athletes face. A member of the coaching staff may be assigned to teach game skills, while another may be assigned to do preventive bandaging, soothe intrateam squabbles, prepare for psychological highs or lows after the "big game," advise on talking with "scouts," and so forth—all of which involve buffering various kinds of stresses.

Stolberg and his colleagues have designed support groups for children of divorce (Stolberg & Garrison, 1985) that distinguish various features of the buffering effects of primary groups. This takes place at a time when adults are less available to help their children given the stresses they themselves are experiencing. First, the children's groups provide emotional support, with the recognition that the members share a common problem. Second, they provide information about what is likely to happen. Third, these groups offer cognitive and behavioral skill training to deal with feelings and events in the divorcing families. In these ways, a support group is created that research has shown to be effective in helping children deal with the stresses of their divorcing families (Bloom & Hodges, 1988).

In general, the following principles seem applicable to the buffering functions of primary groups:

1. Even in a relatively small group without the clear divisions of labor characteristic of larger groups, some individuals perform a buffering function, which involves awareness of the stresses that are placed on members of the group, possibly themselves included. This awareness emerges because of the emotional closeness of the group members and is one of the strengths of the primary group.

2. Buffering involves naming the stress and assessing its implications for the parties involved. Preventive buffering also involves naming the strengths of the group and its environmental contexts. Another characteristic of primary groups is members' closeness to the stressful situation and their ability to be aware of early signs of stress, when members are still functioning effectively.

3. Close sharing of experiences means that early signs of stress can be discussed as common to all members. At the same time, group supports can be exhibited. These supports include bringing out factual information, sharing of emotional stresses, and developing alternative plans of action. With all these, it is likely that a group can generate more ideas than any member can alone.

2. The Promotive Function

In a recent review of 54 social group work research studies, Tolman and Molidor (1994) present data indicating that more than one quarter (28%) were focused on prevention topics, such as teaching children social skills, preventing unwanted teenage pregnancy, teaching parenting skills, and addressing needs of the elderly. Thus social group work has been used in the service of primary prevention across the life course. In this section, I want to illustrate the role of groups to promote stress reduction. Clearly, in training people in social skills, sexual control skills, parenting skills, and the like, people are indirectly aided in reducing the stresses that emerge in the course of these interpersonal behaviors. I would like to focus specifically on group-promoted stress-reduction procedures, recognizing that these inevitably will be blended with other helping activities.

Flowers, Miller, Smith, and Booraem (1994) present a study of single-session groups to promote safe-sex behavior in male at-risk populations. A total of 771 gay and bisexual men voluntarily participated in 117 discussion groups that ran 3 1/2 to 4 hours in length. Trained leaders led these single-session groups over an 18-month period in California. A

IV. The Fourth Dimension

pre- and posttest design was used, augmented by a 3-month follow up. Flowers et al. were able to document that, between pretest and posttest, participants significantly gained in knowledge of AIDS-related problems, in positive attitudes toward the possibility of controlling the spread of HIV infection, and, most important, in safe-sex behavior. These men volunteered for these discussions because HIV infection raises great anxiety within the context of high-risk behaviors. I interpret this study as a promotive effort using the group modality to address stress by providing knowledge, attitudes, and skills to promote behaviors that reduce that stress.

Flowers et al. (1994) showed similar significant results in the 3-month follow-up. Some of these follow-up data included questionnaire results from the primary partner of the participant of the group session. That a large proportion of (unserved) partners cooperated in the research also suggests the power of the stress that high-risk behaviors generate.

A 30-hour leadership training program was employed, along with a supervised apprenticeship program of 8 to 24 hours following a clearly formated psychoeducational model. Clear objectives were identified and measured using the AIDS Prevention Test developed by Flowers et al. (1994). The outline of the discussion group included background and objectives of the STOP AIDS project, the effect of AIDS on each participant's life, methods for engaging in safe sex, HIV antibody testing, community reactions to the AIDS epidemic, and various personal actions in ending the AIDS epidemic. It appears to be possible to convey important and intimate knowledge, attitudes, and behavior change information in a single-session format to relatively large numbers of persons in group settings.

As Moncher and Schinke (1994) note, with the present constriction of funds (for various mental health activities), it seems likely that group intervention as a preventive modality will be the norm for many years. Likewise, the stresses of AIDS will be with us for years to come, suggesting that the use of groups may be a powerful modality in the primary prevention of AIDS.

Other researchers are trying to tease out the contributions that different components make to the overall effectiveness of group training. For example, Magen and Rose (1994) studied parent training groups with regard to the contribution that general problem-solving skills training versus behavioral skills training makes to changes in parental behaviors and attitudes and, consequently, parental interactions with their (aggressive) children. Compared with a waiting-list control group, both the problem-solving training unit and the behavioral skills training unit were found to be significantly effective, but the behavioral skills training was more effective than problem solving alone.

In general, it appears that the group modality is highly versatile as to content and is necessary in the delivery of certain practices, including behavioral rehearsal, skills modeling, brainstorming, observing normative behavior in other members of a group—especially peer groups as they become increasingly important in the lives of adolescents—and the exercise of group sanctions of deviant members (Moncher & Schinke, 1994). I discuss many of these specific practices (behavioral rehearsal, modeling, and communication skills) in other chapters of this book.

C. Secondary Group Aspects

1. Social Action

Stress can be common to many people, as in the situation of racial or gender-based discrimination. Social action projects are often undertaken to reduce the level and type of stress people experience. These projects can be as "simple" as creating flexible work schedules to enable working parents to be with their children (Winett, Leckliter, Chinn, Stahl, & Love, 1985; indirect effects can also be garnered, such as employees working on the flexible schedule driving in nonrush hours, which also reduces the numbers of people driving at peak times). Or they can be as "complex" as actions affecting a whole community, as in the following example.

Galt, a small rural town (population about 5200) in California, was the site of a project seeking to decrease the mental health stresses on various populations at risk and to promote community harmony (Pilisuk, Parks, Kelly, & Turner, 1982). At the time of the project (the early 1980s), there were increasing needs for social services and declining revenue to support them. A project was developed (and funded at a modest level of $70,000 for 2 years) that sought to connect the existing natural helping network with the mental health system in the community. The connection was very sensitive to the nature of this community, where there was a rapid increase in the Mexican American population along with some 250 mentally or developmentally disabled people in local shelters and a proportionately large number of elderly and under-19 population.

The task of the project staff was to identify and gain the cooperation of formal and informal community leaders in community-wide self-help activities. An umbrella group of recognized community leaders helped shape problem-solving forums open to the whole community, which led to the articulation of the concerns of various special groups. These discussions also led to the forming of priorities among these various concerns. Pilisuk et al. suggest that these forums led to the development of a sense of community, a sense that the residents had a stake in the affairs of their town in part because they came to believe that they could influence events (Pilisuk et al., 1982, p. 122; Pilisuk & Parks, 1986; Simon, 1994; Wandersman, 1984).

At the same time, contact was made with informal leaders—"natural community helpers" (Pilisuk et al., 1982, p. 123)—who, without any formal human service role, were consistent providers of assistance to others in the community. Their view of the needs of the community was different from that of the formal leaders. Volunteers were solicited who could provide any kind of help. A *Blue Book* was developed whereby volunteers and people in need could be matched up. No fees were charged, but those helped were expected to volunteer in for whatever services they could provide for someone else. Thus the concept of reciprocity was encouraged in the helping process (Douglas & Jason, 1986, on baby-sitting exchanges; Peterman, 1981, on urban self-help groups).

A variety of other helping arrangements emerged, some of which were successful—such as a community celebration related to the town's growing Latino population—and others that were not—such as use of a "natural helping team" to discuss a person's problems publicly so as to improve communications among helpers. (One interpretation of this failure might be that it reflected the helping professionals' intrusion into sensitive turf of people in need of help who live in a small town and do not want to advertise that they needed help. The helping team concept may have met the needs of the staff of the project more than the needs of the people in the community.)

The proof of the success of these various programs was that they were institutionalized so as to ensure the continuation of their work after the conclusion of the project itself. Such institutionalization (or the taking over of an experimental program to become an established part of the existing helping institutions) should be a goal of every primary prevention program. The cultural celebration (Cinco de Mayo) was particularly important in promoting a sense of community among the previously disaffected minority.

Beyond short-term social action projects like the one described by Pilisuk et al. (1982) are long-term social institutions that have been designed (at least in part) to provide primary prevention services. For example, the community mental health center (CMHC), as a broad concept, was intended to help prevent disorders in people living in the community; because of social conditions such as deinstitutionalization, CMHCs rapidly became involved in treating large number of adults who were seriously psychiatrically disturbed. Berlin (1990) reviews the history of the CMHC in connection with the prevention of infant, child, and adolescent disorders. The Chicago Woodlawn studies (Kellam & Wert- hamer-Larsson, 1986; Schiff & Kellam, 1967) worked with local schools and parent-teacher associations to identify children at risk (and their families) as well as children with potential. With the former, they aided the children to get to school and to master content; with the latter, they helped bright children recognize their self-worth. Most important, this project existed in the local community for many years as a stable addition to institutional supports (see also Comer, 1988; Cowen, Hightower, Johnson, Sarno, & Weissberg, 1989; Cromer & Burns, 1982; Dryfoos, 1994; Porter, 1983).

Stark (1992) describes a social empowerment project in Munich that is based in part on the World Health Organization's health promotion model, the Healthy Cities Project. This is a kind of grassroots and city government cooperation project in which the resources for a healthy future are identified by consumers and ways are found to attain those goals. Helping professionals must learn how to ask questions, not give answers, in enabling people in the community to decrease social stresses and optimize human potential (Rothman, 1979).

The practice principles that appear to underlie these programs include the following:

1. Workers must know the local situation thoroughly from the per- spective of residents, not as outsiders. Part of the process of empowerment involves a community defining for itself the priority concerns for the optimal development of its citizens. This process and the collective

feelings that emerge from it establish a sense of community that is a vital ingredient for persisting empowerment (Wandersman, 1984).

2. Workers must connect potential helpers with those who need help and locate needed resources through which the help can be delivered. In some cases, it may be possible to enable the helpees to become other types of helpers, so that people help each other, each in his or her own way. This kind of exchange system holds enormous potential for primary prevention in many contexts in times of limited funds. (I call attention to the history of the settlement house movement and self-help groups in particular, as decreases in the public welfare system call for adaptive changes in the private sector.) In other cases, resources may be required from government and the private sector to obtain and to sustain a system of helping.

3. As Simon (1994) notes, empowerment involves shaping programs to the expressed ideas and needs of the community members. These programs should be maximally convenient for, and accessible to, these community members.

4. Simon (1994) urges that professional helpers "ask as much from one's clients as from oneself." I interpret this to mean to set high standards for community members and helpers and work toward providing the scarce resources to meet these goals. Build on the strengths of persons, groups, and environments while dealing with their limitations.

5. Simon (1994) cautions workers seeking to facilitate social and community action to be patient because empowerment may take a long time and considerable effort from everyone involved and may generate some determined resistance as well.

6. As workers make their contributions to citizens involved in community action, they need to monitor the process as well as evaluate the outcome. Indeed, this may be one of the distinctive contributions of the helping professional. These kinds of evaluations provide useful feedback for the community members on how they are doing and where they need to devote more time and effort. Workers should be cautious of wanting the action to succeed so strongly that they lose their scientific perspective that can provide the kinds of information that more partisan members may not be able to see. Progress may be slow and there may be setbacks. Interested readers should pursue this complex topic in such works as Bond, Belenky, Weinstock, and Monsey (1992), Kellam and Werthamer-Larsson (1986), Kelly (1988), Porter (1983), and Simon (1994).

2. Social Institutions

By definition, social institutions are created to solve persisting collective problems. For example, schools are established to teach youngsters the massive amounts of formal (and informal) knowledge and skills they will need when they take their places in society. Every so often, though, we need to rethink the nature of these institutional solutions because the nature and scope of problems change, making yesterday's deft innovation tomorrow's unwieldy instrument.

We are in such a crisis time today, when fundamental changes in the American family crash against economic realities, collide into changes in sexual mores and hedonic lifestyles, and career wildly because of the loss of social control. The social landscape is strewn with the "new morbidities" (Dryfoos, 1994, p. 2)—the victims of unprotected sex, drugs, violence, and depression—in contrast with the old morbidities of malnutrition, chronic diseases, and personal hygiene problems. Dryfoos describes the massive poverty in 1991 in stark numbers, with "more than fourteen million children—22 percent of all children—(living) in families below the poverty line. . . . And those children living in mother-only households have become the most deprived of all, with more than 55 percent living in poverty" (p. 2).

Yet out of this dismal social scene, some very important ideas and experiments offer some hope to reclaim society and its future. Dryfoos (1994) suggests the term *full-service schools* as an institutional innovation that may meet the new situation. Full-service schools bring together education, health, mental health, and various welfare services that may be needed in a given locale. The following is an abbreviated version of Dryfoos's idealized full-service school, where everything that might be needed in a particular community is available under one roof, the product of collaboration among many separate agencies:

- Quality education provided by the schools through effective basic skills, individualized instruction, team teaching, cooperative learning, parental involvement, and effective discipline
- Support services provided by community agencies through health, mental health, and dental services; individual counseling, substance abuse treatment, family planning, and family welfare services; housing and food services; recreation; cultural activity; mentoring; job training; and child care

IV. The Fourth Dimension

- Combined training provided by schools and community agencies through health promotion, social skills training, and comprehensive health education

These services provided at the little red schoolhouse sound beyond belief, but Dryfoos provides a broad sampling of schools in settings around the United States that have taken some of these items and adapted them to their local situations. For example, in Washington Heights, New York, a "settlement house in a school" was created for a poor ethnic neighborhood (Hispanic), in part because of the cooperation between the school system and the Children's Aid Society, a nonprofit organization. By a set of fortuitous circumstances, this community was given the opportunity to design a new institution with "education as its centerpiece" (Dryfoos, 1994, p. 107) in combination with health, employment, housing, welfare, and cultural aspects.

The building opens at 7:00 a.m. and runs its various programs until 10:30 p.m., including weekends and during the summer. In the morning, there is a Latin band and recreation, along with breakfast served to about 8% of the student body. Classes during the weekday run alongside the family resource center, where people can get help with public assistance, employment, housing, immigration, crisis intervention, drug prevention, and adult education, served by social workers, paraprofessionals, and volunteers (Dryfoos, 1994). A small number of parent volunteers are on a stipend program learning to become dental assistants, secretaries, and the like. A health and mental health clinic is next to the family resource center and offers a wide range of services, from dealing with minor injuries and illnesses to the provision of primary care for the children (backed up by a community medical clinic). An after-school program offers tutoring and other activities. One adult education program is particularly interesting: teaching Spanish to local police; the "teachers" are students and parents. This is a remarkably different kind of institution that offers its constituents a wide array of services to meet the needs of a new generation. It offers an opportunity to influence change in the community itself, for instance, in police-neighborhood relations.

This full-service school fits well with the model proposed by Zigler and Styfco (1993) for a "comprehensive, integrated, community-based system of family support and child development services located in public school buildings" (quoted in Dryfoos, 1994, p. 58).

Dryfoos's (1994) book is filled with examples of specific innovations carried out in schools around the United States. In each case, a local community is attempting to understand the unique set of stresses facing its children and their families and to make structural changes in the community schools and helping agencies to accommodate these needs. Schools as local institutions are particularly flexible instruments of experimental change, even though one must "do one's homework" thoroughly in making proposals to local boards of education.

Dryfoos (1994) provides ample experiences with some encouraging empirical evidence: "Scattered evidence suggests that school-based clinics have had an effect on delaying the initiation of intercourse, upgrading the quality of contraceptive use, and lowering pregnancy rates, but only in programs that offer comprehensive family planning services" (p. 135).

Other institutions are emerging that are shaped to meet particular needs, such as the hospice, which provides palliative care to the terminally ill and psychosocial services to their survivors (which may be considered a form of primary prevention against a known risk; Clark, 1993). Another phenomenon that may be considered a social institution addressing the needs of groups under stress is the traveling institution, such as mobile library buses bringing educational and recreational materials to distant rural areas and to persons with restricted mobility. Likewise, mobile health and dental clinics deliver screening services to local neighborhoods in rural areas. Access can be facilitated by storefront agencies, neighborhood branch offices of social services, and special meetings with legislators on tour of their districts.

It is possible to take institutional solutions to persisting social problems and make creative adaptations to fit the needs of consumers with the goal of decreasing social stresses and increasing social supports. It is difficult, however, to list a set of principles to achieve complex social system goals, but let me offer the following tentative ideas:

1. Community needs assessment: The professional worker must understand the complex nature of the social situation, both the manifest problems and the strengths it presents. A community comprises many smaller units, including schools, churches, businesses, recreational settings, and governmental units. All of these, one way or another, are involved in the problems and the potentials. Epidemiological information is helpful in making sense of complex data sets, whereas community informants and commentators put flesh on the bare bones of statistics. Just as Pilisuk et al. (1982) began with a community needs assessment,

so every complex project must begin with an orderly understanding of existing conditions, including perceived needs and strengths of all the groups involved.

2. Ideas on goals and objectives: Second only to knowing where the community currently is, is knowing where one would like the community ideally to be. This is a collective musing, where ideas from all constituencies must be melded together and prioritized. The melding together is especially important because a solution to one objective may also be a partial solution for another—or it may raise problems in other contexts. If teens need to have jobs and the elderly need services, is there any way these two community tasks could be creatively combined? Combining known situations may lead to unknown ones, as when the elderly may also need part-time employment, which might be connected to telephone assurance systems for persons needing regular, ongoing monitoring for safety purposes (like latchkey children, handicapped persons, or the retarded). In short, systemic thinking involves interrelated needs and solutions; the glue connecting these is creative thought and imagining how two or more social facts can be connected in constructive ways.

3. Social institutions carry out routinized assignments, which tend to resist change. Every institution has decision makers who can be made sensitive to the changing conditions of the consumers of their services. This requires an organized group to present facts and objectives to meet the perceived preventive or promotive needs. The presentation of new ideas requires considerable planning and fact finding as well as knowing the structure of the decision-making group and its members. Organized assertiveness may be a way of describing how presentation of facts and objectives may best be delivered (Chapter 2, I.E.2). A worker must work through the hierarchical system of the community bureaucracy, presenting information required, applying pressures as needed, all the time assembling a constituency speaking in favor of the preventive or promotive objective (see also Pransky, 1986).

3. Ombudsman Programs

The ombudsman role was originally developed in 19th-century Scandinavia to protect the political rights of individual citizens; the concept has been reintroduced for various purposes in the 20th-century social welfare field. I am concerned here with its preventive, protective, and promotive functions in decreasing stressful situations before they produce psychological disruption and in seeking desired goals, particularly in institutional situations. Wolkon and Moriwaki (1973) describe an ombudsman on a radio station who received letters seeking help. These requests were mainly seeking ways to deal with public or private bureaucracies at legislative or administrative levels that affected the help seekers psychologically. Wolkon and Moriwaki view the ombudsman as attempting to alleviate some reality-based problems so as to help people cope with the hassles of everyday bureaucratic life.

Radio ombudsman services do not allow opportunities for research follow-up. There probably is some satisfaction for the help seeker simply in having an individual offer (free and disinterested) advice in a seemingly heartless world. In any case, similar ombudsman programs have grown in other institutions, schools, large corporations, and government. Affirmative action officers, in-house review boards regarding allegations of sexual harassment, patients' rights representatives (Ziegenfuss, Charette, & Guenin, 1984), networkers (Morris & Frisman, 1987), child advocates (Matsushima, 1990), community information and referral centers, and telephone hot lines are modern-day extensions of the ombudsman idea. To some extent, Ann Landers-type newspaper columns serve a related function on issues of social mores and psychological stresses.

Cherry (1991) presents a study of ombudsmen in the context of nursing home care. He compares ombudsmen with organized volunteer programs. He distinguishes the leverage or watchdog function of ombudsmen with the stimulation function of volunteers and then studies the differential effect of these functions on quality of nursing care in intermediate and skilled care facilities, using concrete measures of care such as presence of decubitus ulcers. The results were complicated by the level of functioning of the residents, who were more or less able to use the services of ombudsmen or volunteers; generally speaking, nursing homes with ombudsmen present showed "less poor care" than homes without these watchdogs present.

Other writers in the gerontological field note the varied outcomes of ombudsmen in nursing home contexts. Sometimes ombudsmen are able to make extensive and constructive changes (Williams, 1986), whereas at other times, confrontational approaches lead to stymied relations with administrators (Barney, 1987). Litwin (1985) proposes that ombudsmen take a stronger stand at the state levels and be more conciliatory at the

IV. The Fourth Dimension

local levels (Cherry, 1991, p. 307; Monk & Kaye, 1982; Netting & Hinds, 1984; Wilson, 1982).

In general, it seems worthwhile to explore the possibilities of an ombudsmen program in a variety of social contexts, partly as a protective device for civil and human rights and partly as a quality control device. Establishing an ombudsmen program requires either a law (as in the case of the 1987 amendment to the 1982 Older Americans Act), government support (as in the case of a national model on preventing drug abuse among students; Kim, 1983), or agreement among parties in a setting (like the radio ombudsmen whose credentials are the force of exposure to public opinion). An ombudsman program provides a degree of flexibility to the bureaucratic structure of modern society that will probably ensure its continuation in many forms. By way of summary, let me offer the following guidelines for ombudsman programs:

1. Identify the institutional context in which an ombudsman program will be placed. What laws or administrative rules are necessary to construct such a program and to relate it organizationally to the rest of the system?

2. Identify the level and range of authority the ombudsman will have within the organization. How much of what powers must the ombudsman have to perform this function in accordance with the ideals leading to its formation? If the minimal amount of power is not present, then it may not be worth setting up this program. What kinds of access, to whom, and on what scheduled or unscheduled basis are critical elements for ombudsmen?

3. Identify the educational task of informing staff and clients about the services and functions of the ombudsman. This is not a familiar role and staff may be resistive to unwanted oversight, whereas clients, especially minorities, may not trust a guardian angel of an institution that heretofore has not been accommodating.

4. Identify procedures for performing the ombudsman role so that all parties involved are clear as to the extent and limits of this service. Make clear that the ombudsman function also protects staff against unwarranted accusations, even though its chief function is to represent the powerless client in an institutional context.

5. Make private efforts to correct problematic situations or to explore enhancing situations, but be prepared to make public reports as a way of reinforcing constructive behavior or changing destructive services.

IV. The Fourth Dimension

4. Information and Referral Systems

One of the major problems in the modern world is the complexity of everyday life. Finding one's way through this social maze is difficult enough under ordinary conditions, but in times of stress or crisis, it becomes very difficult indeed. Yet if information were available, people might be able to head off problems they foresee before the problems overwhelm them. (For various approaches on theory or research guiding practice, see Lorion et al., 1987; Manger, Hawkins, Haggerty, & Catalano, 1992.)

Let me begin by discussing one of the largest information systems in the United States, the Public Health Service, and one of its organizational units, the Centers for Disease Control (CDC). In 1986, the CDC was assigned the lead responsibility for informing and educating the American public about AIDS and HIV. The CDC National AIDS Clearinghouse (NAC) was established, along with the National AIDS Hotline. The NAC had to avoid duplicating a number of other existing bibliographic databases—MEDLINE (the National Library of Medicine), AIDSLINE, and several others. (The volume of information available is enormous and there is a growing electronic linkage among them.) Thus NAC focused on AIDS services and resources and on hard-to-find literature and unpublished reports so as to complement these other databases.

The National AIDS Hotline (NAH) represents another major dimension of information and referral services (Waller & Lisella, 1991). Hot lines in general, especially NAH, have several distinctive characteristics: Callers may remain anonymous, which gives them the liberty and the control to discuss personal and risky matters, and they may call for information at all hours of the day or night, locally or long distance—the NAH, for example, maintains toll-free numbers, including an English-speaking service (1-800-342-2437), one for Spanish speakers (1-800-344-7432), and one for hearing-impaired callers (1-800-243-7889). Because they are speaking privately, responders can converse with the caller with sensitivity and concern.

This does not necessarily mean that the information provided has helped people. Indeed, the research on the effectiveness of hot lines is mixed. Shaffer et al. (1988) review the literature on preventing teenage suicide and report studies with a positive, negative, or no relationship between the presence of crisis centers and the reduction of suicide rates. Miller, Coombs, Leeper, and Barton (1984) suggest a small but significant reduction in suicide rates among young white women, the most frequent users of such services. Yet King (1977) notes that a third of the men and a fifth of the women in a study of telephone counseling reported that the advice given by the hot line made their problems worse. So although hot lines appear to be popular, there is a question about their usefulness.

Information lines take many forms. A county agent receives calls about how people might protect their crops, trees, and flowers from future cycles of pests. Reference librarians enable users to locate needed materials. There are many types of local hot lines related to suicide, substance abuse, poisons, and the like. Here are some examples of frequently called federal information numbers:

AIDS Hot Line: 800-342-AIDS
Auto Safety Hot Line: 800-424-9393
Boating Safety Hot Line: 800-368-5647
Cancer Information Center: 800-253-3496
Energy Conservation Referral Service: 800-523-2929
Fair Housing: 800-424-8590
Firearms Hot Line: 800-ATF-GUNS
Internal Revenue Service: 800-829-1040
Meat and Poultry Safety Hot Line: 800-535-4555
Pesticides Safety Hot Line: 800-858-PEST
Product Safety Hot Line: 800-638-CPSC
Safe Drinking Water Hot Line: 800-426-4791
Social Security Administration: 800-772-1213
Veterans Affairs: 800-827-1000

In addition, the blue pages of the local telephone book should list the 800 numbers of federal senators and members of Congress. These blue pages should also list various offices of the state government, such as the department on aging, child abuse emergency, and a child support hot line.

Another variation of a national information and referral system is a citizens advice bureau (CAB), a system of nationwide offices offering a "window" into the community through person-to-person contacts to aid citizens in finding needed resources or advising them of their rights and responsibilities. Information flows in both directions, however, so that CABs help society to identify social needs and gaps in services. This system originated in England but has spread to other countries. In New Zealand, for example, adaptations have been made to develop mobile bureaus, toll-free numbers, and units in rural areas, prisons, and ethnic minority communities. On a local level, Fawcett et al. (1982) describe the development of an information-referral system in connection with social service agencies in a community. A social services directory was constructed— 154 different services offered by the 62 local agencies, each service entered on a separate Rolodex file card, making the service accessible to each agency, which then had access to knowledge of all the services provided in the community. Periodic updates were easily made.

Coyne (1991) assesses the usage of a statewide toll-free "help line" by adult children of elderly persons with dementia. The categories of information requested primarily deal with information about in-home services and adult day care resources, along with a wide variety of nursing, respite care, legal issues, and like issues (see also Goodman, 1990).

The technology for setting up a hot line is relatively easy, although considerable advertising and training of personnel are required to provide a useful service (Waller & Lisella, 1991). Once in place, the hot line must be maintained, as people come to depend on it as an ongoing source of information.

An important variation of the hot line is the warm line, or perhaps warm-and-friendly line, such as the many kinds of telephone assurance systems that emerge in natural helping networks: "Just calling to find out how you are doing. Need anything?" In countless settings, adult children call aging parents, friends call one another, neighbors make spontaneous calls to neighbors, for whom such a call is like a ray of sunshine: "Just calling to find out how you are doing and if there is anything I can do to be of assistance." Knowing that someone is on the lookout for one provides a reassurance that is a priceless part of being in a primary group. It can head off preventable problems as well as provide aid to those in need.

The notion of a cool line is quite different. Rather than a person calling a professional for information or advice on a topic, the cool line envisions that a helping professional makes a call to a person identified by other sources as needing help, indicating that someone suggested that this person might need some information or advice on dealing with a specific set of stresses. For example, a school nurse or social worker might call the parent or guardian of a child for which there is some question about a need for clothing, food, or sleep. An employee assistance program may operate on the tips provided by fellow employees, who may be aware of on-the-job problems due to at-home concerns.

Another more complicated instance is the situation in which the caller is part of a court-designed control system to delay jailing or detention of a youth at the beginning of a court process. This situation operates on the hypothesis that institutionalization might exacerbate a minor difficulty into a major problem. A citizen volunteer is assigned by officers of the court to call a youth on home detention at random unannounced times to ensure that the youth is obeying instructions to be at home or another known place. The calls are friendly conversations, but the subtext is control. The youth benefits from not being jailed and the community gains both financially—volunteers are cheap—and socially—from the humane treatment of a youth at the beginning of a slippery slope.

A more extreme example is a call to a person who has been talking to friends about a contemplated fight or drive-by shooting or perhaps a planned theft. Obviously, this kind of call to "cool down" someone requires a tip-off from an insider, a person concerned for the safety and well-being of the potential wrong-doer, let alone concern for the potential victims. A cool line (cool-off line) may be subject to prank calls, but it might also pick up some instances of planned violence. The professional makes the proactive call, stating that he or she is from the city cool line office (a well-publicized number that the youth could call back to confirm as an official call) with regard to an anonymous tip that the person being called had committed no crime or offense but was known to be consider-ing some antisocial act. The professional does not know whether this information is correct, but the call is being made to express public concern with this information and to offer assistance to work out problems between conflicting parties or in other ways to express concern for the action that might cause harm to people in the community. The individual being called is thus warned away from that antisocial action and from retribution to persons suspected of calling in the tip. If this individual is not in fact considering any antisocial action, then this first call is one of friendly concern by an official agency of the city. A second call will be made in a few days unless the youth calls the professional himself or herself before that time (so as to confirm that this is an official call). There are many problems with this concept, including invasion of a person's privacy and the likelihood of some false tips. But as a proactive approach to violence, this idea may be worth exploring further.

D. Approaches Involving Sociocultural Contexts

1. The Insurance Principle: Minimizing Individual Loss Through Collective Risk Sharing

The principle behind most types of insurance is as simple as it is ancient: Each person regularly contributes a small amount to a collective fund so that whoever succumbs to the insured hazard (e.g., loss of work, illness) will receive some degree of support as needed. All members of the insured group presumably obtain peace of mind knowing that should they succumb to the hazard, they will be cushioned against the sequelae of that hazard. That is, even though they may suffer from a debilitating illness, they will not starve or go homeless because they cannot get income from their ordinary job. The insurance may also support treatment of that illness. There is a hidden assumption in this principle that the insuring body will have the resources to provide for one—even if one is part of a large group of insured persons who make large claims all at once for a common disaster (see Ginzburg et al., 1993, for related problems).

There is a positive and a negative form of this principle: There is the negative hazards insurance, as described above; but there is also a positive form, such as a group of persons who contribute small sums of money to a common purse so as to accumulate capital in amounts far greater than any one individual could. With this money, the group invests in some enterprise for its collective benefit. Miller (1977) describes such a venture among members of a poor black church group. Church members contributed $10 per month over a 36-month period and enabled the church to invest in business concerns that brought employment and services to the community when there was little likelihood of receiving capital for investment through traditional sources. This principle seems to have many useful variations (see Hraba's, 1979, discussion of the Chinese version of this group accumulation of funds for investment by individuals on a rotating basis). This raising of members of an oppressed group by lifting itself up by its own bootstraps is a classic story of cultural empowerment.

IV. The Fourth Dimension

There are many forms of insurance, from putting small amounts aside each payday in a savings account to betting on horses. At the societal level, there are various kinds of insurance: Human capital expenditures were to be the main thrust of the 1960s War on Poverty, but the war was not funded at the level thought necessary. Such expenditures are lotterylike investments in positive expectations: By training people who otherwise would not likely be able to get a good job, we not only help those individuals but add future tax collections from their expected higher salaries and we are less likely to have to pay for other costs of social failure (e.g., welfare, mental or physical illness, or imprisonment; Bloom, 1990; Ozawa, 1986; Schweinhart & Weikart, 1988).

Either form of the collective principle involves an organization acting as agents who receive some percentage of the profits. Insurance companies have to balance predicted income against predicted expenses (insurance payments of various types). Actuarial tables are essential in making these predictions. Changing events mean that actuarial tables have to be updated continually. Insurance companies plan for small and large contingencies, but they generally cannot plan completely for "the big ones," the once-in-100-years giant flood or earthquake. In those rare occasions, all members of society pays the bill, directly or indirectly.

Government has access to similar predictive tables, but the decisions are much more complex and value-determined. The costs of treating the victims of lead poisoning are enormous, but so are the costs of rehabilitating their environment to prevent lead poisoning (Lin-Fu, 1970, 1979). Governments tend to avoid this issue by treating the small numbers of powerless victims and spending larger sums on other priorities. This is a fact of life that workers in the prevention fields must understand, if only to save themselves the frustration of the zealot. This fact should lead preventers to become more sophisticated in the workings of government and the private sector with regard to the game of allocation of limited resources.

Another form of the insurance principle is in shared costs and benefits from group health programs. Large numbers of subscribers (or their employers) pay small amounts of money on a regular basis so as to receive defined benefits from a health maintenance organization (HMO). Medical personnel receive fixed wages, and the advantages of large-scale purchasing plus a preventive health orientation mean that a reasonable quality of health services can be obtained at an affordable cost. There may be some limitations of choice, as patients have to choose among medical personnel on the staff of the HMO. On the other hand, specialists are often present under one (organizational if not literal) roof so that for a fixed cost patients can have nearly whatever services they need (although there is pressure to control usage of expensive services). In addition, large-scale organizations can afford expensive medical equipment. Whether or not it is possible or desirable to expand this organizational framework to cover all citizens is currently being debated in the United States.

The insurance principle plays out in many sectors of society, offering psychological security if not material advantages over a purely individualistic approach to the hazards of life. As with any business, however, even the insurance industry, with its enormous wealth, can be affected by economic downturns (as in the recession of the early 1990s). There is no absolute guarantee through collective action any more than there is one through individual action. From a configural perspective, both are needed.

2. Social Movements

The very imprecision of the term *social movement* is also its strength. It refers generally to very loosely organized collections of social activities—either in protest or for promotion—that spring up with regard to some social event or change and that exhibit some continuity over time. Because these collections are loosely organized, they are difficult for the powers that be to oppose or support them effectively, whether they be secular or religious movements. Yet social movements are typically noisy and public—that is also one of their strengths. People must respond to them one way or another. Social movements often emerge in times of rapid social change and general upheaval, but not necessarily so. They change as different leaders come and go and as social responses to the movement oppose, agree to, or co-opt the ideals of the movement (Goldstein, 1992).

I distinguish a social movement, which usually has some core of moral ideas, from other collective protests, such as riots, which are intentionally destructive without offering a clear moral alternative. Riots may have positive, if unintended, effects; social movements may fail to attain their goals (such as some health reform movements of the 19th century; Goldstein, 1992). There is no guarantee of success just because the moral core is pure and the volunteers are enthusiastic.

Significant social movements in our times, such as the civil rights movement, the women's movement, and the gay rights movement, have

IV. The Fourth Dimension

developed into more formal collectives that give visibility and leadership to the core ideas. Often several subgroups may be addressing the issues in any movement, such as lesbian groups, gay men's groups, bisexuals, and others for sexual freedom all operating under the banner of gay rights. Such movements are sustained by contributions of members and collateral people.

This section focuses on the health movement in America, a multiple-headed social phenomenon that includes physical exercise, nutrition, and the nonuse of substances such as tobacco and other drugs. A special subset of this health movement involves primary prevention, cross-cutting the exercise, nutrition, and nonuse of substances aspects of the larger movement. Goldstein (1992) discusses the long history of social efforts in regard to mental and social health. Originally, behaviors of any kind were viewed as purely voluntary. When certain behaviors became to be seen as problems, the causes were first attributed to divine or devilish origins (and thus appropriately controlled by religious authorities). Then the causes were viewed as crimes (and thus appropriately controlled by civil authorities). Still later, the causes were viewed as underlying disease entities (and thus appropriately controlled by medical authorities). We are now in a period of medicalization of problem behaviors, and experiencing various kinds of reactions to this pathology-oriented view of aspects of social life—from alcoholism, drug addiction, child abuse, and mental illness to criminal behavior, especially juvenile delinquency. Homosexuality and feminist protest may have escaped from the domination of medical views of these "problem behaviors," thanks to the gay rights and women's liberation movements.

The President's Commission on Mental Health (1978) identified four powerful ideas—described as revolutions in thinking—that mobilized society to act in new ways toward the mentally ill. First came Pinel's humanitarian approach to the insane, treating them as sick people rather than as criminals. Second was Freud's mapping of the subterranean topography of the mind, with its enormous effect on culture and society.

The third revolutionary idea was the concept of the community mental health center that offered comprehensive care in the client's own neighborhood. The fourth health revolution involved major societal efforts at preventing mental illness and emotional disturbance and promoting psychological and social vitality. These movements began the counterreaction against medicalization of problem behaviors and the promotion of socially and personally fulfilling behaviors, which suggests that we may be seeing the first signs of a humanistic movement that returns in part to the individual responsibility theme mentioned above, combined with a caring community and society. We are still too close to these powerful events to examine their dimensions and evaluate their effects clearly, but we can consider some particular instances of the preventive movement as objects of study in their own right—what social strategies can we use to decrease social stresses and optimize human existence?

The holistic health movement fits the general characteristics of social health movements. Emerging apparently spontaneously from many different points of origin, groups reacted against aspects of contemporary medicine and society by offering a different version of health and healthy lifestyle. Often some fringe groups are included under the umbrella of holistic health that "centrists" in the movement try to reject. But because social movements have little organizational structure, there is no way to expel these health groups with seemingly bizarre ideas. Let the buyer beware. The overall effect of the holistic health movement has been salutary. Changes in lifestyle (preventive in nature) are now part of the mainstream of thinking about health. People are assuming more responsibility for their own health, rather than seeing it as a "medical issue." Self-help and health cooperatives (the Boston Women's Health Collective, which publishes *Our Bodies, Ourselves,* 1993, is an important example) have expanded the public's perspective about one's own role in health and care. Pressure for "people's health groups"—meaning democratically organized and run health collectives—probably contributes to, and focuses on, dissatisfaction with the enormous medical empire built up by an entrepreneurial medical profession (see Case & Taylor's, 1979, study of cooperatives, communes, and collectives—including medical groups—as social experiments).

Social empowerment is discussed in Chapter 4 (III.C.1); some forms of social empowerment would qualify as types of social movements (Alinsky, 1972; Joffe & Albee, 1981a, 1981b; Katz, 1993; Rappaport, 1981; Simon, 1994; Solomon, 1976; Swift & Levin, 1987). For primary prevention, the concept of empowerment has two major aspects. The first may be termed *individual* or *interpersonal empowerment,* for example, as in empowering women with knowledge about preterm labor symptoms so as to prevent problems in delivery (Freda, Damus, Andersen, Brustman, & Merkatz, 1990) or empowering teenagers who are at risk of school dropout by giving them a chance to be help givers in a peer tutoring situation rather than help receivers (Allen et al., 1990). When groups of people take up these ideas in many places all at the same time, social movements arise.

Social empowerment occurs when a minority group assembles its individual energies into a collective force (Solomon, 1976) or when a numerical majority attempts to obtain its fair rights in society (Bloom et al., 1975; Brown & Ziefert, 1988; Keller, 1985; Torre, 1988). Social empowerment changes imperceptibly into social movements, particularly through promotive activities as a means to a participatory goal (i.e., participating in some portion of society or activity that is satisfying to the people involved).

Klitzher, Bamberger, and Gruenewald (1990) provide a glimpse into a prevention-oriented social movement, parent-led prevention programs related to substance abuse. This movement can be characterized from its popular literature "as an attempt to reduce [the risk of drug and alcohol use and abuse among their children] through a reinstitution of parental control, attempts to reduce peer influence, and manipulation of peer group and community norms" (Klitzner et al., 1990, p. 112). To achieve these goals that reflect traditional or conservative values, the parent groups advocate four types of change:

1. Changes in the home (such as increased awareness by parents of the youth drug culture, instituting family rules regarding drug use and related behaviors, and the like)

2. Changes in the peer group (e.g., establishing a "parent-peer support group" in which parents of the youths in the peer group meet regularly to discuss the social activities of their children and support one another in enforcing a consistent set of rules)

3. Changes in the schools (like supporting school officials in instituting strict controls of drugs and alcohol use on the school campus)

4. Community-level changes (such as support of enforcement of substance use statutes by local police, vigorous prosecution of suppliers, the development of drug-free alternative social activities such as drug-free concerts, and providing opportunities for youths to have positive community involvement)

Parent-led movements have received considerable publicity in the mass media and have captured the attention of state and federal agencies responsible for preventing drug abuse, who have funded conferences and offered technical assistance to these parent groups.

The Klitzner et al. (1990) study is the first large-scale systematic study describing this social movement. These authors first surveyed 106 programs in 36 states identified by the National Federation of Parents (NFP) and the Parents Resource Institute for Drug Education (PRIDE). From 61 responding programs, the authors conducted on-site and telephone interviews with people nominated by local leaders; this is not necessarily a representative sample of the members.

What Klitzner et al. (1990) found confirms some prior conceptions: Parent-led prevention programs largely involve white middle- or upper-middle-class women participants. Community agency people are involved, but mainly as concerned citizens (i.e., unofficial involvement). The modal age of these programs is 3 to 4 years. These groups appear to be triggered by some common concern, such as drugs or other problems in the schools, although there is a negative association between parent involvement and their child's drug use. Although some aspects of the parent-led programs are decreasing—such as the parent-peer support group, which appears difficult to maintain over time—the programs as a whole are increasing in size.

The most commonly cited activities at the family level are drug education for parents, followed by rule setting and communication skills. At the school and community levels, changes in relevant policies are the primary targets. Perhaps the major finding is that community agencies feel supported by the parent groups and find a "mandate" in this support to "get tough on drugs." I raise the question whether this approach directs community attention to the symptoms of the problem as contrasted with the causal factors. It is always easier to focus community awareness on individual violators than face the broader and more difficult sociocultural conditions, which favor the spread of drug abuse.

Several major commentators on primary prevention direct attention to the root causes of the social-personal problems we seek to prevent, namely, the powerlessness of the poor and the oppressed (Joffe & Albee, 1981a, 1981b) and efforts to interrupt genetic and environmental hazards to lead to the apparent causal factors creating visible social problems (Joffe, 1982). Albee (1986) and Goldston (1986) have written eloquently on the politics of primary prevention; Long (1986) presents an insider's view of how voluntary organizations and energetic leaders may influence political events (see also McElhaney & Barton, 1995, on the advocacy function of the National Mental Health Association). Yet one feels that primary

IV. The Fourth Dimension

prevention is still a "David" in a field of "Goliaths," with much that remains to be done to promote "saving children" (Albee, 1992; Dryfoos, 1994) and a humane and just society in which they and their families may exist.

How does one start a social movement? A person ordinarily does not set out to start a social movement. (Religious prophets who instigate social movements are exceptions.) One is more likely to begin to work toward some specific social goal; in the course of defining one's goals and means, one finds others with similar ideas. There are many who share parts or all of any ideas one may have. The task is to locate these others and to find ways to work collectively toward common goals without being distracted by alternative goals or unacceptable means.

3. Social Justice Mechanisms

Many instances of the use of law, legislative enactments, administrative policies, ordinances, legal decisions, and the like have been mentioned in connection with various primary prevention projects. This section pulls together some of these examples to draw out some implications for primary prevention's use of the law in promoting the health, education, and welfare of citizens. It must be noted immediately that laws can bring people into the preventive or promotive orientation (Nielsen et al., 1981), or it can drive people away. As Coates (1990) notes,

> The law advises, enables programs to be implemented, regulates, and protects (Gostin & Ziegler, 1987). Nonpunitive laws have traditionally been used to contribute to the public health; the HIV epidemic has seen the proliferation of laws at the federal and state levels. The law can assist the public health effort by drawing individuals into programs to monitor their health or help them change their behavior, or it can drive individuals away if the law punishes unfairly or fails to protect from discrimination (Schatz, 1989). (p. 65)

The Constitution guarantees a broad band of basic human rights that has been expanded and contracted over the years of decisions by the Supreme Court and the judicial system. It is important for primary preventers to recognize the power of law in influencing everyday life decisions. To give one example, consider the state of Oregon's approach to health care. In 1989, Oregon passed three pieces of legislation that made up the Oregon Basic Health Services Act (Kaplan, 1993; Ross,

1991). Of relevance here is the establishment of the Oregon Health Services Commission, whose task was to determine priorities on a list of health problems and the costs related to each. Large numbers of persons were involved in establishing this value-laden set of decisions. The final list identified 709 health conditions that would be supported through state funding and drew a sensitive cutoff line between those that the state would support and those that it would not—not an easy decision. Indeed, Ross (1991) points out that this list is based on an illusion of the exactness of scientific knowledge. Kaplan (1993) argues that the process of arriving at these decisions was very democratic, surely more participatory than any other health decision. It is also true that the level of care poor Oregoneans receive would be determined by how much money is available in their fund rather than by medical necessity.

Embedded within this set of decisions was a reallocation from treatment-oriented services that are high tech and expensive (e.g., kidney dialysis) to prevention-oriented services that are low tech and relatively inexpensive (e.g., information services for pregnant women). A court decision to remove discriminatory features put the Oregon proposal on hold, but the issue is of central important to the nation. As with any legal action, one must assess the positive and negative ramifications and either reject the entire package or attempt to make the minor modifications that would make it more equitable and just.

Other states have taken quite different approaches to dealing with primary prevention for their citizens. Tableman (1989) and Tableman and Hess (1985) discuss Michigan's effective statewide planning and actions. Rural areas have their own unique problems and opportunities, which Porter (1983) and his colleagues explore. Let's consider one state in more detail.

Pransky (1986) reports the efforts that went into Vermont's prevention law. Act 79 of 1983, as amended in 1986, reads in part as follows:

Policy and Purpose

It is the policy of the general assembly to encourage community involvement in the development of effective primary prevention programs which promote the health and increase the self-reliance of Vermont children and their families. The general assembly recognizes the far-reaching value, both social and financial, of community-based programs which reduce the need for long-term and costly rehabilitation services. These preventive programs seek

IV. The Fourth Dimension

to eliminate the likelihood of irreparable damage that can arise from interrelated social problems such as child abuse and neglect, domestic violence, alcohol and drug abuse, juvenile delinquency, and other socially destructive behaviors. Therefore a children's trust fund is established for the purpose of providing funds for primary prevention programs.

This reasonable statement took about 4 years to be enacted from start to finish, years in which interested people from various public and private groups met, shaped concept statements, wrote legislative ideas, sought sponsors in the legislature and supporting agencies, responded to opposition (both rational and idiosyncratic), and, with much delay and negotiation, approved a statement (on the last day of the session) and had it signed into law by the governor. Actually, it was 4 years from start to beginning—not finish—for, as Pransky (1986) points out, enactment requires both enforcement and a public belief in those required to obey the law that the law is good, or at least that they will get caught if they do not obey.

On the basis of his experience, Pransky (1986) offers some guidelines to those who wish to develop state prevention legislation:

1. Some policy is required to promote primary prevention in a coherent way; this policy must be translated into state agency duties and responsibilities or else no one will take active responsibility for engaging in primary prevention (Wursten & Sales, 1988).

2. Supporters of primary prevention must collaborate, as no one agency or group has enough power, resources, or capacity to do it alone.

3. Sponsor must do their homework by showing that prevention works and that a state prevention policy development is important in achieving desired results. National data can be helpful; state data are vital. For example, a Vermont school climate improvement project resulted in 90% reduced vandalism in one school.

4. In making a legislative proposal, sponsors must state exactly what it is they wish the state to do. Who is to do what with whom under what conditions (especially, how are the bills to be paid) and with what sanctions?

5. At least one person must be willing to shepherd the idea through the long series of winding paths to the finish (Long, 1986).

6. Sponsors must present testimony before the legislative councils. Pransky (1986) recommends, "Kill them with logic, but understand that it is not logic that will win them over; it is emotion" (p. 20). Sponsors should try to anticipate logical problems as much as possible, as the illogical (emotional) ones will emerge in any case.

7. There is mixed advice on whether to negotiate necessary ingredients (such as operating funds) or whether to let the whole concept stand or fall as a workable entity. Nothing is dead in legislative terms; if rejected once, it may be revised in a new form another day.

8. Never give up. The value of primary prevention in the state is worth continuing efforts.

Weinberg and Levine (1990) present an important overview of a possible future to which we need to pay attention before the problem arises: litigation in primary prevention. Although there are few if any cases in which a primary prevention program has offered objectives by which an individual was to have been benefited but who instead claims to have suffered an injury, the United States is a litigious society (especially in the medical and psychiatric areas). Such a possibility has to be considered. Weinberg and Levine (both lawyers) provide a crash course in law: the meaning of duty of care (the plaintiff is entitled to a measure of legal protection from the defendant's conduct), breech of the standard of care (did the service provider do what a "reasonably prudent person" would have done under similar circumstances?), factual and legal causation (is there a connection between what the service provider did and the plaintiff's injury?), and damages (what compensation is due the plaintiff?). They offer various examples—which come very close to real projects—for which legal claims may be made. Let me offer one illustration.

Hospital ethics committees emerged from a 1976 New Jersey Supreme Court decision in connection with a case that involved removal of life-support systems. More than half of all hospitals in the United States now have ethics committees. Merritt (1987) predicts that such committees may face tort liability for some of their activities. Although currently only doctors are being held liable, the scope of liability may increase, especially as such committees get into the business of formulating policy for primary prevention decisions (Weinberg & Levine, 1990). Such liability might eventually extend to other primary prevention personnel, which in turn might limit preventive proposals. On the one hand, this is a good trend, as the law, ever conservative, tends to err on the side of protecting citizens against rash acts thought to be based on the "best available information," such as early sterilization laws regarding defective or antisocial individuals. On the other hand, fear of personal liability for innovative legislation and action may put a damper on ideas that could in fact help people help

IV. The Fourth Dimension

themselves. We are caught on the horns of a dilemma and must proceed with all due caution—but we must proceed.

Szasz (1986) presents a strong case against suicide prevention. His argument turns on the point that suicide is a mental health problem that helping professionals have a duty to try to prevent. Indeed, if a "patient" (a person defined by the professional as being at risk for suicide) kills himself or herself, then the mental health professional may be sued. Szasz denies the basic premises of this argument. He asserts that a person is a moral agent responsible for his or her actions (including suicide) and that a helping professional cannot prevent a mythological entity—a mentally ill person—from taking leave of this moral responsibility.

For the past 100 years, however, there has been an increasing tendency to define suicide as a mental sickness, which "reinforces the negative valuation of the act, exonerates the suicide from wrongdoing, and excuses the survivors from punishing the deed" (Szasz, 1986, p. 806). Mental health professionals claim competence in treating this mental illness or, in this case, preventing the suicide. Psychiatrists have the legal "duty" to commit the suicidal person to a protective institution, by coercive means if necessary.

Szasz (1986) asserts that mental health professionals who promise to prevent suicide "promise more than they can deliver" (p. 808). To be responsible for preventing suicide, the professional must have control over that person. It is impossible, Szasz asserts, to prevent someone determined to kill himself or herself from doing so, save at the cost of total (institutional) control, which takes away that person's liberty and dignity. But liberty and responsibility are "indivisible" (p. 810), and Szasz seeks to expand both by keeping adults responsible for all behaviors over which they have control. The point of his argument is to prevent helping professionals from claiming (and thus being liable for) too much control over the behavior of a morally responsible adult. The mental health professional can offer (voluntary) help to a person in a state of mental distress, but should not coerce that person, according to Szasz.

In general, laws are instituted to address persistent issues through general guidelines; court decisions address particular problems through specific decisions. Administrative actions to carry out the law and to address particular concerns represent a third way in which government attempts to establish social justice. It is, at best, a continuing quest. For primary prevention, it is important to recognize the part citizens and helping professionals play in shaping laws that in turn influence citizens and helping professionals. If people in primary prevention do not attempt to influence the course of legal developments in ways favorable to their goals for human growth and social development, they will be controlled by the laws. (See Clayton & Leukefeld, 1992, on the issues related to legalization of drugs; Mullooly et al., 1990, on the effects of rule changes in the workplace related to smoking.)

As a last note to this section, I want to highlight a book by Bagwell and Clements (1985), *A Political Handbook for Health Professionals*. This handbook introduces neophytes to the world of politics by summarizing the nature of law and legislative processes and bodies and the art of politics. This art consists of communicating with legislators, lobbying, negotiating, and becoming actively involved with political parties. Let me summarize briefly some major points:

1. Communicating with legislators: One can communicate orally (by phone or in person) or in writing (by letters, telegrams, and other written communiqués). In general, communications that "provide useful information and express an individual opinion" (Bagwell & Clements, 1985, p. 109) are well received; form letters are merely counted or weighed. With information overload facing most legislators, the rule is to be brief, factual, and reasonable. Bagwell and Clements provide sample letters and fact sheets to write good letters. Thank you letters are important, too.

2. Lobbying: Lobbying is a special kind of communication with legislators, either directly (as in face-to-face contacts) or indirectly (as in mass media campaigns, or to instigate other constituents to meet with legislators). Grassroots lobbying can be very effective because it connects to the legislator's political base and political future. Bagwell and Clements (1985) take the reader through the process of lobbying, including the legislation controlling lobbying. The authors list many methods of lobbying (mailgrams, petitions, position papers, testimony before legislative hearings, talk show appearances, litigation) and the strategies by which these may be delivered directly or indirectly to supply information or to seek influence.

3. Negotiating: Bagwell and Clements (1985) define negotiating as "the effort to resolve disagreements on specific issues" (p. 100). This activity moves beyond communicating and lobbying; it involves engagement in a two-directional interchange. Once determining a legislator's

stance (from public records or direct inquiries), a person negotiating for a primary prevention cause must also know his or her own stance and the motivations and social forces driving this position. Bagwell and Clements (1985) offer detailed suggestions for how to prepare, where to negotiate, and how to negotiate.

4. Engaging in political activity: Sometimes more direct action is needed—including taking part in the political process itself, by working in a political party or running for office. Bagwell and Clements (1985) offer many practical suggestions for these activities, including developing networks and coalitions of like-minded persons and groups. In general, the political arena is one that offers immediate contact with that vital fluid, power. It is with social and political power that decisions are made that affect primary prevention and every other aspect of our lives.

METHODS OF PRIMARY PREVENTION

Dimensions V & VI. Increasing Resources and Decreasing Pressures From (and on) the Physical Environment

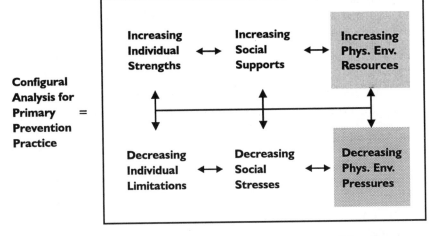

Figure 6.1. The Configural Equation

The physical environment, both in its natural forms of earth, air, water, and animal and plant life and in the many forms of built environments, is a powerful influence in the lives of people whether or not they are aware of this influence. This chapter explores the ways in which the environment may become part of overall primary prevention planning, coequal with the person and the social context. This chapter addresses increasing the renewable resources from the environment and decreasing pressures associated with it—both those from the environment that impinge on people and those from people that affect the physical environment.

279

Dimension V. Increasing Resources From the Physical Environment
A. Aspects Involving People and the Natural Environment
    1. Prevention of Future Despoliation by People
    2. Protected Use of the Present Natural Environment
    3. Promotion of a Healthy Natural Ecology
B. Aspects Involving People and the Built Environment
    1. Prevention of Future Mistakes: The Lessons of Pruitt-Igoe
    2. Protection of the Existing Built Environment
    3. Promotion of a Healthy Built Ecology

Dimension VI. Decreasing the Pressures From (and on) the Physical Environment
A. Aspects Involving People and the Natural Environment
    1. Ordinary Environmental Pressures: Pollution
    2. Extraordinary Environmental Pressures: Natural Disasters
B. Aspects Involving People and the Built Environment
    1. Prevention: Accidents
    2. Protection: The Ordinary Hazards of Modern Life
    3. Promotion: Goodness of Fit Between Person and Environment

V, VI. The Fifth and Sixth Dimensions

The physical environment—as contrasted with the social environment, or the cultural context of human behavior—is occasionally mentioned but little considered in discussions of primary prevention. (See Bloom's, 1965, paper providing a historical perspective on the role of the physical environment in community mental health.) The relative neglect of the physical environment is regrettable for many reasons—we are overpopulating "flagship Earth"; we are "fowling the nest"; we are using up nonrenewable resources at a rapid and senseless rate that will leave our children and their children with an "empty cupboard"; we are misusing space and objects and thereby creating pressures on people that lead to mental and physical morbidity and mortality. Worst of all, we are doing these things knowingly and seem not to have the wits or the will to stop. There is a gross maldistribution of natural and manufactured goods among peoples of the world. Acts of unbounded enjoyment of the good life compete with acts of desperation for survival. The "have" nations offer some aid and much advice to "have-not" nations, but are loath to reduce their own standard of living.

In the past quarter of a century, an increasing number of social scientists and others have rediscovered the physical environment, both the natural places where human behavior occurs (e.g., fields and forests, beaches and bodies of water) and the built environment (e.g., city streets, constructed houses, and modifications to the natural environment that control these situations—such as boardwalks through the Florida Everglades, making them accessible to—but also protected from—human visitors). In the configural model that frames the discussion of this book, I propose coequal dimensions of physical environments, social contexts, and human actors. At one time or another, one of these aspects takes precedence over the others. Consider the effect of a volcanic eruption (such as Mt. Pinatubo affecting world climate) or the collective efforts of the Dutch to reclaim portions of the Atlantic Ocean for farmland. Or consider your feelings the last time you were at the beach with a special friend during a beautiful sunset; perhaps at such moments all three portions of the configuration are equally balanced.

In terms of primary prevention practices, the central question is how all may use the physical environment appropriately for human purposes without abusing it for the other species of life with whom we share it or without using up its resources for present purposes at the expense of later generations. There is an enormous species-level conceit, which many professions unwittingly share, that asks only the first part of this question—how to use the physical environment for human purposes—while neglecting the second part—the appropriate use of the physical environment in relation to neighbors (indeed, relatives) on this planet, now and in the future. We must ask both parts of the question (Gore, 1992).

In this chapter, I first focus on increasing the renewable resources provided by the physical environment; later, I turn to decreasing the pressures that the physical environment may cause for people—or the harm that people may cause to the physical environment. Unlike in the other chapters, I must discuss how humans affect the physical environment as well as how it affects humans—lest we irreparably harm the planet or the objects on it—which then stresses people anew.

The following statements provide guidelines to the relationship between people and the environment. These statements are derived from the writings of environmental psychologists (Ittelson et al., 1974; Wandersman, 1987; Wandersman, Andrews, Riddle, & Fancett, 1983) and community psychologists (Heller, Price, Reinherz, Riger, & Wandersman, 1984; Holahan & Spearly, 1980; Kelly, 1988).

1. The physical environment is a unitary entity, a whole from which one artificially extracts pieces from one's own limited perspectives. One

may see, feel, or hear particular things, but everything in the natural world is systematically interrelated so that a change in one component has differential effects on all the other components. One may not be aware of all these interrelationships, but they occur nonetheless.

2. Sociocultural environments are inextricably related to physical environments. All things are endowed with (sociocultural) meanings. Human actions toward things (natural and social objects) are conducted within these meanings. The person is a dynamic configuration, simultaneously a physical entity, a member of a sociocultural community, and an autonomous individual capable of moving among the physical and the sociocultural events in time and space. To understand human behavior, one needs to understand the person in sociocultural contexts and physical environments over time.

3. Energy is recycled. This refers not only to biological cycles—photosynthesis in plants leading to food for animals leading to nutrients for plants, all of which is set within the physical environment—but to sociocultural cycles as well, such as recycling of reusable resources or community cooperation to sustain organized social life. But as Commoner (1968) notes in one of his "laws of ecology," everything must go somewhere: when, as a part of an overall atomic energy program, a nation creates nuclear wastes that have a half-life of thousands of years, these dangerous energy sources must be put somewhere, which creates problems for a dynamic and changing environment. "There is no free lunch," Commoner reminds us—humans have to pay for whatever ecological change humans make.

4. The perceived environment consists of islands of temporary stability and recurrent change. What one perceives is not likely to be the whole story of the mixture of stability and change, but one acts on these perceptions. People build houses on the San Andreas Fault in California or at the edge of the ocean shore in North Carolina, acts of presumptuous overconfidence in the perceived stability of the built environment over the natural environment, as well as acts of social and personal status.

5. The fundamental law of ecology is adaptive reciprocity, the mutually contingent exchanges that individuals, societies, cultures, and environments forge that maintain some overall balance. Human beings survive by adapting to the physical and sociocultural environments. These adaptive acts, large and small, bring in life-sustaining nutrients and the additional factors (luxuries) that represent quality of life. In a complex

world, reciprocal exchanges are necessary because it is not possible to produce all the things everyone would like to have. The rules of these exchanges change, from raw power and enslavement to the rule of international law. The 1992 Rio Conference on the World Environment was perhaps the most complex discussion on adaptive reciprocity in human history, involving nearly all the nations of the world in discussing effective use and protection of the global environment.

Dimension V. Increasing Resources From the Physical Environment

A. Aspects Involving People and the Natural Environment

1. Prevention of Future Despoliation by People

In a capitalistic society dedicated to the commercial use of natural resources, it has been difficult to gain compliance with the concept that destructive exploitation is a disastrous public policy in both the short and long run. Constructive exploitation is a difficult concept and a more difficult reality to enact. The definition of what is or is not harmful to the environment and people is less clear, however, and becomes a political decision reconsidered with each change of political administration. It is all well and good for conservationists to protect the spotted owl or certain species of fish from the onslaught of forestry or farming interests, but as long as there are increasing numbers of people to feed and house, lumber and agricultural products must come from somewhere. Protecting one area puts pressure on another. Large-scale social decisions often begin concretely with what appears to be a tiny event, such as identifying an endangered species of spotted owls or enjoying a luxury such as baked frogs' legs. Something has to give.

Conservation of public lands is a case in point. Begun with grassroots support that eventuated in laws setting aside certain lands for the perpetual benefit of visitors, debates are now occurring in political and economic circles regarding the degree to which developers should be allowed to extract some of the natural wealth on or under these public lands. As the need for scarce resources increases, so does the pressure on these public properties, just as it did with privately owned lands earlier.

Another difficult situation involves the use of fossil fuels, especially certain types of coal, that leads to acid rain pollution that has killed the fish in thousands of lakes in the United States, Canada, and nations in Europe (Geller, 1986). Industrial accidents and oil spills, the use of pesticides and fertilizers, and pressure from a hungry world to eat fish all reflect an overextended use of the present environment. Given current known reserves of oil, scientists have provided projections on how long this energy resource will be available—it is a matter of years, not centuries. The same is true of various mineral resources. Control of these resources is left to individual nations, some of whom are desperate to "catch up" with the standard of living of the advanced industrial nations (Gore, 1992). The same overuse of fossil fuels may contribute to the greenhouse effect, a global warming trend that could cause such severe climatic changes as flooding or desertization, affecting millions of people. The control of the use of fossil fuels is a critical national and international issue.

Usable water is becoming scarce, with overpopulation and overuse leading to the drying up of major aquifers. Conflicts over water use nationally (in the American West) and internationally (in the Middle East) are very troublesome, with no end or solutions in sight.

The ozone layer is another global environmental problem. Many small actions, such as use of spray cans, and large actions, such as jet travel, produce atmospheric pollution that destroys the protective layer of ozone in the upper atmosphere, leading to skin cancer in humans and other forms of damage to animals and plants (Geller, 1986). International agreements have been reached to phase out some of these destructive elements; whether these phase-outs will be adequate to deal with the problem is questionable.

For each of these large-scale environmental problems, various groups are seeking redress. Some issues are international in scope so international bodies are active in their consideration, from the United Nations to voluntary groups addressing global concerns (e.g., World Wildlife Association and Greenpeace). Other interests are local, for example, a citizens' action group to protest building low-income housing in a green belt that borders a city (Bachrach, Zautra, & Cofresi, 1989; Jansson & Haglund, 1991).

What is fundamentally clear is that each party in these debates has a considerable amount of truth on its side; the parties fight with the passion of feeling that they are in the right. Configural analysis often reveals a fundamental flaw, however: Most of the time, these parties selectively ignore some portions of the ecology in making their argument. Large numbers of species are being obliterated each day for whom there are no specific defenders. If one can see the total configuration of demands and supplies, one has taken the first step toward seeking workable solutions.

There may be some sequence of steps required in gaining control over global ecological gridlock. My guess is that, after recognition of the mutual problems, some form of adaptive reciprocity will eventually be reached. Every side will feel the pain of retrenchment. Without these adaptations, the world is in big trouble. A first major step was taken with the 1992 Rio Conference under United Nations sponsorship.

In addition, individual nations need to assess their own activities—a difficult process. Realistically, this is where large-scale changes will occur, both from world pressure and from social movements and groups within nations. There are various types of social groups, from those led by volunteer organizations of national or international scope (such as Greenpeace) to feminist organizations that attempt to put a caring perspective into a largely exploitative and conflicted male-dominated society (Boston Women's Health Collective, 1993).

The prevention of future despoliation at the hands of people rests in the hands of people, largely the same people. The rationality of individuals, families, communities, and nations is necessary to consider sustainable resources and the need for conservation and recycling, along with the "rationality" of organizations, from businesses using natural resources to the United Nations, which is attempting to supply the present generation while it preserves for future generations the limited bounty of earth. The record of long-term collective rationality versus short-term hedonism does not engender optimism. But it wonderfully focuses the mind.

2. Protected Use of the Present Natural Environment

Table 6.1 presents a set of facts from a United Nations Environment Programme publication, *The State of the Environment* (1989), that provides the basis for understanding our need to protect nature (see also Brown et al., 1994, and all recent publications in this series).

V, VI. The Fifth and Sixth Dimensions

Table 6.1   Profile of the Present State of Nature in the World

- Soil erosion has been reported from almost every country in the world. It has been estimated that humanity causes the loss of about 25,400 million tons of topsoil from world croplands every year.
- Deforestation is the most powerful factor in accelerating the rate of soil degradation. On a global basis, the world's forests are disappearing at the rate of about 15 million hectares each year.
- Animal and plant species are becoming extinct at an unprecedented rate due to the worldwide deterioration of natural environments. Most experts conclude that perhaps a quarter of the earth's total biological diversity, amounting to about 1 million species, is in serious risk of extinction over the next 20 to 30 years. On average 100 species will be lost per day. This is perhaps 1000 times greater than the historical rate of extinction.
- World population continues to grow rapidly. It doubled from 2.5 billion to 5 billion between 1950 and 1987 and is expected to exceed 6 billion by 2000, possibly 8.2 billion by 2025, and stabilizing at 10.5 billion by 2110.
- Growing numbers of people need more food, fuel, and other necessities of life, all of which have to be taken from the earth's limited resources. Agricultural productivity worldwide grew an average of 2.5% over the past 25 years, but differentially: Per capita food production increased 12% between 1980 and 1985 but it fell by 5% in many African nations in the same time period.
- The total forest area in the world is about 4,700 million hectares, or about one third of the total land area in the world. The 15 million hectares disappearing each year are located especially in Africa, Asia, and Latin America.
- About $900 billion are spent each year on global military expenditures. This, plus the Third World debt of about $1,000 billion, are the major obstacles in obtaining funds for sustainable development.
- Manmade changes in the earth's biota—including forest destruction from deforestation and the effects of acidic deposition and the destruction of grassland and other vegetation cover through desertification—result in a net annual release of 1,600 million tons of carbon dioxide emissions into the atmosphere. Estimates project that this will increase to between 6,000 and 10,000 million tons by 2000.
- Hazardous wastes are generated in great volumes, estimated at 300 to 800 million tons a year in Organization for Economic Cooperation and Development countries, with the United States generating an estimated 88% of the whole. America has some 76,000 active landfills, most unlined. The U.S. Environmental Protection Agency has placed nearly 1,000 of these sites on a national priority list as needing urgent attention; this list may grow to 10,000. Costs estimated for cleanup range from $23 billion to $100 billion.

SOURCE: United Nations (1989) and World Health Organization (1988).

In reaction to these kinds of data and projections, the need for conservation on an international scale has become increasingly clear. One response is a global network of gene banks that houses the World Base Collection of crop germplasm (United Nations Environment Programme, 1989, p. 10). More than 100 nations are collaborating in the collection and analysis of plant and animal genes. There are also over 3500 protected areas worldwide, ranging from scientific reserves to national parks. Individuals and groups can support these projects through collective organizations such as the Sierra Club and the Wilderness Society (Moore, 1995). Strategies are generally at the macrolevel, such as political lobbying and acting as watchdogs for events scattered over the globe.

The concept of sustainable development has been emphasized since the late 1960s. Sustainable development means that current practices should not diminish future possibilities of maintaining or improving living standards. This requires economic systems to be managed so as to maintain or improve resources and the environmental base so that future generations can live as well as or better than we do.

Renewable resources are an important part of sustainable development. Wind power, a pure renewable resource, has not yet received concentrated attention to development as a major source of energy, in contrast to coal or oil or atomic energy. Likewise, solar-powered batteries, thermal water, and indeed the ocean tides themselves all represent different approaches to renewable resources. But the costs of research and test programs are so great that all but a few adventures in this territory are unlikely.

Strategies to reduce hazardous wastes include changes in the manufacturing processes and reusing and recycling products. It is also possible to use safer substitutes. The U.S. Environmental Protection Agency (EPA) estimates that existing technologies could reduce the total amount of hazardous wastes generated in the United States by 15 to 30% by the year 2000 (United Nations Environment Programme, 1989, p. 39). Again, strategies to initiate these existing technologies tend to involve governmental watchdogs and volunteer organizations.

The 1985 Vienna Convention for the Protection of the Ozone Layer was a model attempt for coordinating international efforts to reduce the threat of chlorofluorocarbons and related substances. Although the convention depends on the voluntary agreement of participating nations, it also signals global awareness of the problem and the willingness to address these issues.

V, VI. The Fifth and Sixth Dimensions

In general, for each of these horrendous global hazards, groups are attempting to correct them, and other groups are seeking to delay change for their own profit. Primary prevention, as a science-based people-helping enterprise, can contribute by clarifying the configuration of issues involved and aiding relevant groups to be more effective in achieving their ecological goals (Moos, 1985; Moos & Brownstein, 1977).

3. Promotion of a Healthy Natural Ecology

Many people are worried about specific aspects of despoliation of the planet and the totality of the problems. It is equally clear, however, that many people are actively engaged in preventing the predictable problems, protecting our fragile and limited environment, and promoting a balanced use of the environment for all parties concerned (Sawhill, 1995).

One large-scale example has all the ingredients that perplex many around the world: poverty, economic exploitation of the environment, overpopulation pressures, health concerns, educational problems, and the like. Yet this example is an illustration of hope in action. Consider the Brazilian city of Curitiba, with its 1.6 million people. Located 530 miles southwest of Rio de Janeiro, Curitiba is the beneficiary of a master plan from the 1950s and the innovative leadership of its architect-mayor, Jaime Lerner. Brooke's (1992) report of Curitiba's viable, low-cost solutions to supposedly intractable problems illustrates why this city has become a showcase of ideas. Curitiba is a very poor city, with most households averaging less than $100 a week in income, 25,000 shanty dwellers, and a twofold increase in population over the past half century. But there is something so different about this city that boosters and critics alike have to consider it carefully. Brooke (1992) provides some descriptions:

Poor families keep slums clean by exchanging (20-pound) bags of garbage for bags of food (eggs, butter, rice, beans). This is a reciprocal contingency idea, because the two social functions have to occur to some degree; they are linked together, saving the expense of garbage pickup, which can be applied to provision of food, while maintaining the dignity of the poor, who are working for their assistance by providing this service for the community. There are added costs of administering this exchange, but it might be possible to employ citizens for part of this process as well. It may be possible to extend this service to include other kinds of exchanges that may be within the capability of the poor (especially if training were provided)—such as home building for the shanty dwellers. (Compare Jimmy Carter's Habitat for Humanity organization, in which volunteers and some professional builders work with a needy person in building that person's home.) For a historical perspective, consider Robert Owen's New Lanark in the early 19th century—a progressive mill town (Butt, 1971).

Ninety tubular bus stops spaced along 150 miles of express bus lanes are part of a "surface subway." This provides fast mass transportation for a fraction of the cost of digging a subway. Mass transportation is a critical feature of life in large urban areas. Cars carrying one or a few individuals not only cause great amounts of pollution but create congestion as well. Curitiba has 25% fewer cars since this mass transit plan began, which results in an enormous savings on fuel and materials to produce automobiles, and efficient movement. There is no mention of reduced accidents, but this is a possible by-product.

Ninety-three miles of bicycle lanes are being built in Curitiba; to promote their use by rich and poor alike, the mayor began a program to help workers finance bicycle purchases. This will also reduce automobile traffic and provide some exercise for the bicyclists. Probably fewer serious accidents will occur and other savings in nonrenewable resources will take place. The bike paths can be used on off-times for family recreational activities.

Several 19th-century buildings have been recycled: A gunpowder depot is now a theater. A glue factory is a children's art museum. A stove factory is a shopping mall. This gives character to the city. It also saves materials and probably revitalizes portions of the city.

Modern themes are being introduced. The calcadão, or big sidewalk consists of 49 blocks of pedestrian arteries, clogged on any given day with shoppers and strollers. There is a street enclosed in glass with a block-long arcade that contains 80 shops and services and is open day and night. Pedestrian areas humanize large cities, increase safety, and decrease pollution from cars and trucks. They also add to the quality of life of the city because they revitalize commercial areas.

Street people, especially street children, are a serious problem in Brazil, as elsewhere. Curitiba's mayor has started a program in which businesses "adopt" street children through apprentice programs. In addition, Curitiba

V, VI. The Fifth and Sixth Dimensions

has had to deal with the influx of people into the city from farms in the country. This dislocation is due to the mechanization of agriculture, which increases the yield for a hungry nation while it also creates urban refugee problems. To help rural migrants get city jobs, the mayor has converted old buses into mobile classrooms where adults study to become typists, seamstresses, electricians, or auto mechanics. To help youths who turn to the streets for economic survival, the city places them in apprentice programs, where they work in return for meals, a stipend, and schooling.

A vigorous tree planting and parks program provides 62 square yards of green space per inhabitant, one of the highest ratios in the world. Trees revitalize the atmosphere and beautify human settings. Their shade permits people to use the outdoors as part of their living space and thus increases the quality of life in the city. Tree plantings are expensive, but large numbers of persons are employed in their care and tending and costs are repaid in savings from the environment and from a quality of life that is hard to quantify.

Unfortunately, all is not perfect in this Brazilian Eden. Sanitation is not adequate; only 40% of the houses in Curitiba are connected to the city sewer system. The poor, the street people, and the shanty dwellers still exist. These are difficult problems to solve, but one lesson to be derived from Curitiba (and its innovative mayor) is that even large, interrelated problems can be addressed and solved to some degree. It is possible to promote a healthy ecology, even with limited material resources. What is not limited are the ideas that go into making these changes in people and environments (Brooke, 1992).

B. Aspects Involving People and the Built Environment

1. Prevention of Future Mistakes: The Lessons of Pruitt-Igoe

Humans have made mistakes in the past with regard to the environment, especially the built environment in which we create something that is supposed to serve a useful function. But more important than a listing of mistakes are the lessons to be learned from these mistakes, which may be useful in guiding new decisions.

A number of writers have made the association between the quality of housing and various kinds of personal and social pathologies (Newman,

1972; Schorr, 1963; Wilner, Walkley, Pinkerton, & Tayback, 1962). This association is complex, connecting both the physical state of the housing and neighborhood with social status, psychological image, and physical fatigue. Poor and dilapidated housing may not only constitute a physical risk (e.g., rats spread disease and may attack infants), but represent an image of the owner or renter as inadequate or unsuccessful. Limited space or noisy conditions mean that children may have a harder time studying, adults may have less privacy, and the level of interpersonal stress may be high due to continual interaction without relief.

Yet such dwellings in rundown neighborhoods are home to many, and some pleasant associations and commitments arise in every cultural setting. These places become home, where friends are, where the familiar props of life are formed. This may be especially true of oppressed minorities. Thus when the social revolution of the early 1960s called for demolition of slums and the construction of public housing that met health and sanitary codes, there were some mixed feelings but not enough to stop the movement.

Pruitt-Igoe was a low-income housing project in St. Louis (Ittelson et al., 1974; Rainwater, 1970). It consisted of groups of huge, 10-story, high-rise buildings clustered in a former slum area that had been demolished to make way for the public housing. The clusters of buildings were set at different angles from one another, resting on a vast concrete slab. It was a prize-winning architectural structure, a triumph of efficient design. The large number of apartments all had relatively small rooms, large windows to look out over the beautiful St. Louis skyline (or look in at a complex of institutional buildings), and efficient household equipment. Rents in these subsidized buildings were geared to low- to moderate-income families. Yet within 20 years, this multimillion dollar project was dynamited to the ground as a colossal mistake. What happened?

Essentially, the architects ignored the social functions for which this housing project was to serve, as home to large numbers of poor families and children. Ittelson et al. (1974) summarize the problems: Pruitt-Igoe served a largely black population, but was just as much a ghetto as the neighborhoods it had replaced. To save money, the elevators were designed to stop at two-floor intervals. They were slow and unreliable, especially for parents who were trying to watch and care for their children playing on the concrete slab many stories below. The playgrounds were minimal, as was the landscaping in and around the complex, and shops

V, VI. The Fifth and Sixth Dimensions

and other facilities were at some distance from the housing project. The long corridors were minimally lighted, which may have supported the criminal behavior that occurred there. There were few places where people could meet informally so as to establish the supportive helping networks that abounded in the old slum area. Life at Pruitt-Igoe was vertical, institutional, confining, isolating—and unpleasant.

The new facilities quickly deteriorated: windows and screens were broken and not repaired; lights in the halls became nonfunctional; and overall maintenance deteriorated with the city as landlord, just as it did with slum landlords of the past. Morale among the people living at Pruitt-Igoe plummeted; few natural helping networks or public support systems existed to help hold things together. Finally, tenants moved out and apartments went unrented despite the "reasonable" rents. The entire complex began to hang like a millstone around the neck of the city until, with much fanfare, Pruitt-Igoe was blown out of existence—but not out of memory (see Gibbs, 1983, on Love Canal).

What lessons can be learned from this? Clearly, smooth concrete lines do not make an architectural success; this is determined by whether or not the human function is fulfilled. Newman (1972) compares high-rise and low-rise dwellings housing the same types of residents in the same densities and finds significant differences, indicated by the term *defensible space*. Newman makes four points:

1. Territoriality is stronger among low-rise residents because they are more likely than high-rise tenants to know their neighbors and the neighborhood.
2. Low-rise tenants can keep surveillance over their private and public territories—an idea that evolved elsewhere as neighborhood or block-watch groups to reduce crime and to promote solidarity.
3. The human scaling of low-rise apartments is less institutional and rigid than high-rises; people can become involved with one another in neighborly ways.
4. The overall milieu of low-rises makes their integration into the neighborhood more possible, whereas huge high-rise complexes are set apart, continuing social and personal segregation in a new form.

Can one know in advance what needs are present? To a degree. One can identify universal human needs and then ask prospective residents what particular concerns they have for a living environment. Citizen participation (Wandersman, 1984) in its various forms can make a vital contribution to living in social contexts. Allowing citizens to provide their ideas and wishes as input into program and policy planning engenders commitment to the project and a sense of control over it. Citizen participation empowers people to gain some control over their lives. Any program, including primary prevention projects, takes this sense of control away from citizens if they are not allowed to participate in the programs that affect them. Citizen participation is not a perfect solution, as not everyone can contribute and there are costs in time, energy, and frustration. But this democratic process goes to the heart of many problems in social programming (Klein, 1978; Lemkau, 1969; Newman, 1972).

As Wittman (1980) notes, "Physical settings are stages, and physical objects are props, which serve as the medium through which people interact with one another at both social and individual levels" (p. 137). The housing studies by Festinger, Schacter, and Back (1950) found that where people lived in an apartment complex determined to a large extent their friendship patterns. Barker (1968) conducted long-term studies of "behavior settings" in a small Kansas town. These behavior settings were physically circumscribed entities that had associated patterns of social behavior. The local drugstore had certain sets of behaviors that were played out among the physical props of the soda fountain, the magazine rack, and the like. It did not matter what individuals were present; almost all people played out those expected social behaviors in relation to the physical dimensions of the drugstore.

Studies of relocated people, especially the elderly dispersed from their familiar neighborhoods because of urban renewal, show personal disorganization resulting from the break-up of the physical props of existence (Blenkner, Bloom, & Nielsen, 1972). The British experience in building public housing without service amenities after World War II produced a host of antisocial behaviors, crimes, and personal distress. (For a recent attempt to address these issues of defensible spaces, see Cose, 1994. For a historical perspective, see Hall, 1988; Klein, 1978; Lemkau, 1969.)

Could the planners of Pruitt-Igoe have foreseen any of these problems based on the literature existing at that time? It is easy to be a Monday morning quarterback, second guessing the planners of Pruitt-Igoe. But in fact they did not foresee these extreme problems and few social critics raised these issues before the project was built.

Will new Pruitt-Igoes be built in the future? It is possible that they will, because planners still rarely consult with consumers, especially when

V, VI. The Fifth and Sixth Dimensions

public housing is concerned. Economic pressures still drive decisions between social need and physical and fiscal requirements. Ittelson et al. (1974) also describe some success stories, however. The Marcus Garvey Square low-income public housing project in San Francisco consists of townhouses (two-story, two-family dwellings) that are attractive, offer privacy for the families, and permit social contact through common garden areas. One of the unique features of this development is that prospective tenants participated in discussions of the design and the decor. Thus the architects came to understand how the buildings were to be used, whereas prospective tenants came to understand the practical problems in building low-income housing.

Wittman (1980) discusses the history of planning for community mental health settings. Traditionally, hospitals for the physically ill were designed for the physician and staff to have maximal accessibility to the patient. Chairs placed against the walls of long corridors make it easy to sweep the floors but hard to talk with other patients. A different perspective is needed in mental health settings, where clients and staff need opportunities to interact privately and socially over the course of treatment. Grouping chairs in a circle or an arc facilitates conversations among patients, a touch of homelike settings where ordinary behaviors are expected rather than the maddening straight lines of the institution.

Likewise, schoolrooms were traditionally arranged for regimented learning, all instruction flowing from the teacher in the front of the class. More recent thinking of education as involving many kinds of teachers (study groups, peer tutors, places for people to interact as a whole) for many kinds of students has opened up classrooms and provided options in the use of space. These examples demonstrate that it is possible to try to benefit from past experience to construct an environment that is more humanely functional as well as aesthetic, but to prevent future mistakes, it takes the collective wisdom of planners and users.

James Rouse (1978), the developer of Columbia, Maryland, a planned community, writes about its beginnings:

> Our first step in planning . . . was to bring together a work group of people from a variety of disciplines to share ideas on the crucial issues of urban life; to explore in an interdisciplinary way the optimums in education, health, religion, recreation, employment, housing, etc.; to examine successes and

failures in urban and suburban communities; to learn more about how the planning and development of community could contribute to the life and growth of the human individual and the family. . . . At the same time we were recording in detail the physical conditions of the land itself and reporting them in such a way that the land could speak to us about where and how physical development should occur and where it should be protected. (p. 52)

Klein (1978) catalogs the planning of social institutions for Columbia (Shoffeitt & Shoffeitt, 1978; Wastie & Klein, 1978), as well as arrangements to meet the special concerns of women, blacks, and teenagers (Eberhardt, 1978; Karsk & Klein, 1978; Toomer, 1978). A grassroots alternative mental health clinic arose early in Columbia's development, with walk-in service, no fees, peer-style service, and a hot line and outreach program, that eventually emerged as a stable community self-help center (Feinstein, 1978). Although Columbia and other towns of the 1970s have been "researched to death" (Warren, 1978, p. 164), the results are not clear. Satisfaction with the quality of life in Columbia is higher than in comparable cities, but perhaps this is related to having Washington, D.C., and Baltimore just a short drive away from this lovely tree-enveloped village-cluster living place that is home to economically and racially diverse people. The point is that planners and residents and behavioral scientists worked together to address the challenges of the sociocultural and physical environment interchanges as they affect individuals.

2. Protection of the Existing Built Environment

Building a complex civilization brings with it the requirement that its buildings, bridges, and roads be continually maintained through the course of the hard use to which they are put. Such maintenance clearly prevents problems as well as protects the existing state of healthy functioning. But it is not glamorous to do maintenance work, to keep the routine substructures of society in good working order. Especially in times of scarcity, maintenance may be one of the easiest targets for cutbacks. Fortunately, much routine maintenance is done as part of the function of local and state governments. People benefit from pothole-free roads, clean and tended parks, and the timely removal of garbage. Primary prevention does have a proactive role in the protection of the existing built environment. For this discussion, I turn to the work of Scott Geller.

V, VI. The Fifth and Sixth Dimensions

Geller (1986) reviews the many massive and global environmental problems; rather than succumbing to pessimism, he proposes that "many solutions to environmental problems require changes in human behavior" (p. 363) for which the behavioral sciences can contribute to an interdisciplinary systems-level effort in preventing environmental problems. I will present a brief overview of his views, as developed in his extensive research in this area (Geller, 1993).

Geller (1993) takes a behavioral approach, which leads to the position that one can influence environmental protective behavior through relatively simple manipulations of environmental stimuli and response contingencies—and let attitudes and values follow from these behavioral changes. There is ample precedent for this, as when President Dwight D. Eisenhower sent in troops to enforce desegregated schooling at Little Rock—a strong behavior-change mechanism to defend the laws of the land—and then let time and events now in place facilitate gradual changes in attitudes and values. (I should add that the civil rights movement used a combination of change mechanisms, from advocating for changes in the law to the moral example set by nonviolent actions. Each worked in its own way with its differential degrees of risk, as the lives of Martin Luther King, Jr., and Gandhi demonstrate.)

The behavioral approach directs attention to the events that precede an outcome in question—the antecedent stimuli—and the events that follow that outcome, perhaps to act as reinforcer of it—the consequences (see Glenwick & Jason, 1993, for a recent example of this perspective). An early example of this dual antecedent and consequence manipulation is the anti-littering project of Burgess, Clark, and Hendee (1971), who made announcements and provided litter bags (antecedent factors) and gave out movie tickets or 10 cents for appropriate behaviors (consequence factors) to children at matinee theater presentations.

Some environmental actions are relatively simple, like the anti-littering campaign, but others are complicated and require the contributions of several disciplines. For instance, energy-efficient housing involves engineering, landscaping, and behavioral changes to produce optimum outcomes. Some environmental actions need to be repeated over and over for successful completion, whereas others may need to occur only once. Repeated preventive efforts include using contraceptives that must be taken regularly; driving at multiply posted speed limits, which are supposed to reduce accidents, but here, too, engineering technologies of roads and cars have to be added to the preventive equation—see Geller, 1993); and wearing warm clothes on a cold day rather than turning up the thermostat. Other forms of environmental action need to take place only once, such as surgical sterilization, living in a garden city where one can walk to work, and installing a thermostat that keeps the temperature at preprogrammed levels. Of course, one may have to do both single and repetitive acts, such as installing a preprogrammed thermostat and wearing warmer clothes.

Geller (1993) considers a number of antecedent strategies for environmental preservation so as to increase the frequency of desired target behaviors or to decrease undesired ones. He lists several antecedent strategies that have many possible variations:

1. Verbal or written messages in educational packages: Research reviewed by Geller (1993) suggests that

    a. messages should refer to specific behaviors (either desired or undesired behaviors) so that the audience knows what is being addressed

    b. when some undesirable behavior is to be avoided, it is better to specify an alternative desirable behavior in its place

    c. messages should be given in polite language that does not threaten the individual's sense of freedom to choose

    d. the message should be presented in close proximity to the target behavior

2. Modeling and demonstrations: Modeling of some specific behavior (often including the positive or negative consequences to that model) is another approach to influencing behavior regarding the environment. Winett, Leckliter, Chinn, Stahl, and Love (1985) produced large increases in the conservation of electricity among residents who viewed a videotaped presentation of simple conservation efforts by people similar to themselves along with a discussion of the financial benefits accruing to them from these actions.

3. Goal setting and commitment procedures: It is possible to obtain commitments (verbal or in writing) from individuals or groups to perform a desired behavior (e.g., participate in recycling), to avoid undesired behavior (e.g., littering), or to reach a particular goal (e.g., a 25% reduction in energy consumption in an apartment house).

4. Engineering and design strategies for preventing environmental problems: Geller (1986) provides an example of designing large partitioned

receptacles for use with different types of recyclable objects so as to increase participation in recycling campaigns. In another example, Geller (1993) discusses the need to combine technological and behavioral science efforts in prevention. He notes that airbags are maximally effective when used in combination with lap or shoulder belts—it has been estimated that 55% of all fatalities and 65% of all crash injuries could have been prevented using both airbags and lap or shoulder belts—but when drivers stop using this protection, fatalities actually increase by 41%.

Geller (1993) discusses a number of consequence strategies for environmental preservation. Such consequences can be distinct outcomes, such as a monetary rebate or a speeding ticket, or they can involve opportunities, such as appearing on an honor roll or on a most-wanted list at the post office. (Behaviorists discourage the use of punishments as consequences because they are hard to control and have other undesirable sequelae.)

There are two general types of consequences, those related to a given (desired) response and those dependent on a given outcome. An example of the response-contingent consequence is when points are exchangeable for family outings if designated home appliances show reduced usage (Wodarski, 1978). An instance of the outcome-contingent consequence is 75% of energy savings from expected costs returned to the residents of a master-metered apartment complex (Slavin, 1981). Another instance is Geller's (1993) work with the Ford Motor Company to increase seat belt usage among its workers. Geller's training program was measured on a before-and-after basis; overall employee usage went from 12% during baseline to 54%, which translated into at least eight employee lives saved and about 400 serious injuries prevented, as well as reducing company costs by nearly $10 million.

Geller (1993) also reports that feedback aids in achieving desired environmental results. For example, one project on litter control that employed a daily presentation of litter on the front page of a community newspaper resulted in a 35% average reduction (Schnelle, Gendrich, Beegle, Thomas, & McNees, 1980). Technology also provides feedback aids, such as light and sound warning devices that seat belts haven't been activated.

These examples provide the basis for optimism in using behavioral methods in the protection of the environment by modifying human actions. As Geller (1993) points out, however, they are usually short-term and small projects that do not have much hope of affecting the massive problems we face. It is by combining methods into an ecological approach that one can begin to develop preventive or promotive programs appropriate to the scale of the problems involved. Geller, Winett, and Everett (1982) propose some communitywide systems to keep the community clean; these systems have been implemented in more than 200 communities here and abroad.

3. Promotion of a Healthy Built Ecology

Overall Design: Urban Planning

Around the turn of this century, an unsuccessful farmer and businessman eked out a living as a parliamentary reporter until he published a book that brought him fame and wealth: *Garden Cities of Tomorrow* (1902/1965). Ebenezer Howard has since been identified as the father of city planning. I will present his early vision as a brief historical introduction to this discipline. Hall (1988) reviews Howard's precursors and contemporaries in the development of the garden city concept and how the concept was turned into reality.

Howard (1902/1965) recognized the obvious problems of the overcrowded city and the depleted rural areas, but saw something new that could solve many problems at once: The garden city combines the strengths of city life (employment opportunities, rich cultural diversity, and entertainment) with the strengths of country living (clean air, sunshine, open spaces, nature, and low rents) while avoiding the negatives of each (high prices, long hours of work, unhealthy living conditions in the city; lack of social life, entertainment, and the like in the country).

Howard's (1902/1965) plan, which was operationalized to some degree in two towns in England, involved the purchase of 6,000 acres of inexpensive country land of which the central 1,000 acres was the garden city itself, with a population of 30,000. The green belt (i.e., the countryside) surrounds the city like a natural barrier to protect it from encroachment of people overflowing large cities, as well as being a natural limit of construction from the garden city. This city is self-sufficient, with working areas separated from living areas to prevent the polluting atmosphere that British industrial cities of the 19th century knew too well (Butt, 1971;

V, VI. The Fifth and Sixth Dimensions

Morton, 1969). Workers lived close to their employment so they could spend more time with their families and in nearby parks and recreational areas. Cultural opportunities were to be available, such as a museum or library, all within the confines of the small city. The maps of the physical layout of the garden city were sketchy; it seems to have a circular design with several major boulevards. Because of the healthy surroundings, Howard predicted that welfare costs would be low—presuming that poverty and unhealthy surroundings caused illnesses and need for public relief (Petersen, 1977). Most of all, this concept would provide residents with a sense of community, a coherent self-sustaining way of living and working with dignity and health—factors that were desperately missing from the industrial towns of England at that time. The garden city would be economically self-sufficient and " at peace with nature" (Donaldson, 1977, p. 86). Nature would never be lost sight of, even though workers living in these cities would be fully engaged in factories and offices.

Several such communities—Letchworth and Hampstead—were actually constructed during Howard's life (1850-1928), as was the garden village of New Earwick (built for the Rowntree chocolate company workers) and Welwyn Garden City (Hall, 1988). They were fascinating urban-suburban planning attempts, but all had a variety of problems (Donaldson, 1977; Petersen, 1977). New Earwick, for example, was so attractive and so well designed and constructed that the ordinary workers for whom this community was intended could not afford to live there (Hall, 1988).

The concept of the suburban lifestyle—bedroom community to the large city—quickly overtook the garden city ideal, and life has not been the same since (Allen, 1977; Hall, 1988; Insel, 1980; Ittelson et al., 1974). There have been planned cities in the United States, such as Columbia, Maryland (Klein, 1978), but so too do we have Levittowns constructed in the wake of a rapidly expanding housing need after World War II, which enabled many thousands of people to purchase their own small standard-constructed, look-alike homes (in racially segregated areas). This was the American Dream come true—at least for some low-income people.

The underlying pressures that oppose rational planning of urban areas, where now more than 75% of all Americans live, involve both economics and population. Increasing numbers of people want the good life and can afford some variation of it. Thus the places where people want to live and the kinds of housing that they need to fit their varied lifestyles have produced enormous changes across the social and physical landscape. In some areas, local zoning ordinances are attempting to gain control over land use—by restricting who can gain entrance to some desired areas—leading to a new source of conflicts in values. Dense concentrations of peoples in some areas of the country and sparse settlements in others exaggerate the changes occurring. City life may provide freedom (of action and thought), but the city is also a more expensive place to live and may be confining in the sense of creating unsafe areas (Newman, 1972). As other social disruptions occur—deinstitutionalization, increased drug use, unemployment, and higher costs of housing—large numbers of homeless in cities across America (and elsewhere in the world) are a painfully visible symbol of a failure to grasp the dimensions of the environmental factors and exert rational control (see Rivlin & Imbimbo, 1989, for an imaginative self-help project for a homeless group). Much creative thinking is needed in this area.

Large-Scale Building and the Continuum of Supported Living

Architecture and engineering address the built environment and involve creations and modifications made to change the natural environment in ways helpful and pleasing to people. Traditionally, architects and engineers have focused on utility, hygiene, or aesthetics. Rudolph Virchow asserted in the mid-19th century that "medicine is a social science though its methods be those of the natural sciences, its ultimate aim is eminently social" (Rosen, 1958, p. 13). One might also say that architecture and engineering are social sciences, or, more correctly, they may become so as scientists make the connection between the physical environment and human behavior. Let's look at some examples.

Institutional environments have long been constructed for the benefit of staff—long straight corridors to make cleaning easy, chairs against the walls so brooms can make straight sweeps in an orderly, tidy environment, "institutional" drab colors—perhaps not to excite fragile minds—and tough sturdy furniture made to last forever. These are not unreasonable bases for constructing living-working environments, but other considerations may be more important.

V, VI. The Fifth and Sixth Dimensions

For example, consider some appropriate goals in the care of vulnerable people, such as institutionalized aged persons or those suffering from dementia. Environmental changes may be made that support their existing strengths while protecting them against their own limitations. More home-like institutions might ease the tasks of transition into a new assisted living situation, as well as contribute to a sense of comfort of residents and encouragement for the resident's family to visit (Cohen & Weisman, 1991).

The characteristics of the residents must be considered: What strengths and limitations do they have that the physical environment has some chance of helping? What physical features in combination with what sociocultural contextual and organizational features would be helpful for the residents?

Consider basic human functions, from sleeping, eating, toileting, and socializing to engaging in helping or leisure activities. These functions occur at home in familiar places, but also in conventional institutions in places convenient for the staff—sleeping wards, dining areas, and large restrooms. It may be possible to reorganize assembly line mental health institutions into small team organizations, with the same or greater productivity (as has been done with success in automobile manufacturing). Private bedrooms (with mementos as sources of comfort and ties to reality and an all-important sense of control over one's private life), small shared bathrooms (with some responsibilities for cleaning where possible), small clusters of kitchen-dining areas (which become central foci of social interaction and possibly include some contributions in cooking or folding napkins and such, on the grounds that meaningful activities help maintain competence and self-esteem), dens or private spaces, family-size public living rooms (for entertaining guests)—all are possible, but at a cost. The cost is not only financial but is conceptual—seeing residents as human beings in another setting, not as inmates in a totally controlling institution (Goffman, 1961).

Another feature of contemporary thinking regarding environmental supports for persons with special needs is the continuum of supported living idea. In regard to people with dementia, the great majority are maintained at home until stress on caregivers and the lack of proper equipment make other settings necessary. Home aides might be used to augment the home environment and to give support and relief to the family caretaker (Nielsen, Blenkner, Bloom, Downs, & Beggs, 1972). In general, the idea is to support the highest level of mental and physical functioning for as long as possible, working with the strengths of the declining person, not merely working against his or her weaknesses. Prosthetic devices and environments (Lindsley, 1964) can help support limited functions in individuals, even though they cannot replace them completely (see also Chernoff & Lipschitz, 1988; Kennie, 1993).

A first step might be a day-care center where both normal aged and those with Alzheimer's and other diseases may go for a few hours or a whole day to get special care or simply time away from home (and thus provide respite for the home caregiver).

A second step might be a group home where a small number of residents live together with one or two caregivers. The atmosphere is still homelike, but strangers and possibly professionally trained staff provide a higher degree of support and control. A third step could be in an institutional environment, preferably one with modular or cluster living arrangements together with the availability of safe, supportive equipment (e.g., showers with benches). Even in the most extreme change from the home setting, it is helpful to include familiar objects that remind the person of his or her history, selfhood, and continuity as part of the transition from home to institution.

In regard to the prosthetic environment (Lindsley, 1964), the point is to link personal limitations to physical environmental resources. If a person is becoming disoriented in terms of persons, places, and time, then multiple sensory cues and reminders about people (photographs with names and connections), places (photographs of built environments or maps; medicine boxes with spaces for different medicines to be taken at different times; storage compartments with items labeled and accessible), and time (alarm clocks set throughout the day to remind the person to take medicine or calendars and daily diaries with appointment times and visits listed) become sources of support in addition to whatever social arrangements are present—including volunteer telephone callers who remind the person of timed activities as well as provide pleasant social conversation and support. Safety and security measures may also be needed, from bed railing supports to alarm bells on doors to prevent wandering. Unobtrusive enclosures, understandable pathways with familiar landmarks, and activity clusters to facilitate social interactions as well as privacy can be produced by architectural and engineering designs (Cohen & Weisman, 1991).

V, VI. The Fifth and Sixth Dimensions

Just as older persons showing signs of mental decline need familiar landmarks to define themselves and their routines, so these people may need protection from overstimulation that may exaggerate their confusion. The caretaker must modulate the environment (physical and social) to adjust to the capacity of the mentally frail individual to prevent both overload and understimulation. People vary greatly from one to another, but also within the development of any one person, especially as driven by dementia or other conditions of declining function.

This example focuses on the elderly, both the well aging and those with mental or physical limitations. The point, however, is more general: People of every age can benefit from thoughtfully planned physical environments that promote safe and stimulating development. Experiences with the elderly may be generalized to ideas for stimulating the growth of all people (Brett, Moore, & Provenzo, 1993).

Building Design

Weinstein and David (1987) offer several guiding propositions on the interactions between children and built environments; similar points may be made between adolescents and adults and the built environments in which they live.

1. "Built environments have both direct and symbolic affects on children" (Weinstein & David, 1987, p. 6). For example, Ittelson et al. (1974) refer to symbolic associations that may transform objectively poor living environments (i.e., what would conventionally be called "slums") into "home," a rich association of family and friends all living the same way in vibrant interactions (Rivlin & Imbimbo, 1989). This is supportive without denying the squalor. Another example: When an attractive school is built in a slum area, it not only provides a place to educate neighborhood children, but it also represents a source of pride for the people living in the area and may act as a magnet to attract others.

2. Human needs are served in every built environment beyond the institutional purpose of that construction. For example, children play, whether they are at home, in school, at the hospital, or in shopping malls—each of which has its own distinctive institutional purpose—and this common function must be accommodated in one fashion or another. Hospitals and doctors' offices often have a children's section in the waiting

areas, where toys are available. Shopping malls have many accommodations to the developmental needs of all ages of customers, from convenient benches and resting and eating areas for weary adults and the elderly, to amusements like fountains or miniature merry-go-rounds, presumably for the young. Some accommodations may be unintended sources of amusement, such as the down escalator for a youth playing at going up. For adolescents, malls present avenues for observing and being observed, for brief interactions or extended ones (as in movie theaters). Thus whether intended or not, built environments serve multiple and simultaneous—and possibly conflicting—functions.

3. Environments are inevitably linked, although people may not be aware of these linkages. Bell, Fisher, Baum, and Greene's (1990) series of studies linked living place (high-rise apartment houses), noise (from traffic on nearby freeways), and school performance (children living on the lower floors have poorer reading test scores, are more distractible, and show a lack of persistence on cognitive tasks) (Wandersman, 1987; Wandersman et al., 1983). Lead poisoning represents another environmental hazard that is a costly personal and social problem that is invisible unless public health workers bring it to the attention of the nation ("Is There Lead in Your Water?" 1993; Lin-Fu, 1979).

4. For people at different stages of development, built environments serve distinctive functions. Ittelson et al. (1974) present an overview of these stage-related functions. The conception of appropriate hospital environments for the newborn has changed dramatically in recent years from the isolated nursery viewed through a glass window (except for brief feeding periods), to contemporary arrangements where the father is present at the birth and for the immediate parent-infant bonding experience, to rooming-in situations where the mother has continuous access to the newborn. For the young child, the home environment becomes the first source of learning about people, objects, and eventually abstractions (like causation and time). Bell et al. (1990) propose the concept of *place identity* to refer to the physical-world socialization of the child. The child comes to learn who he or she is not only by the continuous transactions between child and caretakers but also by means of the continuous experiences with space and physical objects in space (clothes, toys, beds, chairs, and such) that make up the substratum of existence. Children learn to view themselves as distinct from other people and from the physical environment, but contextual experiences are absorbed within their definitions of

themselves. Sense of self changes with life-course development, becoming more structured and more stable as the social and physical environmental experiences are incorporated into a moving sense of self in relation to familiar or novel settings. Thus place identity is a substructure of self-identity; it has some enduring aspects and some changing aspects as well.

For the school-aged child, Ittelson et al. (1974) note the importance of play and the play settings. A universal experience, play serves many vital functions in growth and development (Erikson, 1963). Because most built environments are constructed for adults, conscious consideration must be given to the needs of children in physical environments not specifically designed for them (such as shopping malls, churches, and recreation areas; Brett et al., 1993). In environments designed for children, such as schools, the manifest function involving education must be considered in combination with other functions perhaps less clearly viewed or accepted, such as the socialization function of being with peers, defensible spaces, and designated study areas.

Environments serving the developmental needs of adolescents have to provide both the privacy and the freedom to explore an increasingly accessible physical environment. Access to cars makes parking lots a necessity in suburban high schools, whereas safety features—seat belts, banked roads, warning signs—attempt to protect or alert the young driver to physical hazards or the social behaviors related to them (like the deadly combination of drinking and driving; see Simpson, 1987).

Environmental aspects of the mature years are varied and manifold. Ittelson et al. (1974) consider issues such as the openness or closeness of family dwellings, neighborhood contacts, accessibility to shopping and other services, and the quality of life within social and cultural norms (see Chapter 6, V.B.3).

The workplace is another important aspect of adult life for which environmental conditions are assuming an increasing concern. Industrial accidents are astronomically high but are essentially invisible to the public. Fox et al. (1987) report a time-series study of accident prevention in open-pit mining. Large numbers of serious and minor accidents had long been noted to occur, presenting significant problems to the people involved and to the mining operation. A complex token economy was initiated in one mine whereby workers and their families received trade stamps as bonuses for safety records (and nonbreakage of equipment). These stamps were exchangeable for a wide range of goods at nearby stores. Apparently the pressure for safety was very powerful, whether exerted by family members or by workers themselves, because results showed significant improvement in safety in this one mine. The entire program was replicated in a different mine with the same results, suggesting that a simple, cost-effective method of promoting safe interactions in a rough working environment could pay off for the workers as well as for the employer. This model of a token economy bears consideration for a much wider variety of settings. How can one reinforce appropriate behavior so that it becomes self-reinforcing, that is, performed automatically without the need of external rewards? This question, in various forms, is the continuing task of socialization at every age (Weinstein, 1987).

In old age, the physical environment seems to reassert itself as a factor to be considered consciously. Lawton (1968) translates Lindsley's (1964) concept of the prosthetic environment into a set of functional areas needed to maintain the aging person in the face of disability and loss of energy. These include

1. A safe physical environment, both a sheltering unit and safety features within that unit, such as nonskid rugs, hand railings on stairs, and good lighting
2. Prosthetic aids for decreasing functions, such as amplifiers in telephones and large-print books
3. Self-maintenance supports, such as hand rails on tubs, wheelchairs, or loops rather than knobs on cupboards

Many of the ideas associated with one age group are applicable to other age groups as well. The major point is that by design of environments and through guided perceptions in the use of those environments, there are many entrance points for primary prevention: What can one do by means of changes in the physical environment (things and spaces between things) that can facilitate (support or promote) some personal attribute without doing harm to the environment at the same time? How can one appropriately (harmlessly) amplify personal or social limitations in sight, hearing, or movement? These are the challenges for people who design ecologically sound environments—as well as for those who advocate for these kinds of designs.

V, VI. The Fifth and Sixth Dimensions

Design of Components

Although one does not often think about it, the world around us, both the natural and the built environments, did not emerge as we live in them by chance. Someone saw possibilities, made plans, implemented decisions, and made changes that led to what we now take for granted. Most people, particularly those who do not possess much status or power in society, accept these environments as givens, figuratively as well as literally cast in concrete. If one's environment is so unchangeable, then a large segment of one's life is unchangeable. Life is thereby diminished for people who hold this belief.

Young people take for granted the adult world of bricks and mortar, as well as social and cultural conventions. For children of the upwardly mobile, this can be an exciting world of change; for children locked in a relatively unchanging and unpleasant world, this can be one source of anomie and learned helplessness. Baldassari, Lehman, and Wolfe (1987) describe a project that challenged these assumptions—Children Creating Alternative Futures—in which inner-city children learned through an action project that they could make changes in social and physical environments and thus control one portion of their future (Freire, 1973, 1990). Some 43 children of different academic and socioeconomic levels, ethnic backgrounds, and gender from two different urban schools met twice a week for 2 hours over a 4-month period to participate in planning and designing changes in their environment. This participatory empowerment not only changed certain portions of the local environment but changed the young people as well. From academic indifference to riveting participation, these young people decided what project to undertake and how to do it; they did it by becoming involved not in fantasy but in the dynamics of their own neighborhood—in one case, clearing an eyesore, an empty lot. They validated their own ethnic identities—for the first time, Spanish-speaking ability became a vital resource in the academic setting as these youngsters interviewed community people. But most of all, they learned that they could affect their current environments, both social and physical, and hence their own futures (Browne et al., 1994; Simon, 1994).

Likewise, it is possible to enhance the lives of disabled children, as well as able children, through designs of playgrounds sensitive to developmental needs. Shaw (1987) illustrates this point in his description of a playground he designed for disabled children. Beyond the describing philosophy of these designs—such as giving the playground a sense of unique and coordinated place, fitting the strengths as well as the limitations of the occupants—Shaw illustrates ways to enhance the growth and development of children through built environments. A variety of spaces and objects in space are needed to provide a rich environment to stimulate play behavior and thus personality and skill development. Shaw notes that children particularly enjoy "defensible spaces," small enclosures with one entrance and exit, close to pathways (through which children move on to adjacent play areas) and activity areas (large spaces for collective or interactive happenings). But with the disabled, one must plan for accessibility (such as by wheelchairs) or activities at different heights (such as a chalk wall for drawing or a raised sandbox). Parallel bars are used to enhance upper-body strength; with creative planning, children in wheelchairs can participate in activities—such as a ladder hung horizontally above a ramp where children pull themselves up to a platform hand over hand. The variety of environments also includes graded challenges, hard enough to be challenging, but easy enough to permit accomplishment.

Fitness trails offer individual choices of what exercises to engage in and how much of the exercise to do at each station. These are usually directed at the very able, but people of many degrees of ability can use one or another aspect of these outdoor exercise points.

All aspects of the physical environment are considered fair game for designing, all textures, all colors or (nonrepresentative) shapes—so as to stimulate imagination, play, and development through modifications in the built environment. All children need to move, to grow, to explore, to touch, to test. Most adults feel concern that children do not harm themselves as they move about and so tend to constrain youngsters. Micro-environmental designs can incorporate adults' concern for safety with children's need for movement and exploration; this is a perfect task for primary prevention in promoting healthy environments. Playgrounds can have woodchips under swings rather than concrete or pebbles (Brett et al., 1993). Safety nets can be used in combination with rappelling exercises. Innovative jungle gyms can be made of durable and soft materials in intriguing combinations (like automobile tires strung across as a bridge). Even helpful gym shoes can be designed (Gardiner et al., 1988). The small details like these can facilitate, rather than inhibit, growth and development in a larger social-physical environment.

V, VI. The Fifth and Sixth Dimensions

One final example: light bulbs. Edison's invention provides the continuous light needed by a 24-hour-a-day world; one could hardly imagine life without light bulbs. But ordinary light bulbs are not energy efficient and so a new generation of Edisons has invented a new lighting device, the compact fluorescent bulb. Industry advertising reports that a single 27-watt compact fluorescent—roughly the equivalent of a 100-watt incandescent bulb—saves 730 kilowatt-hours of electricity and a corresponding reduction in fossil-fuel burning electricity generation plants that provide that energy. As an extra savings, this reduction of fossil-fuel burning keeps about 520 pounds of carbon dioxide out of the air. All this from changing a single light bulb (Northeast Utilities Service Company, 1992).

We are challenged at every turn in our daily lives to enhance human potential and conserve the environment.

Dimension VI. Decreasing the Pressures From (and on) the Physical Environment

---

A. Aspects Involving People and the Natural Environment

1. Ordinary Environmental Pressures: Pollution

The environment is both fragile and strong. It is fragile in the sense that people, alone among the species of the world, are able to make changes on an enormous scale to both the world itself and to people for good or ill. To do harm to the environment may mean to make irreparable damages to some structures and species of the physical and natural world. Farming and deforestation may start desertification, along with climatic conditions that escalate this widespread physical change. Likewise, some practices, like extensive fishing, may kill off whole species.

Yet the physical environment has awesome strength, as witnesses to hurricanes or earthquakes can testify. There is strength in the annual miracle, the birth of spring plants and flowers from the snows of winter. In this section, I consider some ordinary pressures people exert on the environment and the ordinary pressures the environment exerts on human beings. I will also consider the ordinary ways in which humans attempt to live with these pressures.

A good example of the complex relationship between people and the environment involves the human destruction of the ozone layer. Although the chemistry is relatively easy to understand, the effects are far-reaching. As products of human activities, from aerosol sprays to fuel emissions from jumbo jets, chemicals are entering the atmosphere and in effect destroying large patches of the band of ozone. Once destroyed, the gap in the ozone layer permits the sun's rays to penetrate the earth's surface in ways harmful to human beings. Humans harm the ozone layer and the gaps in the ozone layer harm humans. How does one resolve this problem before it gets more serious than it already is? Scientists first noticed the thinning of the ozone layer as a result of by-products of other activities and then began to study the conditions directly. Soon actions of certain chemicals in wide use became recognized as the culprits, and the information was conveyed to decision makers who, as careful politicians, made sure of the facts and the implications, weighed their choices, and finally called international conferences to negotiate control mechanisms. A phase-out of these destructive chemicals was agreed to—with time enough to invent alternatives.

The vital lessons to be learned include these:

1. One must keep scientific tabs on all aspects of ecology to observe any untoward events. (Here is a new possible threat: Frogs are dying throughout the world in sudden and mysterious ways. These hardy survivors from the age of dinosaurs are succumbing to diseases and no one understands why. If frogs become extinct, then insects will thrive, because frogs are one of their major predators. Birds and small animals who feed on frogs will be endangered. So the dominos of ecology fall; Yoffe, 1992.)

2. Decision makers must be notified of the problem; through negotiation processes, some collective response—including sticking one's head in the sand—must be made. Because overlapping events have causes—the frogs of Bangladesh that kept this nation nearly free of insects went to feed the appetite of French connoisseurs for frogs' legs, and the insect population and malaria have escalated rapidly (Yoffe, 1992)—it is likely that some parties profit by the existing state of events. These special interest groups argue to go slowly in making corrective changes—"We don't know all the facts"—while they continue to profit from the wors-

ening state of affairs. Conservation groups and their allies counterattack and seek more rapid analysis and action.

3. One must keep in touch with related phenomena, such as the degradation of environments (like paving over marsh areas to build shopping centers—frogs and other animals die out), or the use of toxic chemicals that are safe for people—without testing their safety for other species. These are part of the same ecological picture, which means that many more people and groups must be called into play to save the environment and people.

People are endlessly adaptive in the face of harsh physical environments. Eskimos have made extraordinary adaptations to the extreme temperatures in which their culture has long existed, just as people of the Amazon jungles have adapted to hot, humid conditions. People in the desserts of Israel have developed new forms of irrigation that support large fruit groves and agriculture—dripping water directly onto plants that are covered to prevent evaporation. Also, the lack of sweet water led to the development of desalinization plants. Like any pioneer group, Israelis worked with their existing environment and nurtured it to expand to include new and useful plants, experimental intensive farming, and ways to conserve resources. Their methods have been widely copied in many different nations. In the American Southwest, people also developed innovative ways of living and farming, but even these extraordinary efforts fell against the intractable limits of nature when irrigation left salt deposits that eventually ruined the soil. Every innovation carries risks.

One final illustration of ordinary environmental events is heating a house. Wood is gathered and burned the world over to provide heat and energy for cooking and for other purposes. Ordinary by-products of burning wood are the chemicals released in the burning process. Yet no other source of heat and energy is as easily and as cheaply available to many people, and so wood continues to be burned. There seems to be no action, however humble, that does not have serious environmental implications when that action is performed by and for 5 billion people. Ordinary actions have extraordinary consequences. Because these actions are so ordinary, so much a part of our everyday lives, we need vision to make headway against that harm we do to ourselves and our world.

The following principles can be derived from this discussion:

V, VI. The Fifth and Sixth Dimensions

1. Private actions multiplied by 5 billion require collective responses proportionate to the projected untoward effects.

2. Once a collective decision is made, the action reverts to the 5 billion people. Such actions have to be clear, decisive, and feasible.

3. Some monitoring system must oversee both collective governmental or business decisions and the individual acts that produce the problem.

These principles describe the working of representative and responsible democratic societies unfettered by greed and collusion. Whether the human race is capable of such utopian acts remains to be seen.

2. Extraordinary Environmental Pressures: Natural Disasters

Natural disasters are out of the control of humans. Events like floods, tornadoes, hurricanes, cyclones, and earthquakes, as well as major climatic changes that produce droughts, occur and people who are in the way get hurt. Primary prevention asks what can be done in advance of the natural disaster. The answer is as old as Joseph in the Bible, who, forecasting 7 years of good harvests and 7 years of lean, suggested to the king that grain be stored during the fat years to prepare for the lean ones. People today do not always read dreams as well as Joseph did, so we have to find other mechanisms to predict the future and plan effective means to address the expected problem.

With 750,000 residential fires, about 75,000 toxic-waste dump sites, property losses due to floods exceeding $4 billion, and nearly 700,000 people who receive emergency care from the American Red Cross annually, disasters, natural and assisted, involve huge efforts. Across all of these, the general strategy is one of

- Anticipation (with smoke alarms and automatic sprinkler systems; scientific study of the natural conditions that presage possible disasters)
- Preparatory training (fire drills in schools and workplaces and recommendations for homes; large-scale training exercises by disaster relief workers along with general directions for the populations likely to be affected)
- Storage of appropriate supplies (fire extinguishers; extra copies of computer disks or duplicate photographs; money in the bank and friends in the neighborhood; provisions)

The Red Cross is instructive with regard to large-scale disasters. The Red Cross prepares for disaster relief with its professional core staff, as well as trains first aiders, who might also double as helpers during a large-scale emergency. During disasters, the Red Cross (and others) attempts to provide organized care for large numbers of persons (Gillespie & Banerjee, 1993; Ginzburg et al., 1993). Think of all the needs and services a community requires each day and the scope of these disaster relief operations will become clearer. The logistics are horrendous, especially when ordinary transport and communication services are not available. Stockpiling vital materials and creating networks of special supplies are part of the overall picture. Wherever disaster hits, the network is called on to supply needed goods. This is very much like a store that is part of a national chain; when it needs certain goods, it calls up a regional supply center and the goods are identified by code numbers and shipped rapidly. The logistics of these operations have been much facilitated by modern computers, as are those of disaster relief.

Beyond the immediate response to natural disaster, there are psychological sequelae (just as the survivors of the Nazi Holocaust were left with deeply disturbing memories and reactions). A study by Echterling (1989) dealt with one such sequela, preventing school absenteeism after a major flood. Echterling volunteered to offer consultation to school officials to help students address their emotional needs after a flood that was provoked by 5 days of rain in order to prevent absenteeism that typically occurs. Four people eventually died, and 4,000 homes were affected. He provided a manual that described typical reactions by children to disasters—sleeping problems, separation anxiety, attention problems, and fears—along with ways of dealing with them. These ways included making time at school to talk about the fears and anxieties related to the flood and setting up crisis counseling and support groups for those identified as being at high risk. Brochures for parents—"After the Flood: Emotional First Aid for Children"—were distributed by the thousands.

Teachers were encouraged to include content on floods in their curricula as appropriate, aiding children to think preventively, for instance by distinguishing between flood watches and flood warnings. Teachers also were instructed to aid students in making positive and realistic self-statements related to their emotions and behavior, especially in connection with fears about similar climatic conditions. Data suggest that there were no differences in student attendance rates before and after the flood; interviews with 400 area households suggest that the brochures were very useful in helping parents deal with their children's responses to the flood.

I highlight this project because its methods are generalizable to other situations, both in making individual contact with at-risk individuals and in supplying the natural family network with written materials on actions to take to prevent predictable problems (see also Bachrach et al., 1989; Jansson & Haglund, 1991).

Gillespie and Banerjee (1993) provide many ideas regarding strategies for disaster preparedness. They conceptualize disaster preparedness as a cycle beginning with preliminary awareness—which a literature review could provide—as well as surviving a natural disaster. One then assesses the situation and by accumulating local and external knowledge, one plans a response to a disaster. The final stage of disaster preparedness is to practice the planned steps, as far as this is possible. Second and later generations in this cycle are anticipated as new information becomes available.

One can plan to minimize damage by judicious choices of where to build (not on a fragile sea coast, not on a fault line), what to build with (using seismic designs for structures and appropriate materials), and how to secure objects in place to prevent injury.

Gillespie and Banerjee (1993) also discuss minimizing social hardships by improving organizational effectiveness to respond to persons in need, such as with early warning systems (radio, TV, sirens), evacuation plans, and back-up communication systems. The social dimension also includes internal coordination procedures (who does what for what purpose) and external linkages (who is called in, in what order, and with what relationship to local leadership). Social preparedness also involves emergency financial aid, liability insurance, medical aid, and continuation of community functions such as education, policing, and social welfare, now rapidly expanded to include temporarily needy people. As this discussion suggests, it is never possible to anticipate every need during a disaster, but it is possible to plan to address many kinds of predictable problems before they occur so as to minimize the untoward effect and to optimize regaining a normal state.

B. Aspects Involving People and the Built Environment

1. Prevention: Accidents

The physical environment of the home is not the safe haven that legend and myth would have us believe. As Tertinger, Greene, and Lutzker

V, VI. The Fifth and Sixth Dimensions

(1984) point out, over 90% of the injuries and more than one half of fatalities to children under the age of 5 occur at home (see also Barone, Greene, & Lutzker, 1986). Homes are dangerous to the elderly as well (Urton, 1991).

Gelles (1982) comments that unsafe physical environments are commonly found in homes of abusive and neglectful families, thus connecting the physical with the psychosocial contexts. Whether strong control methods are used to prevent children from playing with dangerous objects (electrical wires and outlets, cleaning supplies, etc.) or are incidental to this play needs to be studied. Tertinger et al. (1984) attempted to do this, correcting methodological weaknesses of prior studies in this area. The authors developed a Home Accident Prevention Inventory (HAPI) to measure the type and quantity of hazardous items accessible to children in various locations in the home, so as to have a before-and-after measure of the effects of a preventive training program. Six families were invited to participate in childproofing their homes, which included training and several home visits by a counselor. Families provided written permission for these visits, including specifying some off-limit areas that would not be accessed.

The childproofing strategies involved telling parents three ways to make household hazards less accessible to children:

1. Using child-resistant closures, such as caps over electric outlets and safety caps on medicines
2. Locking up items
3. Keeping items out of the reach of children

An analysis of the family's home was made and the family was informed that it had, say, nine hazards in a specific category (the least number of hazards of any of the categories so that clients would be more likely to achieve early success in correcting these hazards). The counselor practiced with the first item, employing one of the three strategies mentioned above, and then asked the client to think of how to handle the other items. In this way, training was provided along with positive reinforcement and instructions to make the corrections on the other hazards before the next weekly visit. On subsequent visits, additional target categories were addressed. Further positive reinforcement was given when parents met a 50% reduction criterion for a given category. Uncorrected targets were added to the next week's list. After criteria had been met in all categories, the counselor terminated the training program but continued to have unannounced follow-up visits. Results show that the education-feedback training package produced gradual reduction of hazards in given categories, but with no generalization to other categories.

On a more general level, Peterson and Mori (1985) and their colleagues (Peterson, Mori, Selby, & Rosen, 1988) describe a general approach to prevention of child injury, using the classic public health triad:

1. Host characteristics: Children most likely to have accidents are boys, active children, children from single-parent families or young mothers, and children from large families.
2. Agent characteristics: Most common agents of child injury are automobile accidents, drowning, burns, ingestion of harmful substances, and falls.
3. Environmental characteristics: The home and the automobile are the most frequent locations for injury, especially under conditions of stress such as relocation or birth of sibling and in absence of appropriate adult supervision.

Peterson and Mori (1985) note, however, that such a model is not useful for individual interventions; they offer a modified model that focuses on the target of intervention, a method for introducing change, and a tactic for connecting the intervention to the target. The methods of introducing change are categorized as *mandated/legislative* or as *educational/persuasive* (p. 587). Either method may be conducted on an active or passive basis—that is, involving some action on the part of the person being protected or involving no action by that person because some aspect of the physical or social environment was modified to be protecting. The tactics for connecting target and intervention have been articulated by Caplan (1964) as (a) population-wide preventive services, (b) services directed only toward those who have reached a certain common milestone of development, or (c) services given to people at high risk (see also American Medical Association Council on Scientific Affairs, 1989, regarding the prevention of firearm injuries. Roberts & Peterson's, 1984, anthology on the prevention of problems in childhood employs this same useful threefold categorization).

Peterson and Mori (1985) note that most preventive services directed toward agents are legislated, employ passive means, are used on a population-wide basis, and are generally effective—the Poison Prevention Packaging

Act of 1981 being a case in point. Education is a common approach taken toward either caretakers or children; population-wide methods (like television messages) tend to be relatively ineffective, whereas milestone approaches show better results (e.g., influencing parents of newborns to use automobile seat restraints).

Some of the greatest areas of need regarding injury prevention are exactly those not shown to employ effective methods, such as a young child crossing a busy intersection by himself or herself or being home alone when a fire breaks out. These are targets requiring active strategies delivered through educational means. Peterson and Mori (1985) use the example of the latch-key child (one with working parents who comes home from school to an empty house). The task is to teach a wide range of safety behaviors to these children in a short time using paraprofessionals so as to be a cost-effective method. Peterson and Mori present evidence that it is possible to teach these skills. It is also possible to add a social dimension to this problem, as in some kind of telephone assurance system whereby children call adults or high school students trained to respond to ordinary and emergency concerns. (Phone-a-friend projects sometimes employ older students who learn to make a valued contribution to the well-being of others. This constitutes a kind of helper principle. See Chapter 4, III.A.1; see also Guyer et al., 1989; Pless & Arsenault, 1987.) For other topics, see preventive efforts related to back injuries among workers (Wollenberg, 1989), airplane safety (Williams, Solomon, & Bartone, 1988), automobile safety (Simpson, 1987; Zador & Ciccone, 1993), safety on playgrounds (Bond & Peck, 1993), safety issues regarding solar protection (Girgis, Sanson-Fisher, & Watson, 1994), mining safety (Fox et al., 1987), and an injury prevention program in an urban black community (Schwartz et al., 1993).

2. Protection: The Ordinary Hazards of Modern Life

One experiences many hazards in the course of daily life that are so much a part of existence that one may not recognize them as problematic. Consider noise. Monahan and Vaux (1980) discuss the effects of noise on human behavior—a "cacophony of sounds from an endless variety of sources" (p. 28), especially in urban environments. Glass and Singer (1972) show that noise is likely to disrupt the performance of complex tasks that require concentration but not the performance of simple tasks

(Ewigman, Kivlahan, Hosokawa, & Horman, 1990). Monahan and Vaux summarize the research of Cohen, Evans, Krantz, and Stokols (1980), who compared elementary school children from four schools that were in the flight path of the Los Angeles International Airport with similar children not in the flight path. The findings:

> Children in the "noise" schools showed elevated blood-pressure levels, were more likely to fail at a cognitive task, and seemed to "give up" trying to solve it, suggesting a reduced motivation and a lessened sense of personal control over events (Seligman, 1975). The children were more susceptible to auditory distraction the longer they had attended the noisy schools. There was no evidence of adaptation with prolonged exposure to noise. (Monahan & Vaux, 1980, p. 29)

Another significant aspect of noise is its insidious effect on a person's hearing. Sustained loud noises, such as those heard in industrial situations, performing in a band, or listening to loud music over long periods of time, can produce irreversible damage to the delicate structure of the inner ear. Protection from excessive noise is useful to reduce these harmful effects, but their awkwardness frequently interferes with people using these precautions. Jazzier designs and marketing are needed, such as "ear-condoms" for "safer listening." In addition, the social skills to be able to turn down amplification can be taught ("Just say No-ise").

Likewise, it is possible to discuss other ordinary features of modern life that present problems, such as population density and crowding (Freedman, 1975; Ittelson et al., 1974; Schorr, 1963); height of living quarters; distance from social facilities; and location in geographic and social areas. In these cases, one can attempt to make changes in the individuals involved, in the environmental factors themselves, or both.

Robertson (1986) has made many contributions to the prevention literature with regard to injury control. He provides a summary of 10 strategies applicable to a wide range of hazards that involve the physical environment and objects in it. He uses the general term *energy* to refer to any kind of activity or behavior that is potentially harmful.

1. Prevent the accumulation of objects that expend energy in hazardous concentrations (i.e., objects whose use is harmful). Examples include large numbers of handguns or hazardous road and off-road vehicles

V, VI. The Fifth and Sixth Dimensions

(motorcycles, minibikes) whose functions raise risk levels to users and others (Bachrach et al., 1989).

2. Reduce the concentrations of hazardous amounts of energy. For example, limit the mass and top-speed capabilities of road vehicles and lower the maximum temperature in water heaters (Katcher, 1987).

3. Prevent the release of energy that has been concentrated in hazardous amounts. For example, increase skid resistance of road surfaces and the breaking capability of vehicles and make matches and containers of flammable liquids difficult for children to use.

4. Modify the rate or spatial distribution of energy from its source. Common examples are use of seat belts and child restraints for all occupants of moving vehicles (Geller, 1990; Zador & Ciccone, 1993) and automatic ventilation in motor vehicles and other structures where poisonous gases may accumulate.

5. Separate in time and space the energy and those to be protected. For instance, remove pedestrian and bike paths from roads; place trees, utility poles, and other rigid objects away from roadsides; evacuate populations when hurricanes or flash floods are predicted.

6. Interpose a physical barrier between the energy and those to be protected. Examples include condoms, air bags in vehicles, crash helmets for motorcyclists and bicyclists ("Protective Role of Bicycle Safety Helmet Confirmed," 1994), and unscalable fences around swimming pools and water-filled quarries.

7. Modify basic qualities of the energy or its exchange with vulnerable populations. For instance, eliminate pointed knobs or edges in interiors or buildings or on transportation vehicles; provide soft floor coverings in housing for the aged and on playgrounds for young children (Bond & Peck, 1993); place free condoms in private restrooms rather than public waiting rooms to increase the chances of their being taken (Amass, Bickel, Higgins, Budney, & Foerg, 1993).

8. Make those to be protected more resistant to energy exchanges. Some examples of these are exercise programs for groups vulnerable to falls, such as the elderly, and providing blood-clotting factors to persons with hemophilia.

9. Begin to counter damage already done. Prevention often slides into early treatment. Although training people to be aware of problematic situations is useful preventive training, they should also be trained to give emergency aid, such as stopping hemorrhaging or not moving people who

may have suffered spinal injuries. But in a direct prevention line, it also means to replace smoke detectors and fire extinguishers after use, require underwater lights in pools, and install roadside emergency telephones at critical areas.

10. Stabilize, repair, and rehabilitate the injured person. In this case, treatment slides into rehabilitation, as when prosthetic devices are used for injured persons or when work and living areas are redesigned for the physically handicapped.

Each of these principles can be used in many different ways to prevent problems when people interact in physical environments, which always occurs. It takes some creative imagination to derive specific instances of the everyday world from these abstract principles, but this translation of theory to practice is exactly what primary prevention is all about.

3. Promotion: Goodness of Fit Between Person and Environment

This final section discussing the dimension of the physical environment will also pull together some of the major themes that have run through these pages.

Although people are intrinsically social animals, we also need time and space to ourselves: privacy. Like sleep, privacy restores individuality, permits a sorting out of the pressures and opportunities of everyday life and long-term decision making, and revitalizes autonomy (self-control) in the face of social control. For these global and philosophical reasons, environments, especially built environments, must exist that permit all persons to have some privacy at some time: The infant needs respite from the stimulation of the doting parent; the child needs relief from the flood of demands made by peers and parents; the adolescent needs privacy to explore the mysteries of growth and development and share these secrets with chums; adults need to get away from their social roles and obligations to rediscover themselves and their personal sense of direction; the elderly who may have too much privacy forced on them by the deaths of friends and the relocation of family need privacy as a mark of independence and a temple for reminiscence.

One finds these private places whenever one can; it behooves planners and builders and social directors of all types to facilitate privacy in a public world, not as an end in itself but to cleanse the palate of sociability.

Healthy functioning may be promoted at a private retreat, a vacation (among crowds of strangers, which is privacy of a different kind, a change of pace), a respite service (baby-sitter or full-fledged service that takes care of a dependent while individuals collect their energies and strengths—see Valentine & Andreas, 1984), a quiet chapel, a room in the house with a door that can be closed, even meditation in a noisy room.

People define defensible space through such measures. They defend what is at their core at this moment. It could be a cardboard box into which the child crawls and permits no one to enter. It could be one person's home (= castle). It could be a housing development with guarded gates keeping out intruders (Newman, 1972). People find or build spaces that they define as worthy of defending in order to defend themselves.

Environmental psychologists, community psychologists, social psychiatrists, social workers, and other helping professionals seek to promote the goodness of fit between the individual and the environment. This fit may be accomplished in many ways, possibly simultaneously. One can change the individual, the social network, and/or the physical environment. Each change in one system will have reverberations in the others, requiring rebalancing the whole. More likely, all these changes will occur by degree, in part because of the interrelatedness of all things in the ecological system.

Goodness of fit is not a final state but a relative homeostatic balance in a sea of change. One must continually reconsider this fit and make suitable adaptations in persons, groups, and environments. With the physical environment, at least, a major element of goodness of fit is more under planned control.

I would like to conclude this chapter by discussing a fascinating paper on creating a good fit between a physical environment and the service goals. Cotton and Geraty (1984) describe their experience in translating clinical concepts into architectural and interior design plans and vice versa. Although this example focuses on a psychiatric unit for youngsters (age 4 to 12 years old) who have serious problems such as suicidal behavior, stealing, and school adjustment difficulties or who have been victims of child abuse, it is so filled with ideas about goodness of fit that it may serve as well to stimulate the imagination of people in primary prevention.

Conventional mental hospital designs often convey negative, antitherapeutic messages according to Cotton and Geraty (1984). These authors and their interdisciplinary colleagues were given the opportunity to design an ideal psychiatric setting for children when the children's unit of a larger hospital was to undergo renovation. They began by using a Design Log Technique (Spivak, 1978), in which clinicians described what behaviors typically occurred in general settings—activities room, quiet room, bedrooms, bathrooms. Designers clarified the priorities and goals of each setting and tried to translate these into space usage. Local codes and federal specifications for building were factored into the designs as well. Observations were collected and reviewed by staff and patients, especially with regard to the feasibility of good ideas.

Cotton and Geraty (1984) used the treatment goals for the psychiatric clients to organize their presentation; primary prevention professionals will have to adapt these goals to their own ends. For example, "Goal 2. To provide spaces that represent a continuum of external controls and can be adapted to the needs of individual patients and groups of patients as they fluctuate in their capacity to use internal controls" (p. 629). To attain this goal, the planners had to resolve the dilemma of providing a safe (controlled) environment versus one that offered freedom and openness. This is both a clinical and an architectural dilemma, to offer protection and safety at the same time as being warm and nonpunitive. For example, the locked door (control) was made of Plexiglas (openness). There was no door for the kitchen on the unit (openness), but the drawers were locked (control). Cabinets with play materials were open—except when the children were out of control. The quiet rooms were designed to be safe (with tamperproof screws, carpet that was glued to the floor, the absence of ingestible, sharp, or throwable objects), but also warm and cozy (warm colors, no bars, cloth hangings on the walls). These quiet rooms served multiple functions so as to avoid association with bad behavior. The layout was planned to enable children to spend time alone (for freedom and privacy) but near the staff space (for security). Closets have air vents (to prevent suffocation) and shower rods break away at 30 pounds (to prevent hanging). Each small component of the therapeutic environment as well as each broad feature of that setting was carefully considered by all relevant parties, discussed, debated for feasibility, and tried in practice—and presumably modified when the unexpected occurred.

It is with such care and attempted foresight that primary prevention must influence the building and use of environments (see also Becker, 1985). Permit me one last speculation, on the prevention-oriented nursery:

V, VI. The Fifth and Sixth Dimensions

The nursery is the baby's special place for care and love, protection and stimulation, rest and restoration. It does not have to be a big and fancy room, but it should have certain features that provide for the prevention of predictable hazards, the protection of existing states of health and healthy functioning, and the promotion of desired developmental objectives.

The crib should contain a hard (very firm) mattress with a thin mattress pad for comfort. A flexible rubber pad should be under a sheet to deal with inevitable wettings. Both sheets and pad should be cleaned periodically. The sides of the crib should be open enough to permit the infant to see out but closed enough not to allow the baby's head from getting caught between the bars. These sides should be firm enough to support the child's attempts to lift himself or herself, but strong and high enough to discourage scaling the walls. The whole crib should be capable of being cleaned and sanitized.

The child will spend a great portion of the day in the crib during the first year of life, and so for the times the child is lying on his or her back, there should be an eye-catching object above the bed. Mobiles are nice, with their constant motion with the air currents, but any object (a stuffed toy, a cloth with varied colors or objects on it mounted as a picture) will attract attention. (Avoid small objects, like Christmas lights or jewelry, which, if they fall into the baby's hands may end up in the baby's mouth.)

The floor is another place where babies spend considerable time. A soft rug or carpet on the floor gives traction to the beginning crawler and is easier on the parents who spend time on the floor with their infant. Whatever the covering, the floor should be clean because babies put their hands into their mouths frequently, along with whatever else happens to be on the floor.

There should be a storage box for toys, both to encourage the future chores of helping to put toys away and to prevent the parents from breaking their necks falling over a toy. Having the toys out should be a sign of play; putting them away should be a sign of rest. Different toys, age graded and childproof (i.e., accident resistant), are stimuli of great importance to a child, but equally so is the interaction that translates a colored object into a meaningful experience (Levenstein, 1988).

There should be wall decorations to please the eye and distract the child during times of diaper changes or dressing. Cloth hangings with clear pictures of animals and things are good for their aesthetics as well as educational potentialities. Whether objects are hand drawn, cut from magazines, or purchased from a specialty store makes little difference to the child new to the experience. Mirrors on the wall hold a special interest for the infant who is coming to distinguish himself or herself from others and has endless fascination with moving people.

Screens should be on the windows, preventing people and insects from going in or out. There should be enough light to see clearly when cleaning child and room and enough subdued light to change day into night when sleep is called for. Nightlights enable parents to peek in without disturbing the child. Caps or coverings should be on the electric wall outlets, and locks should be on the doors of cabinets. Chairs for late-night feedings should be the type that toddlers can safely climb on as they learn the variety of skills of balance and locomotion.

This ideal baby's room I have described is as ordinary as the nursery for my grandson, and yet his parents have thoughtfully arranged these "necessary" things to serve as "preventive, protective, and promotive" things. This was done, not for the sake of primary prevention, but in the name of common sense and a user-friendly arrangement of things in space. It is easy to see how each choice of item in the room has been made with an eye to multiple purposes. There is no conspicuous "prevention" tool in the room (unless it is the intercom that enables the parents to hear the child cry, cough, sneeze, or otherwise to indicate a need for help). They have independently discovered a great truth about primary prevention, that it can be *exhilirating* to protect the baby's existing state of health and healthy functioning and to promote desired growth and development.

V, VI. The Fifth and Sixth Dimensions

7

Systematic Applications of Primary Prevention Methods

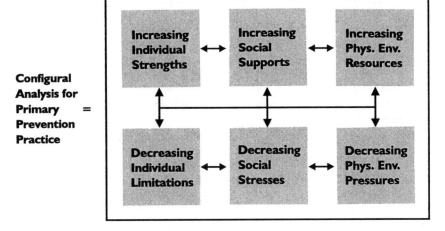

Configural Analysis for Primary Prevention Practice =

Figure 7.1. The Configural Equation

This final chapter presents some general strategies for thinking about the configuration of structures and forces acting on any target of primary prevention and for selecting which of the many tactics are most relevant to the task at hand. This chapter illustrates an approach to systemic thinking that moves away from linear decision making toward a method that incorporates the configuration of relevant events.

A. The Configural Equation as Both a Conceptual and a Practice Tool
B. The Conceptual Task: What Do We Want to Achieve?

A. The Configural Equation as Both a Conceptual and a Practice Tool

Our ordinary language is linear: Words and sentences follow one after the other in a long stream that represents our thoughts and feelings. We often turn to pictures or objects to illustrate simultaneous occurrences; with the advent of computerized drawings, these pictures can also be endowed with movement—the turning, twisting views of a car or rocket as viewed on television, for example. But we face new difficulties when we try to portray complex social interactions that occur over time—the very task we must accomplish when we propose a primary prevention program.

The configural equation may serve as both a conceptual tool and a tool for practice. To support this assertion, I will present the outline of a primary prevention project to emphasize both the conceptual and the practice tasks, each of which employs the configural equation.

Imagine that we want to achieve some goal in primary prevention, for example, preventing unwanted teenage pregnancy. Furthermore, assume that we have applied for and received a modest grant that will supply all the resources we will need (or be able to use) in the project. Say that we received 100 units of energy-purchasing power (EPP), that is, we can pay for the salaries of personnel and the resources they need to perform their services. (For simplicity, I will not include expenditures on routine matters such as office space or secretarial supplies.) The essential point of this illustration is to show how we may spend those 100 units of EPP in the most cost-effective manner possible. This means we will spend it on those aspects of the situation that we think are most important in preventing unwanted teenage pregnancy and are amenable to our efforts at influencing these events.

B. The Conceptual Task:
What Do We Want to Achieve?

The preventive problem-solving process directs us to consider the nature of the problem or potential we seek to understand and to change in some constructive ways. This conceptual question must come before the question of practice because whatever we eventually do will be done on the basis of how we understand the nature of the problem or potential and its causal context. Specifically, What is unwanted teenage pregnancy and what causes it? The way we conceive possible answers to both questions will direct how we look at and act toward adolescents and their contexts.

1. Definition of Terms

What is unwanted teenage pregnancy? The definition seems simple enough but in fact there are gray areas, as with young people who have babies because they see this as a means of getting out of an intolerable living situation (even though they may be getting into an even more intolerable one). And what are teenagers? Is the 11-year-old sexually active girl to be included in the project? Is a 30-year-old man who impregnates teenagers to be included? What if the culture from which these pregnant adolescents come values children highly and does not consider illegitimacy or nonmarriage a problem? For whom is unwanted pregnancy a problem? The distant taxpayer who eventually pays the bills? The "moral community" that disfavors promiscuous, precocious, and unsafe sexuality? The young woman herself, because her life script may be now largely written in negative terms? The biological father who may or may not have intended this outcome? The innocent baby? These are vexing questions but ones that must be resolved before the project begins.

2. Analysis of Causal Context

The next basic question, at the heart of any scientific understanding and action with regard to the event, is about the causal context. Notice that when we consider the conceptual meaning of the term *unwanted teenage pregnancy,* we in effect consider the definition from the point of view of the various parties in the configuration—persons, groups, cultures, society in particular. These questions seem reasonable ones to ask, and this is the point I want to make: The configural equation is a shorthand summary of perspectives that should be considered in understanding a problem conceptually and in planning what strategies to use to influence involved parties and situations in making constructive changes.

Let's apply this configural equation to an analysis of the causal context. Causal contexts are extremely complex; we may know only a small fraction of the relevant structures and forces in a situation. We make use of three sets of experiences to understand the causal factors with regard to a topic: theories about this topic (or about behavior in general, which then are applied to this topic); empirical research; and personal or borrowed experiences. For all three, probably the best source of information comes from a literature search that contains relevant materials on theories, research, and recorded practice wisdom. To begin the literature search, we need a conceptual definition and the understanding of the meaning of the context so as to make sense of what we read others have done.

I will supply a brief literature search derived from the work of McAnarney and Schreider (1984) and others. I read these reviews of possible causal factors and then categorized them by means of the configural equation—which of the proposed causal explanations are related to personal factors, which are related to small or large group factors, which are related to cultural factors, and so on. There has been so much work on teen pregnancy that it is easy to place most of the ideas into one or more categories. But if some category is not filled, then another important use of the configural equation is to try to imagine what events of this categorical type might be involved in causing unwanted teenage pregnancy. Thus the configural equation may serve as a way of categorizing the information one finds in the literature, but it may also prompt one to look for or imagine new ideas as well.

Table 7.1 contains a literature review of factors presumed to be associated with unwanted teenage pregnancy. Note that these 25 factors are divided into the categories of the configural equation but are numbered sequentially for ease of use. It is a mixed bag; some factors appear to be objective empirical statements whereas others are more speculative. This represents the best available information about factors in unwanted teenage pregnancy; we must sort through it to decide which factors, if any, we would consider the most likely causal factors for which we have a chance of making constructive changes.

Table 7.1 Literature Review of Factors Presumed to Be Associated With Unwanted Teenage Pregnancy

A. Personal Factors: Cognitive
1. Teenager may lack knowledge about human anatomy, particularly human sexuality as related to conception and contraception.
2. Teenager may hold "myths" about sexuality (e.g., "use it or lose it" or "pregnancy cannot happen the first time").
3. Teenager's conceptual equipment to see the broader picture or long-range implications of actions may be inadequate or limited.
4. Teenager may not expect to have sex on a given date and hence may not be prepared or have taken precautions.

B. Personal Factors: Affective
5. Teenager may be impulsive in sexual behavior, with limited ability to delay gratification.
6. Teenager may be self-centered in sexual activities, and thus disregard the rights and feelings of the partner.
7. Preparing in advance for sexual behavior may raise self-images of being "sexually active" with its negative cultural (and self) definition, even though not preparing in advance may have very negative implications.
8. Solo masturbation, although widely used to relieve sexual tension, is limited by culturally generated guilt and restrictive social norms.
9. Having a baby may be seen as a way to establish a lasting relationship or to get out of an oppressive home situation.

C. Personal Factors: Behavioral
10. Teenager may lack the interpersonal skills to say "no" in ways that do not cut off desired social contacts.
11. Teenager may have difficulties in obtaining effective contraceptive devices, even after barriers of location, cost, and cultural pressures are considered.
12. Sex may be influenced by the use of illegal or legal substances, thus putting sexually active substance users in double jeopardy.

D. Social Systems: Primary Group Experiences
13. Peers tend to encourage peers in the direction of boundary-pushing autonomy as part of the necessary tasks of becoming an adult, including sexual explorations.
14. Peer groups exert pressure toward conformity to peer norms that may include sexual activity at a rate faster than the individual may wish to proceed.
15. Being away from home (at college, in the army) means that youths are suddenly offered peer group norms as guides to behavior, including active but unsafe sexuality.
16. Homosexual youths encounter negative experiences not only from many of their peers but from a homophobic society, which may lead them into unsafe compensatory heterosexual activities.

(continued)

Table 7.1   Literature Review of Factors Presumed to Be Associated With Unwanted
Teenage Pregnancy (Continued)

E.   Social Systems: Secondary Groups, Institutions, and Society
   17. Mass media glorifies sexual activity in "the young and the restless" without
       portraying the full range of sexual and love relationships and responsibilities.
   18. Culture and society promote differential sexual mores and expectations,
       which produce conflicts in the relationships between young men and
       women.
   19. Sexuality may be caught up in other social factors, such as prostitution for
       drug money.
   20. Sexual violation occurs in large numbers, from date rape to stranger-rape,
       incest, and spousal and child sexual abuse.
   21. Laws and court decisions may affect the social climate about sexual
       behavior in healthy or unhealthy ways.
F.   Physical Environment and Time Factors
   22. The distribution in space of eligible partners may create stresses in
       speeding up or slowing down sexual explorations.
   23. Accessibility to protective devices, along with sociocultural mores, may
       inhibit safe and healthy sexual development.
   24. Access to suitable locations where young people may meet without the
       pressures to engage in sexual activity may be limited.
   25. Historic time periods may be more or less liberal or conservative,
       affecting the experiences and expectations young people have as they
       move into adult sexual roles.

SOURCE: McAnarney and Schrieder (1984).

As you look over Table 7.1, many of the 25 items may seem intuitively appealing; one may be able to think of immediate ways to prevent these from happening or to promote the constructive opposites. But we must suspend these automatic intuitive reactions until we have had time to work through the model I am proposing and then test these results with intuitive responses.

We have been given 100 units of EPP to address one or more of the presumed causal factors. Obviously, we cannot address all of them lest we spread our efforts too thinly. So we must choose major causal factors and then figure out how many EPP units we wish to spend in reducing or eliminating a given factor. For example, if we believe that Factor 1, lack of knowledge about human anatomy, is critical, then we have chosen a conceptual objective to address with regard to the specific content area. That is, we view the way people understand the world as a prime aspect in how they behave in that world. (Again, suspend your active mind from thinking what you will do—that is a question of methods, to which I will return shortly.) Or we may believe that Factor 10, lack of interpersonal skills to say no, is a critical factor and so we may choose to spend some of our EPP on this personal communication skill.

For sake of argument, suppose these are the two major parts of our project. Let's examine what we have done. We have made a conceptual decision on the network of major factors leading to unwanted teenage pregnancy and from this decision will follow the entire set of tactics for dealing with these matters. This is perfectly respectable, although you may be questioning the particular contents of my suggested theory of unwanted teen pregnancy. The point is that it is the prerogative of the theorist or practitioner to make these choices—and live with the consequences that follow in the course of the project.

This seems like a reasonable plan of action, one that may sound familiar to readers of the unwanted teen pregnancy (UTP) literature. But as part of a configural analysis, we can see that the project involves two kinds of personal-oriented factors and ignores the sociocultural aspects and the physical environmental aspects. We cannot be all things to all people, but is the original selection the wisest one possible?

The configural philosophy holds that each category of causal factors is potentially important and should be considered in one's thinking about any primary prevention plan. As with a restaurant menu, you must think about and possibly select at least one item from category A, one from category B, and one from category C to have a well-balanced meal—or a well-balanced project in primary prevention.

Let us go back to the list of possible causal factors and decide whether or not we wish to consider factors from other domains in the configural equation. This time, we find that Factor 14, peer pressure into premature unsafe sexual activity, and Factor 17, mass media glorifying (unsafe) sexual activity, are important enough to consider as part of our project.

Now we have a more complete configural analysis of the causes of unwanted teenage pregnancy in our community. We are saying that personal factors in combination with peer group factors and cultural factors influence the rate of unwanted teenage pregnancy. It would be immodest to call this a theory, but at least it is a set of interrelated hypotheses.

We are not yet ready to go to the large number of strategies and tactics listed in Chapters 2 through 6. Next we need to specify more clearly the conceptual weight each of these presumed causal factors carries with regard to unwanted teenage pregnancy. Some factors may be causally more important than others. It is to these factors that we will use the greater amount of our EPP units, assuming that each factor is equally easy to influence. We have selected these four factors because we believe they are, individually, important in the causal nexus. Now I want to raise a new kind of question: How important are these four factors within this set itself? We take our 100 EPP units and weigh the conceptual importance of these factors in relationship to each other. We could rate them all equally—25 a piece. Or we could rate one or two as more important than the others; for example, Factors 10 and 14 (social skills and peer pressures) might be seen as more immediately connected to the actions related to unwanted pregnancy and thus merit increased attention. The other two are important but less so for this particular project. Perhaps we assign 5 EPP units to join a coalition of agencies trying to modify TV broadcasting in more socially and sexually responsible ways. Maybe the public schools already have a sex education course and only need funds to purchase teaching aids relevant to their curriculum and our project plans as well, and so for 10 EPP units we can address these cultural issues—albeit lightly.

With the remaining 85 EPP units, we could divide them equally or in some other distribution. Let's examine these options. Conceptually, it appears possible to argue that the ability to communicate effectively in groups is both a skill in its own right and an active force in shaping group norms. Thus we have conceptually linked Factors 10 and 14, and might consider spending all 85 EPP units on a program that combines communication skills and group pressures. Or we could spend half on each factor separately on the grounds that they are distinct skills or events. If we thought one were more important than the other, then we might spend the preponderance of the units on that one. The point is that how we define the conceptual situation is the guideline for how we are going to act.

C. The Practice Task: Which Tactics Offer the Best Opportunity for Achieving Objectives?

Assuming we have completed our conceptual task, the next issue concerns selecting the most relevant tactics to achieve these goals and objectives. Chapters 2 through 6 present some 50 major strategies and numerous other minor tactics. How can we review this rich source of methods to best attain our goals?

The answer is partly given to us by the way we conceptualized the problem. First, we discovered we wanted to use personal factors and then we decided on primary group and cultural contexts. The two major causal factors are from personal and primary group domains, and so we can look at those domains as sources of preventive or promotive methods. We want to increase social skills, and so we should look at the dimension of the configural model that addresses increasing individual strengths (Dimension I, Chapter 2), where we find a category on social skills training.

The second major conceptual factor involves reducing the peer group pressures toward unwise sexual activity, which may be conceptually linked to Dimension IV, Chapter 5, or, viewed in another direction, it may be linked to Dimension III, Chapter 4, which addresses increasing social supports (for safer sex). Because the peer group variable does not clearly fall into Dimension III or IV, we should consider them both in looking for methods to decrease group pressures toward unwise sexual behavior or to increase group supports toward wise expression of sexual behaviors.

Let's continue with the peer group variable, because it does not have an immediate home within the list of preventive tactics. We can begin to narrow down what portions of these two dimensions (and chapters) are most relevant to practice considerations. Reviewing the headings, we can see some relevance of Dimension III, A. Interpersonal Aspects, 3. Friendship; B. Primary Group Aspects, 2. Natural Helping Networks. Likewise, Dimension IV, A. Interpersonal Aspects, 1. Aid From Peers; and B. Primary Group Aspects, 1. The Buffering Function, may be useful to consider.

What we want, in effect, is some way to cool off the primary group pressure for premature sexuality while at the same time trying to increase positive peer pressure toward more wholesome activities equally pleasurable but without negative consequences. Positive peer groups are supposed to buffer their members against harmful stresses and pressures from outsiders; somehow, some peer groups deliver the stresses (toward premature unsafe sexuality) rather than buffering members from these pressures. Is there a way to turn this around? What can a group do as a group that gives pleasure to its members without endangering those members? There are examples of efforts to redirect group goals toward social service (helping others, such as in peer tutoring) or toward personal growth and development (as in recreational activities, new experiences with yoga, or biofeedback). Group contingencies may be used to motivate errant members to join in prosocial developments. There are many strategies for increasing (constructive) social supports while decreasing (destructive) social demands. What particular choices one makes depends on the nature of the audience, one's own resources, and related factors.

The general point is that connecting a preventive tactic to a conceptual mapping of the problem is not automatic or mechanical; structured leads use the configural model to focus the search in particular areas.

D. Conclusion

Let's review the whole preventive problem-solving process. We have become aware of a significant social challenge and we have sought to understand what this challenge is and the likely causal factors affecting it. In this, we stand on the shoulders of giants who have provided us with large amounts of information. But we must design our projects to fit local conditions. Let us say, in connection with preventing unwanted teen pregnancy, that we create a special workshop in the school setting on both skills training and the promotion of constructive peer pressure. To do this, we need some umbrella term that deals with the strengths of the teenagers, does not stigmatize those who may be at high risk, and motivates joining and adherence. Suppose we choose the label "Teen Strategies—Good Ways for Better Living"—"Teen Strategies," for short. We set up special workshops after school (but also open during the day, when students may have free time) to deliver strategies that are fun and socially useful. Constructing these takes up 85 points, divided about equally between the personal and peer level targets. We get at the interpersonal skills through the medium of the group and we encourage the group members to be true to their own values as well as be sensitive to the values of others.

We set up the study and pretest a large group of teens invited to the first series of workshops and an equivalent number of teens (selected at random) invited to wait until space opens on these same workshops—and thus who constitute a waiting list type of control group. We implement Phase 1, providing the experimental group with the strategies workshop, and then measure both groups at the conclusion of this phase to see if there are perceptible differences in attitudes and actions between the two groups. Assuming that the experimental group is more able than the controls to say "no" gracefully and to be able to control group pressures, then the waiting list group gets the same workshops and a third testing period occurs, at which time the control group has caught up with the experimental group on these two factors, which are conceptualized as being causally relevant for unwanted teenage pregnancy. (We discover, after the fact, that we cannot control which students get the sex education classes; they all get them at about the same time, and thus experimental and control students learn more about anatomy and other matters. This may produce some changes in earlier measures, but it will be constant between the experiment and control groups.) Thus we have made our selection of causal factors, constructed a practice and evaluation design to see if discernible results emerge as a result of using these assumptions, and are pleased to discover the results support our hypotheses.

The possible permutations on 25 variables are very large, so that the act of constructing a prevention project requires a high degree of creativity and fortitude. We could very well be wrong, which is to say we have selected lesser factors and have not given greater factors the emphasis they require. But we will never know this until we or others test changing the target variables.

The possible permutations on 50 primary prevention practices are also very large and require thoughtful application of the specific method to the specific situation. Again, we may not have selected the best strategy for the given situation, but only time will tell, because our selected strategy showed some empirical support in the literature.

In this book I have tried to illustrate the variety of ways the configural perspective can guide thinking about how to conceptualize and how to practice primary prevention. This approach offers a checklist of possible causal factors based on what the literature and our own background lead us to believe is the best available information. The checklist of system factors is a contribution of the configural approach; the possible causal factors for this specific target is courtesy of the hard work involved in doing a literature review. The configural philosophy of addressing multiple causal influences at different system levels is the product of many observers who recognize the necessity of thinking in a systemic fashion. The specific weighing of factors and how they are implemented in the real world is your contribution.

APPENDIX A

Primary Prevention Sources

I. Bibliographies and Indexes

Biegel, D., Farkas, K. J., Abell, N., Goodin, J., & Friendman, B. (1989). *Social support networks: A bibliography, 1983-1987.* Westport, CT: Greenwood.

Biegel, D. E., McCardle, E., & Mendelson, S. (1985). *Social networks and mental health: An annotated bibliography.* Beverly Hills, CA: Sage.

Bloom, M., & Buckner, J. C. (1989). The Journal of Primary Prevention Cumulative Index Project, 1980-1989. *Journal of Primary Prevention, 10*(1), 67-94.

Buckner, J. C., Trickett, E. J., & Corse, S. J. (1985). *Primary prevention in mental health: An annotated bibliography* (DHHS Publication No. ADM 85-1405). Washington, DC: Government Printing Office.

Kidder, M. G., Tinker, M. B., Mannino, F. V., & Trickett, E. J. (Compilers). (1986). An annotated reference guide to the consultation literature, 1978-1984. In F. V. Mannino, E. J. Trickett, M. F. Shore, M. G. Kidder, & G. Levin (Eds.), *Handbook of mental health consultation.* Washington, DC: U.S. Department of Health and Human Services.

Silverman, P. R. (1978). *Mutual help groups: A guide for mental health workers* (DHEW Publication No. ADM 78-646). Washington, DC: Government Printing Office.

II. Handbooks and Encyclopedias

Berlin, I. N., & Stone, L. A. (Eds.). (1979). *Basic handbook of child psychiatry* (Vol. 4). New York: Basic Books.

Edelstein, B. A., & Michelson, L. (Eds.). (1986). *Handbook of prevention.* New York: Plenum.

Felner, R. D., Jason, L. A., Moritsugu, J. N., & Farber, S. S. (Eds.). (1983). *Preventive psychology: Theory, research, and practice.* New York: Pergamon.

Glenwick, D. S., & Jason, L. A. (Eds.). (1993). *Promoting health and mental health in children, youth, and families.* New York: Springer.

Jeger, A. M., & Slotnick, R. S. (Eds.). (1982). *Community mental health and behavioral-ecology: A handbook of theory, research, and practice.* New York: Plenum.

Mannino, F. V., Trickett, E. J., Shore, M. F., Kidder, M. G., & Levin, G. (1986). *Handbook of mental health consultation* (DHHS Publication No. ADM 86-1446). Washington, DC: Government Printing Office

III. Books and Anthologies Reviewing Given Fields of Study or Methods

Arnowitz, E. (Ed.). (1982). *Prevention strategies for mental health.* New York: Prodist.

Bagwell, M., & Clements, S. (1985). *A political handbook for health professionals.* Boston: Little, Brown.

Biegel, D. E., & Naparstek, A. (Eds.). (1981). *Community support systems and mental health: Research, practice, and policy.* New York: Springer.

Brown, B. (Ed.). (1978). *Long-term gains from early intervention.* Boulder, CO: Westview.

Burchard, J. D., & Burchard, S. N. (Eds.). (1987). *Prevention of delinquent behavior* (Vol. 10). Newbury Park, CA: Sage.

Chernoff, R., & Lipschitz, D. A. (Eds.). (1988). *Health promotion and disease prevention in the elderly.* New York: Raven.

DiClemente, R. J., & Peterson, J. L. (1994). *Preventing AIDS: Theories and methods of behavioral intervention.* New York: Plenum.

Dryfoos, J. (1994). *Full-service schools: A revolution in health and social services for children, youth, and families.* San Francisco: Jossey-Bass.

Gartner, A., & Riessman, F. (1977). *Self-help in the human services.* San Francisco: Jossey-Bass.

Glasscote, R. M., Kohn, E., Beigel, A., Raber, M. F., Roeske, N., Cox, B. A., Raybin, J. B., & Bloom, B. L. (1980). *Preventing mental illness: Efforts and attitudes.* Washington, DC: Joint Information Service.

Gottlieb, B. H. (1983). *Social support strategies.* Beverly Hills, CA: Sage.

Greenspan, S. L. (1980). *Psychopathology and adaptation in infancy and early childhood: Principles of clinical diagnosis and preventive intervention.* Springfield, VA: NTIS.

Hampton, R. L., Gullotta, T. P., Adams, G. R., Potter, E. H., Jr., & Weissberg, R. P. (1993). *Family violence: Prevention and treatment.* Newbury Park, CA: Sage.

Hampton, R. L., Jenkins, P., & Gullotta, T. P. (Eds.). (1996). *When anger governs: Preventing violence in America.* Thousand Oaks, CA: Sage.

Insel, P. M. (1980). *Environmental variables and the prevention of mental illness.* Lexington, MA: Lexington.

Iscoe, I., Bloom, B., & Spielberger, C. (Eds.). (1977). *Community psychology in transition.* New York: Wiley.

Kennie, D. C. (1993). *Preventive care for elderly people.* Cambridge, UK: Cambridge University Press.

Ketterer, R. E., Bader, B., & Levy, M. (1980). *Strategies and skills for promoting mental health.* Beverly Hills, CA: Sage.

Last, J. M. (Ed.). (1980). *Maxey-Roxenau public health and preventive medicine* (11th ed.). New York: Appleton-Century-Crofts.

Lofquist, W. A. (1983). *Discovering the meaning of prevention: A practical approach to positive change.* Tuscon, AZ: AYD Publications.

McCormick, M. (Ed.). (1980). *Prevention of mental retardation and other developmental disabilities.* New York: Marcel Dekker.

Mednick, S. A., Baert, A. E., & Backmann, B. P. (1981). *Prospective longitudinal research: An empirical basis for the primary prevention of psychosocial disorders.* New York: Oxford University Press.

Miller, S. D., O'Neal, G. S., & Scott, C. (Eds.). (1982). *Primary prevention approaches to the development of mental health services for ethnic minorities: A challenge to social work education and practice.* New York: Council on Social Work Education.

Munoz, R. F., Snowden, L. R., & Kelly, J. G. (Eds.). (1979). *Social and psychological research in community settings.* San Francisco: Jossey-Bass.

Ng, L. K. Y., & Davis, D. L. (Eds.). (1981). *Strategies for public health: Promoting health and preventing disease.* New York: Van Nostrand Reinhold.

Oxford, J. (1990). *Community psychology: Theory and practice.* New York: John Wiley.

Perlmutter, F. (Ed.). (1982). *New directions for mental health services: Mental health promotion and primary prevention.* San Francisco: Jossey-Bass.

Ponterotto, J. G., & Pedersen, P. B. (1993). *Prevention prejudice: A guide for counselors and educators.* Newbury Park, CA: Sage.

Price, R. H., Ketterer, R. F., Bader, B. C., & Monahan, J. (Eds.). (1980). *Prevention in mental health: Research, policy, and practice.* Beverly Hills, CA: Sage.

Ritter, D. R. (Ed.). (1982). *Consultation, education, and prevention in community mental health.* Springfield, IL: Charles C Thomas.

Roberts, M., & Peterson, L. (Eds.). (1984). *Prevention of problems in childhood: Psychological research and applications.* New York: Wiley.

Schinke, S. P., & Gilchrist, L. D. (1984). *Life skills counseling with adolescents.* Baltimore: University Park Press.

Seiban, E. (Ed.). (1977). *New trends of psychiatry in the community.* Cambridge, MA: Ballinger.

Sepulveda, J., Fineberg, H., & Mann, J. (Eds.). (1992). *AIDS: Prevention through education: A world view.* New York: Oxford.

Shure, M. B., & Spivak, G. (1978). *Problem-solving techniques in childrearing.* San Francisco: Jossey-Bass.

Simon, B. L. (1994). *The empowerment tradition in American social work: A history.* New York: Columbia University Press.

Sprafkin, J., Swift, C., & Hess, R. (Eds.). (1983). *Rx television: Enhancing the preventive impact of TV.* New York: Haworth.

Weinstein, N. D. (Ed.). (1987). *Taking care: Understanding and encouraging self-protective behavior.* New York: Cambridge University Press.

World Health Organization. (1977). *Primary prevention of schizophrenia in high-risk groups: Report of a working group.* Copenhagen: Author.

Zigler, E., & Styfco, S. J. (1993). *Head Start and beyond: A national plan for extending childhood intervention.* New Haven, CT: Yale University Press.

Zigler, E., & Valentine, J. (Eds.). (1979). *Project Head Start: A legacy of the war on poverty.* New York: Free Press.

IV. Vermont Conferences on Primary Prevention of Psychopathology (in chronological order)

Albee, G. W., & Joffe, J. M. (1977). *Primary prevention of psychopathology* (Vol. 1). Hanover, NH: University Press of New England.

Forgays, D. G. (Ed.). (1978). *Environmental influences and strategies in primary prevention* (Vol. 2). Hanover, NH: University Press of New England.

Kent, M. W., & Rolf, J. E. (Eds.). (1979). *Social competence in children* (Vol. 3). Hanover, NH: University Press of New England.

Bond, L. A., & Rosen, J. C. (Eds.). (1980). *Competence and coping during adulthood* (Vol. 4). Hanover, NH: University Press of New England.

Joffe, J. M., & Albee, G. W. (Eds.). (1981a). *Prevention through political action and social change* (Vol. 5). Hanover, NH: University Press of New England.

Bond, L. A., & Joffe, J. M. (Eds.). (1982). *Facilitating infant and early childhood development* (Vol. 6). Hanover, NH: University Press of New England.

Albee, G. W., Gordon, S., & Leitenberg, H. (Eds.). (1983). *Promoting sexual responsibility and preventing sexual problems* (Vol. 7). Hanover, NH: University Press of New England.

Rosen, J. C., & Solomon, L. J. (Eds.). (1985). *Prevention in health psychology* (Vol. 8). Hanover, NH: University Press of New England.

Kessler, M., & Goldston, S. E. (Eds.). (1986). *A decade of progress in primary prevention* (Vol. 9). Hanover, NH: University Press of New England.

Burchard, J. D., & Burchard, S. N. (Eds.). (1987). *Prevention of delinquent behavior* (Vol. 10). Newbury Park, CA: Sage.

Albee, G. W., Joffe, J. M., & Dusenbury, L. A. (Eds.). (1988). *Prevention, powerlessness, and politics: Readings on social change.* Newbury Park, CA: Sage.

Bond, L. A., & Wagner, B. M. (Eds.). (1988). *Families in transition: Primary prevention programs that work* (Vol. 11). Newbury Park, CA: Sage.

Bond, L. A., & Compas, B. E. (Eds.). (1989). *Primary prevention and promotion in the schools* (Vol. 12). Newbury Park, CA: Sage.

Mays, V. M., Albee, G. W., & Schneider, S. F. (Eds.). (1989). *Primary prevention of AIDS: Psychological approaches* (Vol. 13). Newbury Park, CA: Sage.

Albee, G. W., Bond, L. A., & Monsey, T. V. C. (Eds.). (1992). *Improving children's lives: Global perspectives on prevention* (Vol. 14). Newbury Park, CA: Sage.

Kessler, M., Goldston, S. E., & Joffe, J. M. (Eds.). (1992). *The present and future of prevention: In honor of George W. Albee* (Vol. 15). Newbury Park, CA: Sage.

Bond, L. A., Cutler, S. J., & Grams, A. (Eds.). (1995). *Promoting successful and productive aging* (Vol. 16). Thousand Oaks, CA: Sage.

Journals That Regularly Cover Primary Prevention Topics

American Journal of Community Psychology
American Journal of Epidemiology
American Journal of Orthopsychiatry
American Journal of Public Health

Community Mental Health Journal
Health and Social Work
Health Policy Quarterly
Hospital and Community Psychiatry
Human Ecology
Journal of Community Psychology
Journal of Health and Social Behavior
Journal of Man-Environment Relations
Journal of Preventive Psychiatry
Journal of Primary Prevention
Prevention in Human Services
Preventive Medicine
Public Health Reports
Social Policy

Textbooks and Casebooks

Bloom, B. L. (1977). *Community mental health: A general introduction.* Monterey, CA: Brooks/Cole.

Bloom, M. (1981). *Primary prevention: The possible science.* Englewood Cliffs, NJ: Prentice Hall.

Levine, M., & Perkins, D. V. (1987). *Principles of community psychology: Perspectives and applications.* New York: Oxford University Press.

Perlmutter, F. (1982). *Mental health promotion and primary prevention.* San Francisco: Jossey-Bass.

Price, R. H., Cowen, E. L., Lorion, R. P., & Ramos-McKay, J. (Eds.). (1988). *14 ounces of prevention: A casebook for practitioners.* Washington, DC: American Psychological Association.

Schulberg, H. C., & Killilea, M. (Eds.). (1982). *The modern practice of community mental health.* San Francisco: Jossey-Bass.

Teaching Tools

Bowker, J. (Ed.). (1983). *Education for primary prevention in social work.* New York: Council on Social Work Education.

Downie, R. S., Fyfe, C., & Tannahill, A. (1990). *Health promotion: Models and values.* Oxford, UK: Oxford University Press.

Noble, M. (Ed.). (1981). *Primary prevention in mental health and social work: A sourcebook of curriculum and teaching materials.* New York: Council on Social Work Education.

Perlmutter, A. H. (Prod.). (1992). *An ounce of prevention* (Videotape, part of a telecourse, "The World of Abnormal Psychology"). Washington, DC: T. Levine Communications, Inc., & the Annenberg/Corporation for Public Broadcasting.

Governmental Documents

Bloom, B. L. (1985). *Stressful life event theory and research: Implications for primary prevention* (DHHS Publication No. ADM 85-1385). Washington, DC: Government Printing Office.

French, J. F., Fisher, C. C., & Costa, Jr., S. J. (Eds.). (1983). *Working with evaluators: A guide for drug abuse prevention grant managers* (DHHS Publication No. ADM 83-1233). Washington, DC: Government Printing Office.

French, J. F., & Kaufman, N. J. (Eds.). (1981). *Handbook for prevention evaluation guidelines* (DHHS Pub. No. [ADM] 81-1145). Washington, DC: Government Printing Office.

Goldstein, M. J. (Ed.). (1982). *Preventive intervention in schizophrenia: Are we ready?* (DHHS Publication No. ADM 82-111). Washington, DC: Government Printing Office.

Hinkle, L. E., Jr., & Loring, W. C. (1977). *The effects of the man-made environment on health and behavior*. Washington, DC: Government Printing Office.

Klein, D. C., & Goldston, S. E. (1977). Primary prevention: An idea whose time has come. *Proceedings of the Pilot Conference on Primary Prevention, April 24, 1976* (DHEW Publication No. ADM 77-447). Washington, DC: Government Printing Office.

Manson, S. P. (Ed.). (1982). *New directions in prevention among American Indians and Alaska Native communities*. Portland, OR: Oregon Health Sciences University.

National Institute on Drug Abuse. (1981a). *Vol. 1: Prevention planning workbook* (DHHS Publication No. ADM 81-1061). Washington, DC: Government Printing Office.

National Institute on Drug Abuse. (1981b). *Vol. 2: A needs assessment workbook for prevention planning* (DHHS Publication No. ADM 81-1062). Washington, DC: Government Printing Office.

Peplav, L. A., & Goldston, S. E. (Eds.). (1984). *Preventing the harmful consequences of severe and persistent loneliness* (DHHS Publication No. ADM 84-1312). Washington, DC: Government Printing Office.

Price, R. H., & Smith, S. E. (1985). *A guide to evaluating prevention programs in mental health* (DHHS Publication No. ADM 85-1365). Washington, DC: Government Printing Office.

U.S. Department of Health, Education, and Welfare. (1977). *Summary proceedings. Tripartite conference on prevention* (DHEW Publication No. ADM 77-484). Washington, DC: Government Printing Office.

APPENDIX B

Theories and Models in Primary Prevention

The Health Belief Model (Rosenstock, 1990; Rosenstock, Strecher, & Becker, 1994)

The health belief model (HBM) emerged in the 1950s as scientists tried to figure out why large numbers of people were not taking advantage of free X-rays to detect tuberculosis. Over time, the model has been expanded "to include all preventive actions, illness behaviors, and sick-role behaviors" (Rosenstock, 1990, p. 42). The following summary follows Rosenstock's recent exposition (1990; Rosenstock et al., 1994), but is phrased in the vocabulary of this book (see also Janz & Becker, 1984).

First, some background demographic factors (especially education) influence how people deal with core belief factors.

Second, people will take preventive, protective, or promotive actions with regard to a given health condition:

I. regarding the perceived threat
   a. if they perceive themselves susceptible to it
   b. if they perceive the problem to be serious
II. regarding the expected outcome of a given action
   c. if they believe that a given course of action available to them would be beneficial

   d. if benefits of the action outweigh the costs of, or the barriers to, that
       action
   III. regarding a person's self-efficacy belief if that person believes he or she
       has the requisite knowledge and skill to produce the desired outcome

There may also be cues to action, like information from the media or
personal influences, but this is not a well-developed part of the model.

As a model guiding practice, the HBM seems to be easily translatable
into concrete situations. Consider the example of designing a primary
prevention program to prevent injury and death in adolescents who are
involved with drinking and driving. Let's make the translations:

Adolescents will be more likely to take preventive, protective, or
promotive actions (say a broad spectrum defensive driver course with
segments on driving, substance use, and the law) with regard to the issue
of drinking and driving

   I. if they see drinking and driving as a threat
      a. if they think they (or their friends) could get hurt in an accident caused
         by someone who had been drinking and driving
      b. if they believe that such accidents are very serious (painful, life threaten-
         ing, expensive, loss of driver's license)
   II. if they expect that they could do something about it
      c. if they believe that going to a defensive driver training course with its
         components on driving and drinking will help to control this problem
      d. if they believe that the benefits of taking this program will outweigh the
         costs involved (time, energy, money, status), or the barriers to, that
         action
   III. (in the context of the person's self-efficacy belief) if they believe that they
       can learn the requisite knowledge and skill to control their driving and
       drinking effectively

This translation from the model seems easy, but there are some problems
to be aware of. The HBM provides a framework for conceptualizing about
how people think about healthful behavior, but it does not supply the
weighting—how serious "serious" has to be, how susceptible one has to
be, and so on—before the balance tips in favor of responsible action.
Moreover, reviews of research using the HBM show mixed results,
especially with complex problems such as modifying lifestyle behaviors

related to HIV infection. As Rosenstock et al. (1994) advise, we should test the HBM as a whole, not as a collection of specific variables. They note that perceived threat is a sequential function of perceived severity and then perceived susceptibility; when the perceived threat is high, then perceived benefits and barriers become salient in combination with self-efficacy in performing a complex lifestyle action (cf. Kirscht & Joseph, 1989). Many studies have used this model as a frame of reference in designing their preventive practices. (See Rosenstock et al., 1994, for a review of the research in this area.) The HBM directs the practitioner to several important factors operating in promoting or inhibiting healthy behaviors. This theory, and any theory, requires some creative efforts in its translation: What specific actions could we take that would fulfill the spirit of the theory and the realities of the psycho-sociocultural context in which the preventive effort is taking place?

The Theory of Reasoned Action (Fishbein & Ajzen, 1975; Fishbein, Middlestadt, & Hitchcock, 1994)

One kind of theory of behavior holds that it is rational to take a particular course of action among possible alternatives when that option yields the largest algebraic sum of values the person might obtain. This approach has some parallels to the 19th-century utilitarian theory and its hedonic calculus, but the modern rational theory presumes to supply more of the ingredients in this decision-making process. One widely used form of this approach is the theory of reasoned action (Fishbein, 1979; Fishbein & Ajzen, 1975; Fishbein & Middlestadt, 1989; Fishbein et al., 1994), which applies to any social behavior over which the individual has control.

I will present a brief overview of the whole theory and then connect it to understanding and changing AIDS-related behaviors (Fishbein et al., 1994). The theory of reasoned action is a general theory of human behavior that connects beliefs, attitudes, values, perceived social norms, motivations to comply with social norms, intention to behave, and actual behavior. It is clearer to work backward by asking what led to the actual behavior (Fishbein et al., 1994) and distinguish the overt, specified observable action that is under one's volitional control (e.g., "using a latex condom [the next] time I engage in oral sex with my long-term partner") from a general intention (e.g., "always intending to engage in safe sex") and from the outcome of such acts (e.g., "avoiding AIDS"). The theory predicts only the actual specific behaviors whose full identification requires four ingredients: an action that occurs with regard to some target event in a given context and at a given time (Fishbein et al., 1994). With a problem like AIDS, it is important to identify the risk factors to be changed rather than risk markers (Fishbein et al., 1994). Fishbein et al. note that using a condom is a behavior for men but is a marker goal for women. The behavior for a woman involves either putting a condom on the man or communicating with the man about using a condom.

What leads to such a specified behavior? The critical answer is behavioral intention, which must also be defined in terms of the same four elements of action, target, context, and time that are used to define the behavior (Fishbein et al., 1994). Given the behavior identified above for a gay man, the behavioral intention would be just as specific: to increase his intention to "use a condom for oral sex (the next time when I have sex) with my long-term partner" (Fishbein et al., 1994, pp. 64-65).

This intention, in turn, is influenced by two strings of events. The first string represents the person's own attitudes toward performing the behavior, whereas the second string involves perceived social influence on the person's actions.

Let's examine the first string of events—attitudes toward the behavior in question. These are influenced by the person's belief that the behavior will lead to a specified outcome, plus the person's evaluation of the outcome as desirable or not. Fishbein and Ajzen (1975) write:

> The totality of a person's beliefs serves as the informational base that ultimately determines [a person's] attitudes, intentions, and behaviors. Our approach thus views [a person] as an essentially rational organism, who uses the information at [his or her] disposal to make judgments, form evaluations, and arrive at decisions. (p. 14)

Beliefs are formed by direct observation, by inference, or from outside sources (as in education) and link attributes to the object. Attitudes are affective in nature: the general feelings of favorableness or unfavorableness toward an object. Thus both beliefs and attitudes influence behavioral intentions.

The second string deals with the person's appraisal of how important persons in his or her life view this same behavior and its outcomes. This perception of the collective attitudes of others about whether the person should or should not perform the action is called a subjective norm. It is influenced by the perceived beliefs and values of these others and by the individual's motivation to comply.

For example, the subjective norm might be "Most people who are important to me think I should/should not use a latex condom every time I engage in sexual intercourse"; the motivation to comply might be "With respect to health matters, I want to do what people who are important to me want me to do" (Fishbein & Middlestadt, 1989, p. 104). There may be more than one reference group with different views, so that the individual in effect calculates the weightings in a "generalized normative belief" (Fishbein & Ajzen, 1975, p. 302).

When comparing these two strings, one has to determine the relative strength of one's attitudes and beliefs versus one's perceptions of subjective norms. The relative strength will differ for different groups at different times. Fishbein et al. (1994) note research that suggests that U.S. college students' intentions always to use a condom appear to be under normative control, whereas the same behavioral intention appears to be under attitudinal control for sexually active Mexican college students.

A primary preventer would further need to know what a person or group considers the relevant costs and benefits of the behavior and who is being considered for their opinions on the matter. These factors presumably could be influenced through appropriate information, once they were known as salient to a given person or group.

Thus the theory of reasoned action views behavior change as essentially a matter of changing the cognitive structure underlying that behavior, but one needs to know a great deal of information to apply the theory most effectively. (See also Ajzen, 1985; Ajzen & Fishbein, 1977, 1980; Ajzen & Timko, 1986.)

The Social Stress Approach

If this is the age of anxiety, then this is also the era of research on social stress. Cox and Ferguson (1991) describe three different approaches to the study of stress:

1. The engineering or stimulus-response approach emphasizes that a given level of stress (like a noxious environmental event) produces a proportional level of strain reaction.

2. The medico-physiological approach defines stress as a "generalized and nonspecific" physiological response to aversive environmental stimuli (Selye, 1956).

3. The interactional or appraisal theories of stress view stress as an internal representation of a problematic transaction between the person and the environment where pressures meet capability to cope. Stress is viewed as existing when pressure exceeds capability.

I will use the third approach as the exemplar for the social stress model.

Israel and Schurman (1990) present a conceptual framework of the stress process that is useful for this discussion, with some modifications:

1. Objective conditions place people at risk for physical, physiological, or behavioral disorders. This beginning stems from the mountain of research linking problems in major life events with disorders (Holmes & Rahe, 1967), with daily hassles that have an independent effect on disorders (Wagner, Compas, & Howell, 1988), or with chronic strains, cataclysmic events, and ambient stressors (Israel & Schurman, 1990).

2. People perceive these objective conditions in different ways. The same event may be viewed by two individuals differently, and two different events may be interpreted in the same way by two individuals.

3. Important components of the perceived stress are the contributions of individual and situational characteristics, such as biological health, psychological coping skills, feeling in control of the situation through one's actions, and social support or other resources from others. Important distinctions have been made in the process of coping. One function of coping is to deal with the problem, whereas another function is to regulate the emotions (Folkman, 1991). Research suggests that people use both functions together.

4. The individual makes some short-term responses viewed in a multidimensional way, such as physical blood pressure level, psychological tenseness, or a behavioral change (e.g., drinking to reduce tension). Depending on the set of events, these short-term responses may or may not resolve the stress. This is the definitional point of where capabilities either exceed or do not exceed the stressful demands, producing a no-stress or a stressful situation, respectively.

5. There may be a long-term consequence of these repeated responses, such as physiological cardiovascular disease, psychological anxiety disor-

der, or behavioral alcoholism. In these cases, there is feedback to the beginning of the cycle of stress, another set of objective conditions that presents stresses for the individual in question (Israel & Schurman, 1990).

6. Awareness of this natural history of stress permits one to take preventive as well as ameliorative steps.

a. Beginning with objective stressors, one can avoid or reduce them or strengthen oneself to withstand them. One should be especially careful when there is a string of untoward events (losing a job, having to move, getting a traffic ticket) because the accumulative effect of such stressors is a predictor of some physical or emotional problems.

b. One can attempt to redefine untoward events in a constructive way, such as seeing the closing of a factory as being an opportunity to go back to school or take up another occupation one had always wanted to do.

c. One can consider the sources of one's strength throughout the social configuration: one's own physical strengths, the support of one's family and friends, the resources in the community, and the like. Then, combining strengths with limitations, one can put together a package of actions to achieve a given objective while making ample use of emotional coping mechanisms to keep one on an even keel while the problem-solving efforts have a chance to work.

In general, this stress model provides ample warnings and predictors, as well as guides toward other preventive tactics, to rise above the challenges of modern life.

Social Cognitive Theory (Bandura, 1986, 1989a, 1989b, 1994)

Bandura's conceptual framework provides a well-developed theory regarding the nature of behavior and of behavior change. It is an extensive theory with a great deal of conceptual discussion and empirical testing (Bandura, 1986). It has been widely used in many contexts (e.g., Botvin & Tortu, 1988; Lawrence & McLeroy, 1986; Maccoby & Altman, 1988). It may be helpful to present an overview first and then discuss some relevant details.

Bandura (1989a) rejects both the operant view of human behavior as mechanically responding to environmental forces and the autonomous (or free will) view that human actors are entirely independent agents in choosing their behavior. Rather, Bandura presents a triadic view of reciprocal causation (mutual actions among causal factors):

1. human behavior is viewed as an emergent and interactive product of
2. personal factors (cognitive and affective components) and
3. environmental factors (externally existing social and physical environments)

Not only does each of the three influence each other (although the strength of that bidirectional influence varies in each situation) but there are reciprocal influences within each of the three. Let's look at the three major components:

The nature of the person is defined in terms of six capabilities:

1. Symbolizing capability, which enables the person to test possible solutions to problems symbolically and act on the basis of the estimated outcome
2. Forethought capability, in which people set future goals and anticipate future consequences so that the "future" becomes a current motivator by being represented symbolically in the present
3. Vicarious capability, or learning by observing other people's behavior and its consequences for them
4. Self-regulatory capability, in which one's own behavior "is motivated and regulated by internal standards and self-evaluative reactions" (Bandura, 1986, p. 20) to one's own behaviors
5. Self-reflective capability, in which people's thoughts about their own thought processes affect their actions; this includes the central concept of self-efficacy, to which I will return
6. The biological limits of the vast potentiality stemming from direct (operant) and observational learning

Bandura emphasizes the centrality of cognitive factors. Even objective environmental factors are modified into "situations," that is, how the individual perceives the external social and physical environments. (This is like Lewin's concept of the psychological environment, a phenomenological term.) For present purposes, Bandura's social cognitive theory as a guide to behavior change can best be described as efforts to influence the core cognitive agent, the person's perceived self-efficacy, which is a personal judgment of one's capacity to accomplish a certain level of performance (Bandura, 1986). Efficacy, Bandura notes, involves a generative capability in which cognitive, social, and behavioral subskills must be organized into integrated courses of action to serve specific—not global—purposes. Bandura (1989b, 1994) notes, with reference to effective self-protection against AIDS, "The major problem is not teaching people safer sex guidelines, which is easily achievable, but equipping them with skills, and self-beliefs that enable them to put the guidelines consistently into practice in the face of counteracting influences" (p. 26). He continues, "To be most effective, health communications should instill in people the belief that they have the capacity to alter their health habits and should instruct them on how to do it. . . . Success requires perseverant effort" (p. 33).

Bandura emphasizes the special power of modeling complex information as on videotape modeling related to the prevention of risky sexual behavior. He describes the video product by Winett, Neale, and Williams (1982) in which a videotape models self-protective behaviors for teenagers and their parents. This technique not only helped increase knowledge about HIV risky behaviors, but it also improved communications and problem solving between parents and children. These materials provided parents with sound teaching materials, especially in cases where parents may have been unsure of information and effective approaches to adolescents. Home-based information and modeling systems have a wide variety of possible uses.

Self-knowledge about one's efficacy is based on four main sources, which may increase or decrease that perception and may be accurate or erroneous as sources of information. Bandura (1986) notes that the first source—the outcomes of one's own performances in a given area—is the strongest base for perceived self-efficacy because it builds on actual mastery experiences. (This is essentially an operant perspective, that the consequences of actions affect future behaviors.) Success raises efficacy expectations and the likelihood of repeated behaviors, whereas failure lowers them, "especially if the failures occur early in the course of events and do not reflect lack of effort or adverse external circumstances" (p. 399). In a Piagetian sense, new experiences must be blended with the existing mental state of the person. Once a strong sense of self-efficacy is developed through repeated successes, occasional lapses will not have much effect on the enduring sense of one's competencies. When people have built up a strong sense of self-capacity, failure experiences lead them to look at the situation, insufficient effort, or poor strategies—not a personal incapacity for achieving the goal. Once established in a given area, a strong perceived self-efficacy will generalize to other situations, especially those that are similar to the first area.

The second main source of perceived self-efficacy stems from vicarious experiences. Seeing other people similar to oneself performing some task successfully can raise one's own self-efficacy to an extent that the person "should be able to achieve at least some improvement in performance" (Bandura, 1986, p. 399). Models can be quite influential, especially when the individual has had little prior experience, when the criteria of successful performance are clear, and if better ways to achieve the same goal are modeled. Likewise, observations of the failure of others on specific tasks may decrease one's own self-efficacy in the same area. Modeling is especially useful with complex social tasks.

The third way to influence self-efficacy is through verbal persuasion that one has the requisite ability. This common approach to helping—for example, the "talking therapies"—is relatively weak; it essentially encourages people to try harder with existing skills and knowledge or to attain new resources. If people do not have the requisite knowledge and skills, then urging them to go forward is setting them up for failure as well as discrediting the therapist.

The fourth source of information on self-efficacy stems from physiological states to help individuals judge their capability. People tend to read high physiological arousal, such as nervousness or fatigue, as indications of low efficacy—which thus become self-fulfilling prophecies. Actions taken to limit emotional arousal (e.g., taking deep breaths before meeting a client for the first time or going on stage) or to put these events into perspective (e.g., recognizing that the client is likely to be too nervous to notice one's nervousness) will heighten self-efficacy, or at least not let it spiral downward. (Novice interviewers are instructed to get into a relaxed sitting position and listen to the client rather than do all the talking to cover their own initial nervousness.)

In general, primary prevention projects would apply this theory by arranging to instill in individuals beliefs of positive self-efficacy by means of one or a combination of the four approaches described above. Botvin and Tortu (1988) and their colleagues have implemented a life-skills training program that seeks to provide training in self-efficacy, among other skills, leading to the point where the individual can say, "I can do what I want and what I know is good for me."

By way of summary, let's follow Bandura (1989b, 1994) as he applies his theory to the specific question of using perceived self-efficacy in the exercise of control over behaviors that could lead to HIV infection. There are four programmatic components for a prevention program:

First, information must be created and disseminated that increases people's awareness and knowledge of health risks, including candid presentations of the facts of sexual life and drug use, as needed. Bandura recognizes that there will be stiff ideological opposition.

Second, social and self-regulatory skills are needed to translate informed concern into effective preventive action. Social modeling could be especially helpful in this regard, along with a strong sense of self-efficacy (the self-belief in one's capability to use given skills well). This modeling can be maximized if the model has similar characteristics as the observer—age, sex, status, type of problem involved, and situations in which they apply these skills. This is where home videos may be especially useful (Bandura, 1994).

Third, enhancing skills and building resilient self-efficacy are taught by means of opportunities for guided practice and corrective feedback on the application of these skills in high-risk situations. Bandura (1989b) notes that proficiency requires extensive practice, especially in situations like those found in the real world. Being able to control these practice situations adds to self-efficacy, as well as to the ability to bounce back rapidly in the face of setbacks.

Fourth, social support for personal change is enlisted and is needed in the face of interpersonal, sociocultural, religious, and economic factors that may be operating against self-protective behavior. Bandura (1989b) notes that a major benefit of community-mediated programs is that they can bring together both formal and informal networks of influence to transmit information and to model effective behaviors. He concludes by noting that "multifaceted psychosocial programs that equip people with protective knowledge, with the means and self-beliefs to exercise effective personal control, and provide social supports for their efforts at personal change can achieve highly beneficial results" (p. 140).

Recurrent Themes Model of Primary Prevention (Caplan, 1989)

Gerald Caplan (1989) recently reassembled the many facets of his contribution to primary prevention theory, research, and practice into what he terms a *recurrent themes model of primary prevention*. The themes of which he speaks are taken up separately in various chapters of this book, but I would like to summarize his overview to give the reader a sense of the whole model.

Unlike the theories described previously, where the relationships among components are described in detail, Caplan's approach involves a general perspective of ingredients, each one of which has internal dynamics. Caplan begins with a list of biopsychosocial hazards that are either traumatic episodes or continuing problems (such as genetic defects, birth traumas, and poverty). These are related to intermediate variables such as competencies, crises, and biosociocultural supplies, which increase or decrease the likelihood of positive outcomes. For each of these variables, Caplan (1989) proposes various preventive actions, including social action and consultation for the basic hazards of life, and different forms of education, crisis intervention, and social support related to the intermediate variables. Most of these points are discussed in relevant places throughout the book, but some comments on the whole model may be helpful.

The recurrent themes model of primary prevention can be described as a developmental description and incremental action approach. Caplan reminds us to consider past risk factors and competence factors that affect a current situation:

> The hazardous circumstances of past risk factors reappear as the current stressor that precipitates a crisis; the elements of competence that enable an individual to master both a past hazard and a current stress recur in a modified form in the outcome . . . and adequate social supports not only buffer reaction to current stress but also were probably a crucial element in determining whether a past risk factor led to a current unhealthy outcome. (p. 4)

Under competence, Caplan places "self-efficacy," a concept that Bandura considers. Under crisis, Caplan points to the many possible biopsychosocial hazards to which one is subject and the requirement that one learns to adapt actively (rather than passively surrender). One deals quickly with the crisis, which is viewed as a period of opportunity as well as angst. (A great deal of research has been done in connection with the crisis concept, from Lindemann, 1944, to Caplan, 1961, 1989, to Roberts, 1991. Bloom & Klein, 1995, seek to relate the crisis model directly to primary prevention.)

Under social supports, Caplan (1989) hints at his earlier model of physical, psychosocial, and sociocultural supplies that people need to develop in a healthy manner and to avoid mental illness. Handal and Moore (1987) conducted a study to test this model and found general supporting evidence. Caplan (1989) states the basic hypothesis of this portion of his work: "That individuals exposed to a particular level of stress, who concomitantly benefit from a high level of social support, have less risk of subsequent mental and physical illness than do similar individuals exposed to similar stress who do not have such support" (p. 7).

The outcome of these past and present factors can be a sense of well-being and the capacity to study, work, love, and play—which adds to Freud's definition of mental health as the ability to work and to love. Competence may be enhanced or diminished as a result of these causal factors or the individual may take on psychiatric symptoms.

Caplan has contributed to a number of other basic primary prevention methods, such as consultation (Caplan, 1970), and more recently, collaboration. Each of the intermediate variables has some distinctive preventive services. Yet how these are to be orchestrated remains to be described. Caplan and his colleagues continue to develop these themes; one hopes they will address the vital issues of the interrelationships among these concepts and models of practice.

Social Models for Changing Behavior

Many writers have pointed to obvious limitations of the purely individualistic theories of human behavior and the need to consider social groupings, organizations, and cultures in understanding and changing behavior (Albee et al., 1988; Alinsky, 1969, 1972; Allen, 1986; Aronson & Bridgeman, 1979; Coates, 1990). Fishbein et al. (1994) offer the theory of reasoned action that takes half of its force from perceived social influences. Other theorists develop the social models for change fully and explicitly; workers in primary prevention should consider their ideas. I will follow the work of Friedman, Des Jarlais, and Ward (1994) to develop this line of thinking.

It is widely known that peer groups and subcultures influence what individuals choose to do; that is exactly the nature of the effect on their members. Parents socialize children; peers often initiate youths into the pleasures of smoking, drinking, and sex. Drug subcultures teach compatriots how to use and enjoy self-harming substances. Cultural majorities may spread prejudices and discrimination. The question for primary prevention is how groups and cultures can change or be helped to change to prevent untoward behavior, protect current strengths, and promote desired enhancements.

The answers lead us into vast domains of considerations of social structures, social dynamics, and the development of social groups of every scale. I will follow the lead of Friedman et al. (1994) in discussing several specific social models of change.

Diffusion Theory

This socio-anthropological model of cultural change is adapted to the public health context by suggesting four steps or principles (Friedman et al., 1994):

1. Understand the subculture well enough to make informed guesses as to what innovation might be accepted by it.
2. Devise a way to make the innovation acceptable by users.
3. Monitor the reactions.
4. Adapt the innovation as needed.

Friedman et al. describe the innovation of using bleach to clean intravenous drug equipment as effective, acceptable, and widely available. Preventers modified their word-of-mouth campaign to include the giving away of bleach as well to facilitate its use. Results appear to indicate the successful slowing down of HIV infection among San Francisco drug injectors.

Leadership-Focused Models

Friedman et al. (1994) characterize leadership-focused models as ways to influence actual leaders—not just formal leaders,who may be removed from everyday concerns of the group—to adopt some innovation so as to have an impact on their followers. The vital issues of this model are how to locate these actual leaders, how to enlist them to one's point of view, how to motivate them to take the steps (and risks) of advocating for the innovation, and how to prepare them (education, support, and materials) for the task. These authors report research that located local leaders among gays who were invited to help their friends with safer sex methods. The leaders received appropriate education and support and then returned to their local groupings. Results show declines in risky sexual behavior.

Social Movement Theory

Social movements are discussed in Chapter 5 of this book, but I will review some major points here as well, because this has been an effective public health vehicle. Social movements usually develop from the efforts of local leaders, but sometimes they develop as part of larger social movements with regional or national leaders. Friedman et al. (1994) argue that social movements in public health become necessary when either or both of the following are true: a high degree of local popular involvement is needed to implement a change and opposition to change is strong. One needs to discover if there are current efforts to mobilize locals against some concern, if the participants (and others) are well informed, and the nature of the opposition.

Working with preexisting social movements is preferable, even though additional training of leaders may be needed on the new specific topic. Methods of delivery of the social movement message may range from word of mouth to print media to public announcements and even to demonstrations against the powers that be.

Friedman et al. (1994) point out that when special groups, such as ethnic minorities within the gay and lesbian community, lack the organized networks of communication, it becomes increasingly difficult to use these social movement methods, and other methods of social change have to be considered.

Changing the Social Environment

Friedman et al. (1994) recognize that social environments color the prioritizing of objectives. Living in a violent inner-city area appears to reduce the priority of safer sexual behaviors, exercising for one's health, eating certain foods low in sugar, and the like, in favor of actions to stay alive from day to day. Preventers have to address these larger issues with larger social tools, such as policy formation, law, the administration of such rules, and various forms of social advocacy (cf. Rothman, 1979).

For example, counties and states vary on their policies on syringe exchange programs, sexual education in the public schools, and presentation of HIV-related prevention practices on public television. Research information on the effects of existing experiments may be helpful in influencing policy changes.

Friedman et al. (1994) also discuss changes in social structures. For example, in a sexist society where women have less power and status, women find it difficult to express their views with male partners to use condoms. Thus working for equality of rights will have a broad spectrum of effects, including the change in the power structure and its implications for equality of protection in sexual areas. See Chapter 5 for methods for increasing social supports for primary prevention purposes.

REFERENCES

Abbott, M. W. (1992). Television violence: A proactive prevention campaign. In G. Albee, L. A. Bond, & T. Cook Monsey (Eds.), *Improving children's lives: Global perspectives on prevention*. Newbury Park, CA: Sage.

Adelman, H. S. (1989). Prediction and prevention of learning disabilities: Current state of the art and future directions. In L. A. Bond & B. E. Compas (Eds.), *Primary prevention and promotion in the schools*. Newbury Park, CA: Sage.

Adler, A. (1959). *The practice and theory of individual psychology*. Totowa, NJ: Littlefield Adams.

Agras, W. S., Schneider, J. A., Arnow, B., Raeburn, S. D., & Telch, C. F. (1989). Cognitive-behavioral and response-prevention treatments for bulimia nervosa. *Journal of Consulting and Clinical Psychology, 57*(2), 215-221.

Ainsworth, M. D. S. (1991). Attachment and other affectional bonds across the life cycle. In C. M. Parkes, J. Stevenson-Hinde, & P. Marris (Eds.), *Attachment across the life cycle*. London: Tavistock/Routledge.

Ainsworth, M. D. S., Blehar, M. C., Waters, E., & Wall, S. (1978). *Patterns of attachment: A psychological study of the strange situation*. Hillsdale, NJ: Lawrence Erlbaum.

Ajzen, I. (1985). From intentions to actions: A theory of planned behavior. In J. Kuhl & J. Beckman (Eds.), *Action control: From cognition to behavior*. New York: Springer-Verlag.

Ajzen, I., & Fishbein, M. (1977). Attitude-behavior relations: A theoretical analysis and review of empirical evidence. *Psychological Bulletin, 84*, 888-918.

Ajzen, I., & Fishbein, M. (1980). *Understanding attitudes and predicting social behaviors.* Englewood Cliffs, NJ: Prentice Hall.

Ajzen, I., & Timko, C. (1986). Correspondence between health attitudes and behavior. *Basic and Applied Social Psychology, 7,* 259-276.

Albee, G. W. (1981). The prevention of sexism. *Professional Psychology, 12,* 20-28.

Albee, G. W. (1983). Psychopathology, prevention, and the just society. *Journal of Primary Prevention, 4*(1), 5-40.

Albee, G. W. (1986). Advocates and adversaries of prevention. In M. Kessler & S. E. Goldston (Eds.), *A decade of progress in primary prevention.* Hanover, NH: University Press of New England.

Albee, G. W. (1990). Suffer the little children. *Journal of Primary Prevention, 11*(1), 69-82.

Albee, G. W. (1992). Saving children means social revolution. In G. W. Albee, L. A. Bond, & T. V. C. Monsey (Eds.), *Improving children's lives: Global perspectives on prevention.* Newbury Park, CA: Sage.

Albee, G. W., Bond, L. A., & Monsey, T. V. C. (Eds.). (1992). *Improving children's lives: Global perspectives on prevention* (Vol. 14). Newbury Park, CA: Sage.

Albee, G. W., Gordon, S., & Leitenberg, H. (Eds.). (1983). *Promoting sexual responsibility and preventing sexual problems* (Vol. 7). Hanover, NH: University Press of New England.

Albee, G. W., & Joffe, J. M. (1977). *Primary prevention of psychopathology* (Vol. 1). Hanover, NH: University Press of New England.

Albee, G. W., Joffe, J. M., & Dusenbury, L. A. (Eds.). (1988). *Prevention, powerlessness, and politics: Readings on social change.* Newbury Park, CA: Sage.

Albino, J. E. (1984). Prevention by acquiring health-enhancing habits. In M. Roberts & L. Peterson (Eds.), *Prevention of problems in childhood.* New York: John Wiley.

Albritton, R. B. (1978). Cost-benefits of measles eradication: Effects of a federal intervention. *Policy Analysis, 4,* 1-21.

Alcalay, F., Ghee, A., & Scrimshaw, S. (1993). Designing prenatal care messages for low-income Mexican women. *Public Health Reports, 108*(3), 354-362.

Aledort, L. M., Weiss, H., Parker, C., Levi, J., & Simon, R. (1990). Life-style interventions in the young. In S. Shumaker et al. (Eds.), *The handbook of health behavior change.* New York: Springer.

Alinsky, S. (1969). *Reveille for radicals.* New York: Vintage.

Alinsky, S. (1972). *Rules for radicals.* New York: Vintage.

Allen, I. L. (Ed.). (1977). *New towns and the suburban dream: Ideology and utopia in planning and development.* Port Washington, NY: Kennikat.

Allen, J. (1986). Achieving primary prevention program objectives through culture change systems. *Journal of Primary Prevention, 7*(2), 91-107.

Allen, J. P., Philliber, S., & Hoggson, N. (1990). School-based prevention of teen-age pregnancy and school dropouts: Process evaluation of the national replication of the Teen Outreach Program. *American Journal of Community Psychology, 18*(4), 505-524.

Allport, G. W. (1954a). *The nature of prejudice.* Cambridge, MA: Addison-Wesley.

Allport, G. W. (1954b). Techniques for reducing group prejudice. In P. A. Sorokin (Ed.), *Forms and techniques of altruistic and spiritual growth.* Boston: Beacon.

Allport, G. W. (1989). *The nature of prejudice.* Cambridge, MA: Addison-Wesley.

Altman, D. C., Flora, J., Fortmann, S., & Farquhar, J. (1987). The cost-effectiveness of three smoking cessation programs. *American Journal of Public Health, 77*(2), 162-165.

Altman, D. G. (1990). The social context and health behavior: The case of tobacco. In S. A. Shumaker, E. Schron, & J. Ockene (Eds.), *The handbook of health behavior change.* New York: Springer.

Alvy, K. T. (1988). Parenting programs for black parents. In L. A. Bond & B. M. Wagner (Eds.), *Families in transition: Primary prevention programs that work*. Newbury Park, CA: Sage.

Amass, L., Bickel, W. K., Higgins, S. T., Budney, A. J., & Foerg, F. E. (1993). The taking of free condoms in a drug abuse treatment clinic: The effects of location and posters. *American Journal of Public Health, 83*(10), 1466-1468.

American Medical Association, Council on Scientific Affairs. (1989). Firearms injuries and deaths: A critical public health issue. *Public Health Reports, 104*(2), 111-120.

American Red Cross. (1979). *Advanced first aid and emergency care*. Garden City, NY: Doubleday.

American Red Cross. (1993). *Community first aid and safety*. St. Louis, MO: Mosby.

Anderson, E. E., & Quast, W. (1983). Young children in alcoholic families: A mental health needs-assessment and an intervention/prevention strategy. *Journal of Primary Prevention, 3*(3), 174-187.

Anthony, E. J. (1974). The syndrome of the psychologically invulnerable child. In E. Anthony & C. Koupernik (Eds.), *The child and his family* (Vol. 3). New York: John Wiley.

Anthony, E. J., & Cohler, B. J. (Eds.). (1987). *The invulnerable child*. New York: Guilford.

Aoki, B., Ngin, C. P., Mo, B., & Ja, D. Y. (1989). AIDS prevention models in Asian-American communities. In V. M. Mays, G. W. Albee, & S. F. Schneider (Eds.), *Primary prevention of AIDS: Psychological approaches*. Newbury Park, CA: Sage.

Arbuthnot, J. (1992). Sociomoral reasoning in behavior-disordered adolescents: Cognitive and behavioral change. In J. McCord & R. E. Tremblay (Eds.), *Preventing antisocial behavior from birth through adolescence*. New York: Guilford.

Archer, D. L. (1989). Food counseling for persons infected with HIV: Strategy for defensive living. *Public Health Reports, 104*(2), 196-198.

Arcus, M. E., Schvaneveldt, J. D., & Moss, J. J. (Eds.). (1993a). *Handbook of family life education: Foundations of family life education* (Vol. 1). Newbury Park, CA: Sage.

Arcus, M. E., Schvaneveldt, J. D., & Moss, J. J. (Eds.). (1993b). *Handbook of family life education: The practice of family life education* (Vol. 2). Newbury Park, CA: Sage.

Are you eating right? (1992, October). *Consumer Reports, 57*, 644-655.

Arkin, E. B. (1990). Opportunities for improving the nation's health through collaboration with the mass media. *Public Health Reports, 105*(2), 219-223.

Arnold, C. B., & Cogswell, B. E. (1971). A condom distribution program for adolescents: The findings of a feasibility study. *American Journal of Public Health, 61*(4), 739-750.

Arnold, W. B. (1981). Employee fitness in today's workplace. In L. K. Y. Ng & D. L. Davis (Eds.), *Strategies for public health: Promoting health and preventing disease*. New York: Van Nostrand Reinhold.

Arnowitz, E. (Ed.). (1982). *Prevention strategies for mental health*. New York: Prodist.

Aronson, E., & Bridgeman, D. (1979). Jigsaw groups and the desegregated classroom: In pursuit of common goals. *Personality and Social Psychology Bulletin, 5*(4), 438-446.

Asch, S. (1952). *Social psychology*. Englewood Cliffs, NJ: Prentice Hall.

ASH Smoking and Health Review [Entire issue]. (1995, January-February).

Auslander, G. K. (1988). Social networks and health status of the unemployed. *Health and Social Work, 13*(3), 191-200.

Azrin, N. H., & Besalel, V. A. (1980). *Job club counselor's manual: A behavioral approach to vocational counseling*. Austin, TX: PRO-ED.

Azrin, N. H., & Holz, W. C. (1966). Punishment. In W. K. Honig (Ed.), *Operant behavior*. New York: Appleton-Century-Crofts.

Bachrach, K. M., Zautra, A. J., & Cofresi, A. V. (1989). Minimizing the negative impact of a planned hazardous waste facility on the surrounding community. *Journal of Primary Prevention, 10*(2), 133-147.

Backer, T. E., Liberman, R. P., & Kuehnel, T. G. (1986). Dissemination and adoption of innovative psychosocial interventions. *Journal of Consulting and Clinical Psychology, 54,* 111-118.

Baenen, R. S., Stephens, M. A. P., & Glenwick, D. S. (1986). Outcome in psychoeducational day school programs: A review. *American Journal of Orthopsychiatry, 56*(2), 263-270.

Bagwell, M., & Clements, S. (1985). *A political handbook for health professionals.* Boston: Little, Brown.

Bahr, H. M. (1988). Family change and the mystique of the traditional family. In L. Bond & B. Wagner (Eds.), *Families in transition: Primary prevention programs that work.* Newbury Park, CA: Sage.

Baker, S. A. (1988). *An application of the Fishbein model for predicting behavioral intention to use condoms in a sexually transmitted disease clinic population.* Unpublished doctoral dissertation, University of Washington.

Baker, S. B., & Butler, J. N. (1984). Effects of preventive cognitive self-instruction training on adolescent attitudes, experiences, and state anxiety. *Journal of Primary Prevention, 5*(1), 17-26.

Baldassari, C., Lehman, S., & Wolfe, M. (1987). Imagining and creating alternative environments with children. In C. Weinstein & T. David (Eds.), *Spaces for children.* New York: Plenum.

Bandura, A. (1977). Self-efficacy: Toward a unifying theory of behavioral change. *Psychological Review, 84*(2), 191-215.

Bandura, A. (1986). *Social foundations of thought and action: A social cognitive theory.* Englewood Cliffs, NJ: Prentice Hall.

Bandura, A. (1989a). Human agency in social cognitive theory. *American Psychologist, 44*(9), 1175-1184.

Bandura, A. (1989b). Perceived self-efficacy in the exercise of control over AIDS infection. In V. M. Mays, G. Albee, & S. Schneider (Eds.), *Primary prevention of AIDS: Psychological approaches.* Newbury Park, CA: Sage.

Bandura, A. (1994). Social cognitive theory and exercise of control over HIV infection. In R. J. DiClemente & J. L. Peterson (Eds.), *Preventing AIDS: Theories and methods of behavioral interventions.* New York: Plenum.

Barker, R. G. (1968). *Ecological psychology.* Stanford, CA: Stanford University Press.

Barker, R. L. (1987). *The social work dictionary.* Silver Spring, MD: National Association of Social Workers.

Barnett, W. S. (1993a). Benefit-cost analysis of preschool education: Findings from a 25-year follow-up. *American Journal of Orthopsychiatry, 63*(4), 500-508.

Barnett, W. S. (1993b). New wine in old bottles: Increasing the coherence of early childhood care and education policy. *Early Childhood Research Quarterly, 8,* 519-558.

Barnett, W. S., & Escobar, C. M. (1989). Research on the cost-effectiveness of early educational intervention: Implications for research and policy. *American Journal of Community Psychology, 17*(6), 677-704.

Barney, J. L. (1987). Community presence in nursing homes. *Gerontologist, 27*(3), 367-369.

Barone, V. J., Greene, B. F., & Lutzker, J. R. (1986). Home safety with families being treated for child abuse and neglect. *Behavior Modification, 10,* 93-114.

Barratt, A., Reznik, R., Irwig, L., Cuff, A., Simpson, J. M., Oldenburg, B., Horvath, J., & Sullivan, D. (1994). Work-site cholesterol screening and dietary intervention: The staff health heart project. *American Journal of Public Health, 84*(5), 779-782.

Barrera, M., Jr. (1986). Distinctions between social support concepts, measures, and models. *American Journal of Community Psychology, 14*(4), 413-445.

Barth, R. P., Derezotes, D. S., & Danforth, H. E. (1991). Preventing adolescent abuse. *Journal of Primary Prevention, 11*(3), 193-206.

Barth, R. P., Hacking, S., & Ash, J. R. (1988). Preventing child abuse: An experimental evaluation of the child parent enrichment project. *Journal of Primary Prevention, 8*(4), 201-217.

Baruch, G. K., & Barnett, R. C. (1980). On the well-being of adult women. In L. A. Bond & J. C. Rosen (Eds.), *Competence and coping during adulthood.* Hanover, NH: University Press of New England.

Battistich, V. A., Elias, M. J., & Branden-Muller, L. R. (1992). Two school-based approaches to promoting children's social competence. In G. Albee, L. A. Bond, & T. C. Monsey (Eds.), *Improving children's lives.* Newbury Park, CA: Sage.

Beardslee, W. R. (1989). The role of self-understanding in resilient individuals: The development of a perspective. *American Journal of Orthopsychiatry, 59*(2), 266-278.

Beck, A. T. (1984). Cognitive approaches to stress. In R. Woolfolk & P. Lehrer (Eds.), *Principles and practices of stress management.* New York: Guilford.

Beck, A. T., Rush, J., Hollon, S., & Shaw, B. (1979). *Cognitive therapy of depression.* New York: Guilford.

Becker, F. D. (1985). Quality of work environment (QWE): Effects on office workers. *Prevention in Human Services, 4*(1 & 2), 35-57.

Becker, M. H. (1990). Theoretical models of adherence and strategies for improving adherence. In S. Shumaker, E. Schron, & J. Ockene (Eds.), *The handbook of health behavior change.* New York: Springer.

Begab, M. J. (1974). The major dilemma of mental retardation: Shall we prevent it? (Some social implications of research in mental retardation). *American Journal of Mental Deficiency, 78*(5), 519-529.

Begley, C. E., & Biddle, A. K. (1988). Cost-benefit analysis of safety belts in Texas school buses. *Public Health Reports, 103*(4), 479-485.

Beiser, M. (1982). Evaluating primary prevention programs: Models and measures. In S. M. Manson (Ed.), *New directions in prevention among American Indian and Alaskan Native communities.* Portland: Oregon Health Sciences University.

Bell, P. A., Fisher, J. D., Baum, A., & Greene, T. C. (1990). *Environmental psychology* (3rd ed.). Fort Worth, TX: Holt, Rinehart & Winston.

Bell, R. Q. (1986). Age-specific manifestations in changing psychosocial risk. In D. C. Farran & J. D. McKinney (Eds.), *The concept of risk in intellectual and psychosocial development.* New York: Academic Press.

Belsky, J., & Benn, J. (1982). Beyond bonding: A family-centered approach to enhancing early parent-infant relations. In L. Bond & J. M. Joffe (Eds.), *Facilitating infant and early development.* Hanover, NH: University Press of New England.

Bem, S. L. (1975/1985). Beyond androgyny: Some presumptuous prescriptions for a liberated sexual identity. In M. Bloom (Ed.), *Life span development: Bases for preventive and interventive helping.* New York: Macmillan.

Benard, B. (1992). Fostering resiliency in kids: Protective factors in the family, school, and community. *Prevention Forum, 12*(3), 1-16.

Benson, H. (1975). *The relaxation response.* New York: Avon.

Benson, H. (1992). *The relaxation response* (2nd ed.). New York: Random House.

Berger, B. G. (1983/1984). Stress reduction through exercises: The mind-body connection. *Motor Skills: Theory into Practice, 7*(2), 31-46.

Berger, B. G. (1986). Use of jogging and swimming as stress reduction techniques. In J. H. Humphrey (Ed.), *Human stress: Current selected research in human stress* (Vol. 1). New York: AMS.

Berkman, L. F., & Syme, S. L. (1979). Social networks, host resistance, and mortality: A nine year followup study of Alameda County residents. *American Journal of Epidemiology, 109,* 186-204.

Berlin, I. N. (1990). The role of the community mental health center in prevention of infant, child and adolescent disorders: Retrospect and prospect. *Community Mental Health Journal, 26*(1), 89-106.

Berlin, I. N., & Stone, L. A. (Eds.). (1979). *Basic handbook of child psychiatry* (Vol. 4). New York: Basic Books.

Berlin, J. A., & Colditz, G. A. (1990). A meta-analysis of physical activity in the prevention of coronary heart disease. *American Journal of Epidemiology, 132*(4), 612-628.

Berlin, R., & Davis, R. (1989). Children from alcoholic families: Vulnerability and resilience. In R. Coles (Ed.), *The child in our times.* New York: Brunner/Mazel.

Berman, J. S., & Norton, N. C. (1985). Does professional training make a therapist more effective? *Psychological Bulletin, 98,* 401-407.

Bernard, J. (1972). *The future of marriage.* New York: Bantum.

Berrueta-Clement, J. R., Schweinhart, L., Barnett, W., & Weikart, D. (1987). The effects of early educational intervention on crime and delinquency in adolescence and early adulthood. In J. Burchard & S. Burchard (Eds.), *Prevention of delinquent behavior.* Newbury Park, CA: Sage.

Bessell, H. (1972). Human development in the elementary classroom. In L. Solomon & B. Berzon (Eds.), *New perspectives in encounter groups.* San Francisco: Jossey-Bass.

Better food labels—at last. (1993, February). *Consumer Reports, 58,* 65.

Betz, N. E., & Hackett, G. (1986). The relationship of career-related self-efficacy expectations to perceived career options in college women and men. *Journal of Counseling Psychology, 23,* 399-410.

Bickman, L. (1983). The evaluation of prevention programs. *Journal of Social Issues, 39,* 181-194.

Biegel, D., Farkas, K. J., Abell, N., Goodin, J., & Friendman, B. (1989). *Social support networks: A bibliography, 1983-1987.* Westport, CT: Greenwood.

Biegel, D. E., Magaziner, J., & Baum, M. (1991). Social support networks of white and black elderly people at risk for institutionalization. *Health and Social Work, 16*(4), 245-257.

Biegel, D. E., McCardle, E., & Mendelson, S. (1985). *Social networks and mental health: An annotated bibliography.* Beverly Hills, CA: Sage.

Biegel, D. E., & Naparstek, A. (Eds.). (1981). *Community support systems and mental health: Research, practice and policy.* New York: Springer.

Biegel, L. (Ed.). (1984). *Physical exercise and the older person: A guide to exercise for health care professionals.* Rockville, MD: Aspen.

Birch, H. (1972). Malnutrition, learning, and intelligence. *American Journal of Public Health, 62*(6), 773-784.

Birch, H., & Gussow, J. D. (1970). *Disadvantaged children: Health, nutrition, and school failure.* New York: Harcourt Brace.

Birkel, R. C., & Reppucci, N. D. (1983). Social networks, information seeking, and the utilization of services. *American Journal of Community Psychology, 11*(2), 185-205.

Blanchard, F. A., & Cook, W. (1976). Effects of helping a less competent member of a cooperating interracial group on the development of interpersonal attraction. *Journal of Personality and Social Psychology, 34*(6), 1245-1255.

Blenkner, M., Bloom, M., & Nielsen, M. (1972). A research and demonstration project of protective services. *Social Casework, 52*(8), 483-499.

Block, J., & Block, J. (1980). The role of ego control and ego-resiliency in the organization of behavior. In W. A. Collins (Ed.), *Minnesota symposia on child psychology.* Hillsdale, NJ: Lawrence Erlbaum.

Bloom, B. L. (1965). The "medical model," miasma theory and community mental health. *Community Mental Health Journal, 1,* 333-338.

Bloom, B. L. (1977). *Community mental health: A general introduction.* Monterey, CA: Brooks/Cole.

Bloom, B. L. (1985). *Stressful life event theory and research: Implications for primary prevention* (DHHS Publication No. ADM 85-1385). Washington, DC: Government Printing Office.

Bloom, B. L., & Hodges, W. F. (1988). The Colorado separation and divorce program: A preventive intervention for newly separated persons. In R. Price, E. L. Cowen, R. P. Lorion, & J. Ramos-McKay (Eds.), *14 ounces of prevention.* Washington, DC: American Psychological Association.

Bloom, L. Z., Coburn, K., & Pearlman, J. (1975). *The new assertive woman.* New York: Delacorte.

Bloom, M. (1981). *Primary prevention: The possible science.* Englewood Cliffs, NJ: Prentice Hall.

Bloom, M. (1984). *Configurations of human behavior: Life span development in social environments.* New York: Macmillan.

Bloom, M. (1986). Hygenia at the scales: Weighing the costs and effectiveness of prevention/promotion, with special reference to mental retardation. *Journal of Primary Prevention, 7*(1), 27-48.

Bloom, M. (1990). *Introduction to the drama of social work.* Itasca, IL: F. E. Peacock.

Bloom, M. (1993). Toward a code of ethics for primary prevention. *Journal of Primary Prevention, 13*(3), 173-182.

Bloom, M. (1996). Primary prevention and resilience: Changing paradigms and changing lives. In R. Hampton, T. Gullotta, & P. Jenkins (Eds.), *Preventing violence in America.* Thousand Oaks, CA: Sage.

Bloom, M., & Buckner, J. C. (1989). The Journal of Primary Prevention Cumulative Index Project, 1980-1989. *Journal of Primary Prevention, 10*(1), 67-94.

Bloom, M., & Halsema, J. (1983). Survival in extreme conditions. *Journal of Suicide and Life-Threatening Behavior, 13*(3), 195-206.

Bloom, M., & Klein, W. C. (1995). Crisis prevention and crisis treatment. *Crisis Intervention, 1*(3), 167-176.

Bloom, M., & Penn, M. (1991). Primary prevention and state government. In C. G. Hudson and A. J. Cox (Eds.), *Dimensions of state mental health policy.* New York: Praeger.

Blum, G. J. (1983). Self-esteem and knowledge: Primary requisites to prevent victimization. In G. W. Albee, S. Gordon, & H. Leitenberg (Eds.), *Promoting sexual responsibility and preventing sexual problems.* Hanover, NH: University Press of New England.

Blumenkrantz, D. G., & Gavazzi, S. M. (1993). Guiding transitional events for children and adolescents through a modern day rite of passage. *Journal of Primary Prevention, 13*(3), 199-212.

Blythe, B. J., & Erdahl, J. C. (1986). Using stress inoculation to prepare a patient for open-heart surgery. *Health and Social Work, 11*(4), 265-274.

Bolton, Jr., F. G., Charlton, J. K., Gai, D. S., Laner, R. H., & Shumway, S. M. (1985). Preventive screening of adolescent mothers and infants: Critical variables in assessing risk for child maltreatment. *Journal of Primary Prevention, 5*(3), 169-187.

Bond, L. A. (1982). From prevention to promotion: Optimizing infant development. In L. A. Bond & J. M. Joffe (Eds.), *Facilitating infant and early childhood development.* Hanover, NH: University Press of New England.

Bond, L. A., Belenky, M. F., Weinstock, J. S., & Monsey, T. V. C. (1992). Self-sustaining powers of mind and voice: Empowering rural women. In M. Kessler, S. Goldston, & J. Joffe (Eds.), *The present and future of prevention*. Newbury Park, CA: Sage.

Bond, L. A., & Compas, B. E. (Eds.). (1989). *Primary prevention and promotion in the schools* (Vol. 12). Newbury Park, CA: Sage.

Bond, L. A., Cutler, S. J., & Grams, A. (Eds.). (1995). *Promoting successful and productive aging* (Vol. 16). Thousand Oaks, CA: Sage.

Bond, L. A., & Joffe, J. M. (Eds.). (1982). *Facilitating infant and early childhood development* (Vol. 6). Hanover, NH: University Press of New England.

Bond, L. A., & Rosen, J. C. (Eds.). (1980). *Competence and coping during adulthood* (Vol. 4). Hanover, NH: University Press of New England.

Bond, L. A., & Wagner, B. M. (Eds.). (1988). *Families in transition: Primary prevention programs that work* (Vol. 11). Newbury Park, CA: Sage.

Bond, M. T., & Peck, M. G. (1993). The risk of childhood injury on Boston's playground equipment and surfaces. *American Journal of Public Health, 83*(5), 731-733.

Boruch, R. F. and other participants. (1991). Violence prevention strategies targeted at the general population of minority youth. *Public Health Reports, 106*(3), 247-250.

Boston Women's Health Collective. (1993). *Our bodies, ourselves* (2nd ed.). New York: Simon & Schuster.

Boswell, J. (1988). *The kindness of strangers: The abandonment of children in Western Europe from late antiquity to the Renaissance*. New York: Pantheon.

Botvin, G. J., & Dusenbury, L. (1989). Substance abuse prevention and the promotion of competence. In L. Bond & B. Compas (Eds.), *Primary prevention and promotion in the schools*. Newbury Park, CA: Sage.

Botvin, G. J., & Tortu, S. (1988). Preventing adolescent substance abuse through life skills training. In R. Price, E. L. Cowen, R. P. Lorion, & J. Ramos-McKay (Eds.), *14 ounces of prevention*. Washington, DC: American Psychological Association.

Bower, E. M. (1972). K.I.S.S. and kids: A mandate for prevention. *American Journal of Orthopsychiatry, 42*, 556-565.

Bowker, J. (Ed.). (1983). *Education for primary prevention in social work*. New York: Council on Social Work Education.

Bowlby, J. (1951). *Maternal care and mental health*. Geneva: World Health Organization.

Bowlby, J. (1969). *Attachment and loss*. New York: Basic Books.

Bowlby, J. (1988). *A secure base: Parent-child attachment and healthy human behavior*. New York: Basic Books.

Brazelton, T. B. (1973). *Neonatal behavioral assessment scale*. London: Heineman.

Brazelton, T. B. (1986). Issues for working parents. *American Journal of Orthopsychiatry, 56*(1), 14-25.

Brett, A., Moore, R. C., & Provenzo, E. F., Jr. (1993). *The complete playground book*. Syracuse, NY: Syracuse University Press.

Brigham, J., Gross, J., Stitzer, M. L., & Felch, L. J. (1994). Effects of a restricted work-site smoking policy on employees who smoke. *American Journal of Public Health, 84*(5), 773-778.

Brodsky, S. L., & Miller, K. S. (1981). Coercing changes in prisons and mental hospitals: The social scientist and the class action suit. In J. Joffe & G. Albee (Eds.), *Prevention through political action and social change*. Hanover, NH: University Press of New England.

Bronfenbrenner, U. (1979). *The ecology of human development: Experiments by nature and design*. Cambridge, MA: Harvard University Press.

Bronstein, P. (1984). Promoting healthy emotional development in children. *Journal of Primary Prevention, 5*(2), 92-110.

Brooke, J. (1992, May 28). Curitiba journal: The secret of a livable city? It's simplicity itself. The road to Rio. Setting an agenda for the earth. *New York Times,* p. A4.

Broussard, E. R. (1989). The Infant-Family Resource Program: Facilitating optimal development. *Prevention in Human Services, 6*(2), 179-224.

Brown, B. (Ed.). (1978). *Long-term gains from early intervention.* Boulder, CO: Westview.

Brown, C. (1987). Literacy in 30 hours: Paulo Freire's process in Northeast Brazil. In I. Shor (Ed.), *Freire for the classroom.* Portsmouth, NH: Boynton/Cook.

Brown, G. (1971). *Human teaching for human learning.* New York: Viking.

Brown, K. S., & Ziefert, M. (1988). Crisis resolution, competence, and empowerment: A service model for women. *Journal of Primary Prevention, 9*(1 & 2), 92-103.

Brown, L. R., Durning, A., Flavin, C., French, H., Lenssen, N., Lowe, M., Misch, A., Postel, S., Renner, M., Starke, L., Weber, P., & Young, I. (Eds.). (1994). *State of the world.* New York: Norton.

Brown, P. (1981). Women and competence. In A. Maluccio (Ed.), *Promoting competence in clients: A new/old approach to social work practice.* New York: Free Press.

Browning, C. R. (1992). *Ordinary men: Reserve Police Battalion 101 and the final solution in Poland.* New York: Aaron Asher Books/HarperCollins.

Brownmiller, S. (1975). *Against our will: Men, women, and rape.* New York: Bantam.

Bruvold, W. H. (1993). A meta-analysis of adolescent smoking prevention programs. *American Journal of Public Health, 83*(6), 872-880.

Buckner, J. C., Trickett, E. J., & Corse, S. J. (1985). *Primary prevention in mental health: An annotated bibliography* (DHHS Publication No. ADM 85-1405). Washington, DC: Government Printing Office.

Budin, L. E., & Johnson, C. F. (1989). Sex abuse prevention programs: Offenders' attitudes about their efficacy. *Child Abuse & Neglect, 13,* 77-87.

Burchard, J. D., & Burchard, S. N. (Eds.). (1987). *Prevention of delinquent behavior* (Vol. 10). Newbury Park, CA: Sage.

Burgess, R. L., Clark, R. N., & Hendee, J. C. (1971). An experimental analysis of anti-littering procedures. *Journal of Applied Behavior Analysis, 4,* 71-75.

Burros, M. (1994, December 5). Former surgeon general begins push for Americans to slim down. *New York Times,* p. A20.

Butler, C., Rickel, A. U., Thomas, E., & Hendren, M. (1993). An intervention program to build competencies in adolescent parents. *Journal of Primary Prevention, 13*(3), 183-198.

Butt, J. (Ed.). (1971). *Robert Owen: Prince of cotton spinners.* Newtown Abbot, Devon, UK: David & Charles Publishing.

Cairns, R. B., et al. (1991). Violence prevention strategies directed toward high-risk minority youth. *Public Health Reports, 106*(3), 250-254.

Canfield, J., & Wells, H. (1976). *100 ways to enhance self-concept.* Englewood Cliffs, NJ: Prentice Hall.

Cantebury, R. J., & Lloyd, E. (1994). Smart drugs: Implications of student use. *Journal of Primary Prevention, 14*(3), 197-208.

Caplan, G. (1961). *An approach to community mental health.* New York: Grune & Stratton.

Caplan, G. (1964). *Principles of preventive psychiatry.* New York: Basic Books.

Caplan, G. (1970). *Theory and practice of mental health consultation.* New York: Basic Books.

Caplan, G. (1974). *Support systems and community mental health.* New York: Behavioral Publications.

Caplan, G. (1989). Recent developments in crisis intervention and the promotion of support services. *Journal of Primary Prevention, 10*(1), 3-25.

Caplan, G. (1993). Organization of preventive psychiatry programs. *Community Mental Health Journal, 29*(4), 367-395.

Caplan, R. D., Vinokur, A. D., Price, R., & van Ryn, M. (1989). Job-seeking, reemployment and mental health: A randomized field experiment in coping with job loss. *Journal of Applied Psychology, 74,* 759-769.

Cappelleri, J. C., Eckenrode, J., & Powers, J. L. (1993). The epidemiology of child abuse: Findings from the second national incidence and prevalence study of child abuse and neglect. *American Journal of Public Health, 83,*1622-1624.

Carter, C., & Reichman, M. (1987). Genetics and cancer prevention. *Evaluation and the Health Professions, 10*(3), 359-364.

Carter, W. B. (1990). Health behavior as a rational process: Theory of reasoned action and multiattribute utility theory. In K. Glanz, F. M. Lewis, & B. K. Rimer (Eds.), *Health behavior and health education.* San Francisco: Jossey-Bass.

Case, J., & Taylor, R. C. R. (1979). *Co-ops, communes, and collectives: Experiments in social change in the 1960s and 1970s.* New York: Pantheon.

Cassel, J. (1976). The contribution of the social environment to host resistance. *American Journal of Epidemiology, 104,*107-123.

Catania, J. A., Coates, T. J., Golden, E., Dolcini, M., Peterson, J., Kegeles, S., Siegel, D., & Fullilove, M. T. (1994). Correlates of condom use among black, Hispanic, and white heterosexuals in San Francisco: The Amen longitudinal survey. *AIDS Education and Prevention, 6*(1), 12-26.

Catania, J. A., Coates, T. J., Kegeles, S. M., Ekstrand, M., Guydish, J. R., & Bye, L. L. (1989). Implications of the AIDS risk-reduction model for the gay community: The importance of perceived sexual enjoyment and help-seeking behaviors. In V. Mays, G. Albee, & S. Schneider (Eds.), *Primary prevention of AIDS.* Newbury Park, CA: Sage.

Cauce, A. M., & Srebnik, D. S. (1989). Peer networks and social support: A focus for preventive efforts with youths. In L. Bond & B. Compas (Eds.), *Primary prevention and promotion in schools.* Newbury Park, CA: Sage.

Cedar, R. B. (1985). *A meta-analysis of the parent effectiveness outcome research literature.* Ed.D. Dissertation, Boston University.

Chafetz, J. S. (1988). *Feminist sociology: An overview of contemporary theories.* Itasca, IL: F. E. Peacock.

Chafetz, M. E., Blane, H. T., & Hill, M. J. (1970). *Frontiers of alcoholism.* New York: Science House.

Chambliss, C. A., & Murray, E. J. (1979). Efficacy attribution, locus of control, and weight loss. *Cognitive Therapy and Research, 3,* 349-354.

Chen, W. W. (1995). Enhancing of health locus of control through biofeedback training. *Perceptial and Motor Skills, 80,* 395-398.

Cherniss, C. (1977). Creating new consultation programs in community mental health centers: Analysis of a case study. *Community Mental Health Journal, 13*(2), 133-141.

Chernoff, R., & Lipschitz, D. A. (Eds.). (1988). *Health promotion and disease prevention in the elderly.* New York: Raven.

Cherry, L., & Redmond, S. P. (1994). A social marketing approach to involving Afgans in community-level alcohol problem prevention. *Journal of Primary Prevention, 14*(4), 289-310.

Cherry, R. L. (1991). Agents of nursing home quality of care: Ombudsmen and staff ratios revisited. *The Gerontologist, 31*(3), 384-388.

Chesney, M. A., Frautschi, N. M., & Rosenman, R. H. (1985). Modifying Type A behavior. In J. C. Rosen & L. J. Solomon (Eds.), *Prevention in health psychology.* Hanover, NH: University Press of New England.

Chess, S., & Thomas, A. (1986). *Temperament in clinical practice.* New York: Guilford.

Children and the environment: The state of the environment, 1990. (1990). New York: United Nations Environment Programme, UNICEF.

Cialdini, R. B. (1984). *How and why people agree to things.* New York: Morrow.

Clabby, J. F., & Elias, M. J. (1986). *Teach your child decision making.* New York: Doubleday.

Clark, D. (Ed.). (1993). *The future of palliative care: Issues of policy and practice.* London: Open University Press.

Clark, K. B. (1981). Community action programs—an appraisal. In J. Joffe & G. Albee (Eds.), *Prevention through political action and social change.* Hanover, NH: University Press of New England.

Clayton, R. R., & Leukefeld, C. G. (1992). The prevention of drug use among youth: Implications of "legalization." *Journal of Primary Prevention, 12*(4), 289-302.

Clements, G., Krenner, L., & Mölk, W. (1988). The use of the transcendental meditation programme in the prevention of drug abuse and in the treatment of drug-addicted persons. *Bulletin on Narcotics, 40*(1), 51-56.

Clinton, B., & Larner, M. (1988). Rural community women as leaders in health outreach. *Journal of Primary Prevention, 9*(1 & 2), 120-129.

Coate, D. (1993). Moderate drinking and coronary heart disease mortality: Evidence from NHANES I and the NHANES I follow-up. *American Journal of Public Health, 83,* 888-890.

Coates, T. J. (1990). Strategies for modifying sexual behavior for primary and secondary prevention of HIV disease. *Journal of Consulting and Clinical Psychology, 58*(1), 57-69.

Cobb, S. (1974). A model for life events and their consequences. In B. S. Dohrenwend & B. P. Dohrenwend (Eds.), *Stressful life events: Their nature and effects.* New York: John Wiley.

Cochran, M. (1990). Personal social networks as a focus of support. *Prevention in Human Services, 9*(1), 45-68.

Cochran, S. D. (1989). Women and HIV infection: Issues in prevention and behavior change. In V. Mays, G. Albee, & G. Schneider (Eds.), *Primary prevention of AIDS: Psychological approaches.* Newbury Park, CA: Sage.

Cohen, A. Y. (1975). *Alternatives to drug abuse: Steps toward prevention* (DHEW Publication No. ADM 75-79). Washington, DC: Government Printing Office.

Cohen, C. I., & Adler, A. (1986). Assessing the role of social network interventions with an inner-city population. *American Journal of Orthopsychiatry, 56*(2), 278-288.

Cohen, S., Evans, G. W., Krantz, D. S., & Stokols, D. (1980). Physiological, motivational and cognitive effects of aircraft noise on children. *American Psychologist, 35,* 231-243.

Cohen, S., & Wills, T. A. (1985). Stress, social support, and the buffering hypothesis. *Psychological Bulletin, 98*(2), 310-357.

Cohen, U., & Weisman, G. D. (1991). *Holding on to home: Designing environments for people with dementia.* Baltimore: Johns Hopkins University Press.

Colan, N. B., Mague, K. C., Cohen, R. S., & Schneider, R. J. (1994). Family education in the workplace: A prevention program for working parents and school-age children. *Journal of Primary Prevention, 15*(4), 161-172.

Cole, S. S., & Cole, T. M. (1983). Disability and intimacy: The importance of sexual health. In G. Albee, S. Gordon, & H. Leitenberg (Eds.), *Promoting sexual responsibility and prevention of sexual problems.* Hanover, NH: University Press of New England.

Collins, A. H., & Pancoast, D. L. (1976). *Natural helping networks: A strategy for prevention.* Washington, DC: National Association of Social Workers.

Comer, J. P. (1988). Educating poor minority children. *Scientific American, 259*(5), 42-48.

Commoner, B. (1968). *Closing the circle: Nature, man, technology.* New York: Knopf.

Compas, B. E., Phares, V., & Ledoux, N. (1989). Stress and coping preventive interventions for children and adolescents. In L. Bond & B. E. Compas (Eds.), *Primary prevention and promotion in the schools.* Newbury Park, CA: Sage.

Compas, B., & Phares, V. (1991). Stress during childhood and adolescence: Sources of risk and vulnerability. In E. Cummings, A. L. Greene, & K. H. Karraker (Eds.), *Life-span developmental psychology.* Hillsdale, NJ: Lawrence Erlbaum.

Conner, R. F. (1990). Ethical issues in evaluating the effectiveness of primary prevention programs. *Prevention in Human Services, 8*(2), 89-110.

Conte, J. R., Wolf, S., & Smith, T. (1989). What sexual offenders tell us about prevention strategies. *Child Abuse & Neglect, 13,* 293-301.

Cooper, S., Munger, R., & Ravlin, M. M. (1980). Mental health prevention through affective education in schools. *Journal of Prevention, 1*(1), 24-34.

Cooper, S., & Seckler, D. (1973). Behavioral science in primary education: A rationale. *People Watching, 2,* 37-39.

Coopersmith, S. (Ed.). (1976). *Developing motivation in children.* San Francisco: Albion.

Cormier, W. H., & Cormier, L. S. (1979). *Interviewing strategies for helpers: A guide to assessment, treatment, and evaluation.* Monterey, CA: Brooks/Cole. (Also see 3rd edition, 1991.)

Cose, E. (1994, July 11). Drawing up safer cities. *Newsweek,* p. 57.

Cotton, D. H. G. (1990). *Stress management: An integrated approach to therapy.* New York: Brunner/Mazel.

Cotton, N. S., & Geraty, R. G. (1984). Therapeutic space design: Planning an inpatient children's unit. *American Journal of Orthopsychiatry, 54*(4), 624-636.

Cousins, N. (1979). *Anatomy of an illness as perceived by the patient.* New York: Norton.

Cowen, E. L. (1985). Person-centered approaches in primary prevention in mental health: Situation-focused and competence-enhancement. *American Journal of Community Psychology, 13*(1), 31-48.

Cowen, E. L., Hightower, A. D., Johnson, D. B., Sarno, M., & Weissberg, R. P. (1989). State-level dissemination of a program for early detection and prevention of school maladjustment. *Professional Psychology: Research and Practice, 20*(5), 309-314.

Cowen, E. L., & Work, W. C. (1988). Resilient children, psychological wellness, and primary prevention. *American Journal of Community Psychology, 16*(4), 591-607.

Cowen, E. L., Work, W. C., & Wyman, P. A. (1992). Resilience among profoundly stressed urban schoolchildren. In M. Kessler, S. Goldston, & J. Joffe (Eds.), *The present and the future of prevention.* Newbury Park, CA: Sage.

Cowen, E. L., Wyman, P. A., Work, W. C., & Iker, M. R. (1995). A preventive intervention for enhancing resilience among highly stressed urban children. *Journal of Primary Prevention, 15*(3), 247-260.

Cox, T., & Ferguson, E. (1991). Individual differences, stress, and coping. In C. Cooper & R. Payne (Eds.), *Personality and stress: Individual differences in the stress process.* New York: John Wiley.

Coyne, A. C. (1991). Information and referral service usage among caregivers for dementia patients. *The Gerontologist, 31*(3), 384-388.

Crawford, R. (1978). You are dangerous to your health. *Social Policy, 8*(4), 10-20.

Cromer, W. J., & Burns, B. J. (1982). A health center response to community crisis: Some principles of prevention and intervention. *Journal of Primary Prevention, 3*(1), 35-47.

Cross, W. E. (1991). *Shades of black: Diversity in African-American identity.* Philadelphia: Temple University Press.

Crowther, T. (1993). Euthanasia. In D. Clark (Ed.), *The future of palliative care*. London: Open University Press.

Cummings, E. M., Greene, A. L., & Karraker, K. H. (Eds.). (1991). *Life-span developmental psychology: Perspectives on stress and coping*. Hillsdale, NJ: Lawrence Erlbaum.

Cummings, K. M., Pechacek, T., & Shopland, D. (1994). The illegal sale of cigarettes to U.S. minors: Estimates by state. *American Journal of Public Health, 84,* 300-302.

Danish, S. J. (1983). Musings about personal competence: The contributions of sport, health, and fitness. *American Journal of Community Psychology, 11*(3), 221-240.

Danish, S. J., Pettipas, A. J., & Hale, B. D. (1990). Sport as a context for developing competence. In T. P. Gullotta, G. R. Adams, & R. Montemeyer (Eds.), *Developing social competence in adolescence*. Newbury Park, CA: Sage.

Danish, S. J., Pettipas, A. J., & Hale, B. D. (1993). Life development intervention for athletes: Life skills through sports. *The Counseling Psychologist, 21,* 352-385.

Dannenberg, A. L., Gielen, A., Beilenson, P. L., Wioson, M. H., & Joffe, A. (1993). Bicycle helmet laws and educational campaigns: An evaluation of strategies to increase children's helmet use. *American Journal of Public Health, 83,* 667-684.

D'Augelli, A. R. (1993). Preventing mental health problems among lesbian and gay college students. *Journal of Primary Prevention, 13*(4), 245-262.

Davidson, L. L., Durkin, M. S., Kuhn, L., O'Connor, P., Barlow, B., & Hergarty, M. C. (1994). The impact of the safe kids/healthy neighborhoods injury prevention program in Harlem, 1988 through 1991. *American Journal of Public Health, 84,* 580-586.

Davidson, W. S., & Redner, R. (1988). The prevention of juvenile delinquency: Diversion from the juvenile justice system. In R. Price, E. L. Cowen, R. P. Lorion, & J. Ramos-McKay (Eds.), *14 ounces of prevention*. Washington, DC: American Psychological Association.

Davis, L., & Proctor, E. K. (1989). *Race, gender, and class: Guidelines for practice with individuals, families, and groups*. Englewood Cliffs, NJ: Prentice Hall.

Davis, R. M. (1987, March 19). Current trends in cigarette advertising and marketing. *New England Journal of Medicine, 316,* 725-732.

Dearing, J. W., Meyer, G., & Rogers, E. M. (1994). Diffusion theory and HIV risk behavior change. In R. J. DiClemente & J. L. Peterson (Eds.), *Preventing AIDS*. New York: Plenum.

Deering, M. J. (1993). Designing health promotion approaches to high-risk adolescents through formative research with youth and parents. *Public Health Reports, 108*(Suppl. 1), 68-77.

DeJong, W., & Winsten, J. A. (1990). The use of mass media in substance abuse prevention. *Health Affairs, 9*(2), 30-46.

DeJong, W., & Winsten, J. A. (1992). The strategic use of the broadcast media for AIDS prevention: Current limits and future directions. In J. Sepulveda, H. Fineberg, & J. Mann (Eds.), *AIDS: Prevention through education: A world view*. New York: Oxford University Press.

De La Rosa, M. (1988). Natural support systems of Puerto Ricans: A key dimension for well-being. *Health and Social Work, 13*(3), 181-190.

Des Jarlais, D. C., & Friedman, S. R. (1988). The psychology of preventing AIDS among intravenous drug users: A social learning conceptualization. *American Psychologist, 43*(11), 865-870.

Devin-Sheehan, L., Feldman, R. S., & Allen, V. L. (1976). Research on children tutoring children: A critical review. *Review of Educational Research, 46*(3), 355-385.

DeVito, P. J., & Karon, J. P. (1984). *Final report, parent-child home program, chapter 1*. Pittsfield, MA: ECIA, Pittsfield Public Schools.

Devore, W., & Schlesinger, E. G. (1987). *Ethnic-sensitive social work practice* (2nd ed.). Columbus, OH: Merrill.

deVries, H. A., & Adams, G. M. (1972). Comparison of exercise response in old and young men. *The Gerontologist, 11*(3), 29.

Dew, M. A., Bromet, E. J., Brent, D., & Greenhouse, J. B. (1987). A quantitative literature review of the effectiveness of suicide prevention centers. *Journal of Consulting and Clinical Psychology, 55*(2), 239-244.

Dewey, J., & McLellan, J. (1895/1964). The psychology of number. In R. Archambault (Ed.), *John Dewey on education: Selected writings.* New York: Random House.

Dickinson, N. S., & Cudaback, D. J. (1992). Parent education for adolescent mothers. *Journal of Primary Prevention, 13*(1), 23-36.

DiClemente, R. J., & Peterson, J. L. (Eds.). (1994). *Preventing AIDS: Theories and methods of behavioral intervention.* New York: Plenum.

Dohrenwend, B. P. (1986). Social stress and psychopathology. In M. Kessler & S. Goldston (Eds.), *A decade of progress in primary prevention.* Hanover, NH: University Press of New England.

Donaldson, S. (1977). City and country: Marriage proposals. In L. L. Allen (Ed.), *New towns and the suburban dream.* Port Washington, NY: Kennikat.

Dorfman, L., & Wallack, L. (1993). Advertising health: The case for counter-ads. *Public Health Reports, 108*(6), 716-726.

Douglas, J. A., & Jason, L. A. (1986). Building social support systems through a babysitting exchange program. *American Journal of Orthopsychiatry, 56*(1), 103-108.

Downie, R. S., Fyfe, C., & Tannahill, A. (1990). *Health promotion: Models and values.* Oxford, UK: Oxford University Press.

Downing, A. B., & Smoker, B. (Eds.). (1986). *Voluntary euthanasia: Experts debate the right to die.* Atlantic Highlands, NJ: Humanities Press International.

Drolen, C. S. (1990). Community mental health: Who is being served? What is being offered? *Journal of Mental Health Administration, 17*(2), 191-199.

Dryfoos, J. (1988). School-based health clinics: Three years of experience. *Family Planning Perspectives, 20*(4), 193-200.

Dryfoos, J. (1993). Preventing substance use: Rethinking strategies. *American Journal of Public Health, 83*(6), 793-795.

Dryfoos, J. (1994). *Full-service schools: A revolution in health and social services for children, youth, and families.* San Francisco: Jossey-Bass.

Dumas, J. E. (1989). Primary prevention: Toward an experimental paradigm sensitive to contextual variables. *Journal of Primary Prevention, 10*(1), 27-40.

Dumont, M. P. (1967). Tavern culture: The sustenance of homeless men. *American Journal of Orthopsychiatry, 37,* 938-945.

Dunajcik, L. (1994). Biofeedback for headaches. *American Journal of Nursing, 94,* 17-18.

Dunbar, J. (1990). Predictors of patient adherence: Patient characteristics. In S. A. Shumaker, E. Schron, & J. Ockene (Eds.), *The handbook of health behavior change.* New York: Springer.

Durkheim, E. (1951). *Suicide: A study in sociology.* Glencoe, IL: Free Press.

Durlak, J. A. (1979). Comparative effectiveness of paraprofessional and professional helpers. *Psychological Bulletin, 86,* 80-92.

Durlak, J. A. (1983). Social problem-solving as a primary prevention strategy. In R. Felner, L. A. Jason, J. N. Moritsugu, & S. S. Farber (Eds.), *Preventive psychology.* New York: Pergamon.

Durlak, J. A., & Jason, L. A. (1984). Prevention programs for school-aged children and adolescents. In M. C. Roberts & L. Peterson (Eds.), *Prevention of problems in childhood.* New York: John Wiley.

Dusenbury, L., & Botvin, G. J. (1992). Applying the competency enhancement model to substance abuse prevention. In M. Kessler, S. Goldston, & J. Joffe (Eds.), *The present and future of prevention*. Newbury Park, CA: Sage.

Early, C. J. (1968). Attitude learning in children. *Journal of Educational Psychology, 59*(3), 176-180.

Easley, M. W. (1990). The status of community water fluoridation in the United States. *Public Health Reports, 105*(4), 318-323.

Eberhardt, L. Y. (1978). Developing a support base for women. In D. C. Klein (Ed.), *Psychology of the planned community: The new town experience*. New York: Plenum.

Echterling, L. G. (1989). An ark of prevention: Preventing school absenteeism after a flood. *Journal of Primary Prevention, 9*(3), 177-184.

Edelman, E. M., & Goldstein, A. P. (1981). Moral education. In A. P. Goldstein, E. G. Carr, W. S. Davidson, & P. Wehr (Eds.), *In response to aggression*. New York: Pergamon.

Edelstein, B. A., & Michelson, L. (Eds.). (1986). *Handbook of prevention*. New York: Plenum.

Edmondson, J. E., Holman, T. B., & Morrell, W. R. (1984). The need for and effectiveness of surrogate role models among single-parent children. *Journal of Primary Prevention, 5*(2), 111-123.

Edwards, J., Tindale, R. S., Heath, L., & Posavac, E. J. (1990). *Social influence processes and prevention*. New York: Plenum.

Elder, J. P., Wildey, M., de Moor, C., Sallis, J., Eckhardt, L., Edwards, C., Erickson, A., Golbeck, A., Hovell, M., Johnston, D., Levitz, M., Molgaard, C., Young, R., Vito, D., & Woodruff, S. (1993). The long-term prevention of tobacco use among junior high school students: Classroom and telephone interventions. *American Journal of Public Health, 83*(9), 1230-1244.

Elders, M. J., Perry, C. L., Eriksen, M. P., & Giovino, G. A. (1994). The report of the Surgeon General: Preventing tobacco use among young people. *American Journal of Public Health, 84*, 543-547.

Elias, M. J. (1987). Establishing enduring prevention programs: Advancing the legacy of Swampscott. *American Journal of Community Psychology, 15*(5), 539-553.

Elias, M. J. (1989). Schools as a source of stress in children: An analysis of causal and ameliorative factors. *Journal of School Psychology, 27*, 393-407.

Elias, M. J. (1993). Educating students, the public, decision makers, and professionals about prevention: A special review section on the video "An ounce of prevention." *Journal of Primary Prevention, 14*(2), 129-131.

Elias, M. J., & Clabby, J. F. (1984). Integrating social and affective education into public school curriculum and instruction. In C. Maher, R. Illback, & J. Zins (Eds.), *Organizational psychology in the schools: A handbook for professionals*. Springfield, IL: Charles C Thomas.

Elias, M. J., & Clabby, J. F. (1992). *Building social problem-solving skills: Guidelines from a school-based program*. San Francisco: Jossey-Bass.

Elias, M. J., Gara, M. A., Schuyler, T. F., Branden-Muller, L. R., & Sayette, M. A. (1991). The promotion of social competence: Longitudinal study of a preventive school-based program. *American Journal of Orthopsychiatry, 61*(3), 409-417.

Elias, M. J., & Weissberg, R. P. (1990). School-based social competence promotion as a primary prevention strategy: A tale of two projects. In R. Lorion (Ed.), *Protecting the children: Strategies for optimizing emotional and behavioral development*. New York: Haworth.

Ellickson, P. L., Bell, R. M., & McGuigan, K. (1993). Preventing adolescent drug use: Long-term results of a junior high program. *American Journal of Public Health, 83*, 856-861.

Ellis, A. (1974). *Humanistic psychotherapy.* New York: McGraw-Hill.

Ellis, A. (1983). The use of rational-emotive therapy (RET) in working for a sexually sane society. In G. Albee, S. Gordon, & H. Leitenberg (Eds.), *Promoting sexual responsibility and preventing sexual problems.* Hanover, NH: University Press of New England.

Ellis, A. (1985). Rational-emotive therapy and its application to emotional education. In M. Bloom (Ed.), *Life-span development* (2nd ed.). New York: Macmillan.

Ellis, L., & Roe, D. A. (1993). Home-delivered meals programs for the elderly: Distribution of services in New York State. *American Journal of Public Health, 83,* 1034-1036.

Eng, E., & Hatch, J. W. (1991). Networking between agencies and black churches: The lay health advisor model. *Prevention in Human Services, 10*(1), 123-146.

Englander-Golden, P., Elconin, J., Miller, K. J., & Schwarzkopf, A. B. (1986). Brief SAY IT STRAIGHT training and follow-up in adolescent substance abuse prevention. *Journal of Primary Prevention, 6,* 219-230.

Englander-Golden, P., Elconin, J., & Satir, V. (1986). Assertive/ leveling communication and empathy in adolescent drug abuse prevention. *Journal of Primary Prevention, 6*(4), 231-243.

Erickson, A. C., McKenna, J. W., & Romano, R. M. (1990). Past lessons and new uses of the mass media in reducing tobacco consumption. *Public Health Reports, 105*(3), 239-244.

Erikson, E. H. (1963). *Childhood and society* (2nd ed.). New York: Norton.

Erikson, E. H., Erikson, J. M., & Kivnick, H. Q. (1986). *Vital involvement in old age.* New York: Norton.

Eron, L. D. (1982). Parent-child interaction, television violence, and aggression of children. *American Psychologist, 37*(2), 197-211.

Etzioni, A. (1979). How much is a life worth? *Social Policy, 9*(5), 4-8.

Evans, G. W., Jacobs, S. V., Dooley, D., & Catalano, R. (1987). The interaction of stressful life events and chronic strain on community mental health. *American Journal of Community Psychology, 15*(1), 23-34.

Evans, R. L. (1976). Smoking in children: Developing a social psychological strategy of deterrence. *Preventive Medicine, 5*(1), 122-127.

Evans, R. L., & Raines, B. E. (1990). Applying a social psychological model across health preventions: Cigarettes to smokeless tobacco. In J. Edwards, R. S. Tindale, L. Heath, & E. J. Posavac (Eds.), *Social influence processes and prevention.* New York: Plenum.

Evans, R. L., Rozelle, R. M., Mittlemark, M. B., Hansen, W. B., Bane, A., & Havis, J. (1978). Deterring onset of smoking in children—Knowledge of immediate physiological effects, and coping with peer pressure, media pressure, and parent modeling. *Journal of Applied Social Psychology, 8*(2), 126-135.

Ewigman, B. G., Kivlahan, C. H., Hosokawa, M. C., & Horman, D. (1990). Efficacy of an intervention to promote use of hearing protection devices by firefighters. *Public Health Reports, 105*(1), 53-58.

Eyer, D. (1992). *Mother-infant bonding: A scientific fiction.* New Haven, CT: Yale University Press.

Fagan, J. (1987). Neighborhood education, mobilization, and organization for juvenile crime prevention. *The ANNALS, 494,* 54-70.

Fagan, S., Long, N., & Stevens, D. (1975). *Teaching children self-control: Preventing emotional and learning problems in elementary school.* Columbus, OH: Merrill.

Farquhar, J. E. (1978). The community-based model of life-style intervention trials. *American Journal of Epidemiology, 108*(2), 103-111.

Farquhar, J. W., Fortmann, S. P., Maccoby, N., Haskell, W. L., Williams, P. T., Flora, J. A., Taylor, C. B., Brown, W. B., Jr., Solomon, D. S., & Hulley, S. B. (1985). The Stanford Five City Project: Design and methods. *American Journal of Epidemiology, 122,* 323-343.

Farran, D. C., & Haskins, R. (1980). Reciprocal influence in the social interactions of others and three-year-old children from different socioeconomic backgrounds. *Child Development, 51*(3), 254-257.

Fawcett, S. B., Fletcher, R. K., Mathews, R., Whang, P., Seekins, T., & Nielsen, L. (1982). Designing behavioral technologies with community self-help organizations. In A. Jeger & R. Slotnick (Eds.), *Community mental health and behavioral-ecology: A handbook of theory, research, and practice*. New York: Plenum.

Feindler, E., & Fremous, W. (1983). Stress inoculation training for adolescent anger problems. In D. Meichenbaum & M. Jaremko (Eds.), *Stress reduction and prevention*. New York: Plenum.

Feinstein, A. (1978). From counterculture self-help to community self-help. In D. C. Klein (Ed.), *Psychology of the planned community: The new town experience*. New York: Plenum.

Felner, R. D. (1984). Vulnerability in childhood: A preventive framework for understanding children's efforts to cope with life stress and transitions. In M. Roberts & L. Peterson (Eds.), *Prevention of problems in childhood*. New York: John Wiley.

Felner, R. D., & Adan, A. M. (1988). The school transitional environment project: An ecological intervention and evaluation. In R. Price, E. L. Cowen, R. P. Lorion, & J. Ramos-McKay (Eds.), *14 ounces of prevention*. Washington, DC: American Psychological Association.

Felner, R. D., Brand, S., Mulhall, K. E., Counter, B., Millman, J. B., & Fried, J. (1994). The parenting partnership: The evaluation of a human service/corporate workplace collaboration for the prevention of substance abuse and mental health problems, and the promotion of family and work adjustment. *Journal of Primary Prevention, 15*(2), 123-146.

Felner, R. D., Jason, L. A., Moritsugu, J. N., & Farber, S. S. (Eds.). (1983). *Preventive psychology: Theory, research, and practice*. New York: Pergamon.

Ferre, M. I. (1987). Prevention and control of violence through community revitalization, individual dignity, and personal self-confidence. *ANNALS, 494,* 27-36.

Festinger, L., Schacter, S., & Back, K. (1950). *Social pressures in informal groups*. Stanford, CA: Stanford University Press.

Field, D., & Weishaus, S. (1992). Marriage over half a century: A longitudinal study. In M. Bloom (Ed.), *Changing lives*. Columbia: University of South Carolina Press.

Fields, S. (1978). Seeking new prescriptions to heal the whole person. *Innovations, 5*(3), 2-10.

Fine, G. A. (1988). Good children and dirty play. *Play and Culture, 1,* 43-56.

Fischoff, B., Furby, L., & Morgan, M. (1987). Rape prevention: A typology of strategies. *Journal of Interpersonal Violence, 2*(3), 292-308.

Fishbein, M. (1979). A theory of reasoned action: Some applications and implications. In H. E. Howe & M. M. Page (Eds.), *Nebraska symposium on motivation*. Lincoln: University of Nebraska Press.

Fishbein, M., & Ajzen, I. (1975). *Belief, attitude, intention and behavior: An introduction to theory and research*. Reading, MA: Addison-Wesley.

Fishbein, M., & Middlestadt, S. E. (1989). Using the theory of reasoned action as a framework for understanding and changing AIDS-related behaviors. In V. M. Mays, G. Albee, & S. Schneider (Eds.), *Primary prevention of AIDS: Psychological approaches*. Newbury Park, CA: Sage.

Fishbein, M., Middlestadt, S. E., & Hitchcock, P. J. (1994). Using information to change sexually transmitted disease-related behaviors: An analysis based on the theory of reasoned action. In R. J. DiClemente & J. L. Peterson (Eds.), *Preventing AIDS*. New York: Plenum.

Fisher, J. D., & Misovich, S. J. (1990). Evolution of college students' AIDS-related behavioral responses, attitudes, knowledge, and fear. *AIDS Education and Prevention, 2*(4), 322-337.

Flay, R. B. (1987). Mass media and smoking cessation: A critical review. *American Journal of Public Health, 77,* 153-160.

Flay, R. B., Koepke, D., Thomson, S. J., Santi, S., Best, J. A., & Brown, K. S. (1989). Six-year follow-up of the first Waterloo School Prevention Trial. *American Journal of Public Health, 79*(10), 1371-1376.

Flora, J. A., & Thoresen, C. E. (1989). Components of a comprehensive strategy for reducing the risk of AIDS in adolescents. In V. Mays, G. Albee, & S. Schneider (Eds.), *Primary prevention of AIDS.* Newbury Park, CA: Sage.

Flowers, J. V., Miller, T. E., Smith, N., & Booraem, C. D. (1994). The repeatability of a single-session group to promote safe sex behavior in a male at-risk population. *Research on Social Work Practice, 4*(2), 240-247.

Folkman, S. (1991). Coping across the life span: Theoretical issues. In E. Cummings, A. L. Greene, & K. H. Karraker (Eds.), *Life-span developmental psychology.* Hillsdale, NJ: Lawrence Erlbaum.

Fonagy, P., Steele, M., Steele, H., Higgitt, A., & Target, M. (1994). The theory and practice of resilience. *Journal of Child Psychology and Psychiatry, 35*(2), 231-257.

Foote, A., Googins, B., Moriarty, M., Sandonato, C., Nadolski, J., & Jefferson, C. (1994). Implementing long-term EAP follow-up with clients and family members to help prevent relapse—with implications for primary prevention. *Journal of Primary Prevention, 15*(2), 173-191.

Forehand, R. L., Walley, P. B., & Furey, W. M. (1984). Prevention in the home: Parent and family. In M. Roberts & L. Peterson (Eds.), *Prevention of problems in childhood.* New York: John Wiley.

Forgays, D. G. (Ed.). (1978). *Environmental influences and strategies in primary prevention* (Vol. 2). Hanover, NH: University Press of New England.

Forman, S. G. (1993). *Coping skills interventions with children and adolescents.* San Francisco: Jossey-Bass.

Forster, J. L., Jeffery, R. W., Schmid, T. L., & Kramer, F. M. (1988). Preventing weight-gain in adults: A pound of prevention. *Health Psychology, 7*(6), 515-525.

Forti, T. J., & Hyg, M. S. (1983). A documented evaluation of a primary prevention through consultation. *Community Mental Health Journal, 19*(4), 290-304.

Fortmann, S. P., Williams, P. T., Haskell, W. L., Hulley, S. D., & Farquhar, J. W. (1981). Effects of health education on dietary behavior—The Stanford Three Community Study. *American Journal of Clinical Nutrition, 34*(10), 2030-2038.

Fox, D. K., Hopkins, B. L., & Anger, W. K. (1987). The long-term effects of a token economy on safety performance in open-pit mining. *Journal of Applied Behavior Analysis, 20*(3), 215-224.

Frankenburg, W. K., Van Doorninck, W. J., Liddell, T. N., & Dick, N. P. (1976). The Denver Prescreening Developmental Questionnaire (PDQ). *Pediatrics, 57,* 744-753.

Freda, M. C., Damus, K., Andersen, H. F., Brustman, L. E., & Merkatz, I. R. (1990). A "PROPP" for the Bronx: Preterm birth prevention education in the inner city. *Obstetrics & Gynecology, 76*(Suppl. 1), 93S-96S.

Freedman, J. L. (1975). *Crowding and behavior.* New York: Viking.

Freimuth, V. S., Hammond, S. L., & Stein, J. A. (1988). Health advertising: Prevention for profit. *American Journal of Public Health, 78*(5), 557-561.

Freire, P. (1970). *Pedagogy of the oppressed.* New York: Continuum.

Freire, P. (1973). *Education for critical consciousness.* New York: Continuum.

French, J. F., Fisher, C. C., & Costa, Jr., S. J. (Eds.). (1983). *Working with evaluators: A guide for drug abuse prevention grant managers* (DHHS Publication No. ADM 83-1233). Washington, DC: Government Printing Office.

French, J. F., & Kaufman, H. J. (Eds.). (1981). *Handbook for prevention evaluation: Prevention evaluation guidelines* (DHHS Publication No. ADM 81-1145). Washington, DC: Government Printing Office.

Freudenberg, N., & Golub, M. (1987). Health education, public policy, and disease prevention: A case history of the New York Coalition to End Lead Poisoning. *Health Education Quarterly, 14*(4), 389-401.

Friedan, B. (1981). Women—New patterns, problems, possibilities. In J. Joffe & G. Albee (Eds.), *Prevention through political action and social change*. Hanover, NH: University Press of New England.

Friedman, S. R., DesJarlais, D. C., & Ward, T. P. (1994). Social models for changing health-relevant behaviors. In R. J. DiClemente & J. L. Peterson (Eds.), *Preventing AIDS*. New York: Plenum.

Fuentes, E. G., & LeCapitaine, J. E. (1990). The effects of a primary prevention program on Hispanic children. *Education, 110*(3), 298-303.

Furby, L., Fischhoff, B., & Morgan, M. (1989). Judged effectiveness of common rape prevention and self-defense strategies. *Journal of Interpersonal Violence, 4*(1), 44-64.

Furby, L., Fischhoff, B., & Morgan, M. (1991). Rape prevention and self-defense: At what price? *Women's Studies International Forum, 14*(1 & 2), 49-62.

Gaboury, A., & Ladouceur, R. (1993). Evaluation of a prevention program for pathological gambling among adolescents. *Journal of Primary Prevention, 14*(1), 21-28.

Gambrill, E., Thomas, E., & Carter, R. (1971). Procedures for sociobehavioral practice in open settings. *Social Work, 16,* 51-62.

Garbaino, J. (1988). Preventing childhood injury: Development and mental health issues. *American Journal of Orthopsychiatry, 58*(1), 25-45.

Garber, J., & Seligman, M. E. P. (Eds.). (1980). *Human helplessness: Theory and applications*. New York: Academic Press.

Gardiner, L. L., Dziados, J. E., Jones, B. H., Brundage, J. F., Harris, J. M., Sullivan, R., & Gill, P. (1988). Prevention of lower extremity stress fractures: A controlled trial of a shock absorbent insole. *American Journal of Public Health, 78*(12), 1563-1567.

Garland, A., Shaffer, D., & Whittle, B. (1989). A national survey of school-based, adolescent suicide prevention programs. *Journal of the American Academy of Child and Adolescent Psychiatry, 28*(6), 931-934.

Garmezy, N. (1971). Vulnerability research and the issue of primary prevention. *American Journal of Orthopsychiatry, 41*(1), 101-116.

Garmezy, N., & Masten, A. (1991). The protective role of competence indicators in children at risk. In E. Cummings, A. L. Greene, & K. H. Karraker (Eds.), *Life-span developmental psychology*. Hillsdale, NJ: Lawrence Erlbaum.

Garmezy, N., Masten, A., Nordstrom, L., & Ferrarese, M. (1979). The nature of competence in normal and deviant children. In M. W. Kent & J. E. Rolf (Eds.), *Social competence in children*. Hanover, NH: University Press of New England.

Garmezy, N., Masten, A., & Tellegen, A. (1984). Studies of stress-resistant children: A building block for developmental psychopathology. *Child Development, 55,* 97-111.

Gartner, A., & Riessman, F. (1977). *Self-help in the human services*. San Francisco: Jossey-Bass.

Geismar, L. L. (1971). Implications of a family life improvement project. *Social Casework, 1971,* 455-465.

Geller, E. S. (1986). Prevention of environmental problems. In B. Edelstein & L. Michelson (Eds.), *Handbook of prevention*. New York: Plenum.

Geller, E. S. (1990). Preventing injuries and deaths from vehicle crashes: Encouraging belts and discouraging booze. In J. Edwards, R. S. Tindale, L. Heath, & E. J. Posavac (Eds.), *Social influence processes and prevention*. New York: Plenum.

Geller, E. S. (1993). Increasing road safety behaviors. In D. Glenwick & J. Jason (Eds.), *Promoting health and mental health in children, youth, and families*. New York: Springer.

Geller, E. S., & Hahn, H. A. (1984). Promoting safety belt use at industrial sites—An effective program for blue collar employees. *Professional Psychology, 15*(4), 553-564.

Geller, E. S., Winett, R. A., & Everett, P. B. (1982). *Preserving the environment: New strategies for behavior change*. Elmsford, NY: Pergamon.

Gelles, R. J. (1982). Problems in defining and labeling child abuse. In R. Starr (Ed.), *Child abuse predictions: Policy implications*. Cambridge, MA: Ballinger.

Gensheimer, L. K., Roosa, M. W., & Ayers, T. S., (1990). Children's self-selection into prevention programs: Evaluating an innovative recruitment strategy for children of alcoholics. *American Journal of Community Psychology, 18*(5), 707-723.

George, L. K., & Gwyther, L. P. (1988). Support groups for caregivers of memory-impaired elderly: Easing caregiver burden. In L. Bond & B. Wagner (Eds.), *Families in transition*. Newbury Park, CA: Sage.

Gerbert, B., & Maguire, B. (1989). Public acceptance of the Surgeon General's brochure on AIDS. *Public Health Reports, 104*(2), 130-133.

Germain, C., & Gitterman, A. (1995). Ecological perspective. In R. L. Edwards & others (Eds.), *Encyclopedia of social work* (19th ed.). Washington, DC: National Association of Social Workers.

Gerrard, M., McCann, L., & Fortini, M. (1983). Prevention of unwanted pregnancy. *American Journal of Community Psychology, 11*(2), 153-167.

Gibbs, L. M. (1983). Community response to an emergency situation: Psychological destruction and the Love Canal. *American Journal of Community Psychology, 11*(2), 116-125.

Gilchrist, L. D., Schinke, S., Snow, W., Schilling, R., & Scnechal, V. (1988). The transition of junior high school: Opportunities for primary prevention. *Journal of Primary Prevention, 8*(3), 99-108.

Gillespie, D. F., & Banerjee, M. M. (1993). Prevention planning and disaster preparedness. *Journal of Applied Social Science, 17*(2), 237-250.

Gilligan, C. (1982). *In a different voice: Psychological theory and women's development*. Cambridge, MA: Harvard University Press.

Gillmore, M. R., Hawkins, J. D., Day, L. E., & Catalano, R. F. (1992). Friendship and deviance: New evidence on an old controversy. *Journal of Early Adolescence, 12*(1), 80-95.

Ginter, P. M., Duncan, W. J., & Capper, S. A. (1991). Strategic planning for public health practice using macroenvironmental analysis. *Public Health Reports, 106*(2), 134-141.

Ginzburg, H. M., Jevec, R. J., & Reutershan, T. (1993). The public health services' response to Hurricane Andrew. *Public Health Reports, 108*(2), 241-248.

Girgis, A., Sanson-Fisher, R. W., & Watson, A. (1994). A workplace intervention for increasing outdoor workers' use of solar prevention. *American Journal of Public Health, 84*(1), 77-81.

Glanz, K., Lewis, F. M., & Rimer, B. K. (Eds.). (1990). *Health behavior and health education: Theory, research, and practice*. San Francisco: Jossey-Bass.

Glass, D. C., & Singer, J. E. (1972). *Urban stress*. New York: Academic Press.

Glasscote, R. M., Kohn, E., Beigel, A., Raber, M. F., Roeske, N., Cox, B. A., Raybin, J. B., & Bloom, B. L. (1980). *Preventing mental illness: Efforts and attitudes*. Washington, DC: Joint Information Service.

Glasser, W. (1969). *Schools without failure*. New York: Harper & Row.

Glenwick, D. S., & Jason, L. A. (Eds.). (1993). *Promoting health and mental health in children, youth, and families.* New York: Springer.

Glidden, L., & Whigam, K. (1987). Smokeless tobacco reduction program. *Public Health Reports, 102*(1), 90-95.

Glynn, T. J. (1989). Essential elements of school-based smoking prevention programs. *Journal of School Health, 59*(5), 181-188.

Goffman, E. (1961). *Asylums: Essays on the social situation of mental patients and other inmates.* Garden City, NY: Anchor.

Golann, N. (1986). *The perilous bridge: Helping clients through mid-life transitions.* New York: Free Press.

Goldstein, A. P. (1983). Behavior modification approaches to aggression prevention and control. In A. P. Goldstein (Ed.), *Prevention and control of aggression.* New York: Pergamon.

Goldstein, M. J. (Ed.). (1982). *Preventive intervention in schizophrenia: Are we ready?* (DHHS Publication No. ADM 82-111). Washington, DC: Government Printing Office.

Goldstein, M. S. (1992). *The health movement: Promoting fitness in America.* New York: Twayne.

Goldston, S. E. (1986). The federal scene: Ten years later. In M. Kessler & S. Goldston (Eds.), *A decade of progress in primary prevention.* Hanover, NH: University Press of New England.

Goldston, S. E. (1991). A survey of prevention activities in state mental health authorities. *Professional Psychology: Research and Practice, 22*(4), 315-321.

Gomel, M., Oldenburg, B., Simpson, J. M., & Owen, N. (1993). Work-site cardiovascular risk reduction: A randomized trial of health risk assessment, education, counseling, and incentives. *American Journal of Public Health, 83*(9), 1231-1238.

Gondolf, E. W. (1987). Changing men who batter: A developmental model for integrated interventions. *Journal of Family Violence, 2*(4), 345-359.

Goodman, C. (1990). Evaluation of a model self-help telephone program: Impact on natural networks. *Social Work, 35*(6), 556-562.

Gordon, S. (1983). The politics of prevention and sex education. In G. Albee, S. Gordon, & H. Leitenberg (Eds.), *Promoting sexual responsibility and preventing sexual problems.* Hanover, NH: University Press of New England.

Gordon, T. (1970). *Parent effectiveness training.* New York: Wyden.

Gordon, T. (1974). *Teacher effectiveness training.* New York: Wyden.

Gordon, T. (1977). *Leader effectiveness training.* New York: Putnam.

Gordon, T. (1989). *Teaching children self-discipline . . . at home and at school: New ways for parents and teachers to build self-control, self-esteem, and self-reliance.* New York: Random House.

Gordon, V. C., & Ledray, L. E. (1985). Depression in women: The challenge of treatment and prevention. *Journal of Psychosocial Nursing, 23*(1), 26-34.

Gore, A. (1992). *Earth in the balance: Ecology and the human spirit.* Boston: Houghton Mifflin.

Gostin, L., & Ziegler, A. (1987). A review of AIDS-related legislation and regulatory policy in the United States. *Law, Medicine, and Health Care, 15,* 5-15.

Gottlieb, B. H. (Ed.). (1981). *Social networks and social supports.* Beverly Hills, CA: Sage.

Gottlieb, B. H. (1983). *Social support strategies.* Beverly Hills, CA: Sage.

Gottlieb, B. H. (1987). Using social support to protect and promote health. *Journal of Primary Prevention, 8*(1 & 2), 49-70.

Graham, J. W., Collins, L. M., Wugalter, S. E., Chung, N. K., & Hansen, W. B. (1991). Modeling transitions in latent stage-sequential processes: A substance use prevention example. *Journal of Consulting and Clinical Psychology, 59*(1), 48-57.

Gray, J. J., & Hoage, C. M. (1990). Bulimia nervosa: Group behavior therapy with exposure plus response prevention. *Psychological Reports, 66,* 667-674.

Green, J. W. (1982). *Cultural awareness in the human services.* Englewood Cliffs, NJ: Prentice Hall.

Green, R.-J. (1995). High achievement, underachievement, and learning disabilities: A family systems model. In B. A. Ryan, G. R. Adams, T. P. Gullotta, R. P. Weissberg, & R. L. Hampton (Eds.), *The family-school connection: Theory, research, and practice.* Thousand Oaks, CA: Sage.

Greenspan, S. I. (1980). *Psychopathology and adaptation in infancy and early childhood: Principles of clinical diagnosis and preventive intervention.* Springfield, VA: NTIS.

Grobstein, R. (1979). Amniocentesis counseling. In S. Kessler (Ed.), *Genetic counseling: Psychological dimensions.* New York: Academic Press.

Group for the Advancement of Psychiatry. (1989). *Psychiatric prevention and the family life cycle: Risk reduction by frontline practitioners.* New York: Brunner/Mazel.

Grozuczak, J. (1981). Health promotion strategies for unionized workers. In L. Ng & D. Davis (Eds.), *Strategies for public health.* New York: Van Nostrand Reinhold.

Guerney, B. G., Jr. (1988). Family relationship enhancement: A skill training approach. In L. Bond & B. Wagner (Eds.), *Families in transition.* Newbury Park, CA: Sage.

Gullotta, T. P. (1982). Easing the distress of grief: A selected review of the literature with implications for preventive programs. *Journal of Primary Prevention, 3*(1), 6-17.

Guyer, B., Gallagher, S. S., Chang, B., Azzara, C. V., Cupples, L. A., & Colton, T. (1989). Prevention of childhood injuries: Evaluation of the statewide childhood injury prevention program (SCIPP). *American Journal of Public Health, 79*(11), 1521-1527.

Hall, P. (1988). *Cities of tomorrow.* Oxford, UK: Basil Blackwell.

Halpern, R., & Covey, L. (1983). Community support for adolescent parents and their children: The parent-to-parent program in Vermont. *Journal of Primary Prevention, 3*(3), 160-173.

Hampton, R. L., Gullotta, T. P., Adams, G. R., Potter, E. H., & Weissberg, R. P. (Eds.). (1993). *Family violence: Prevention and treatment.* Newbury Park, CA: Sage.

Hampton, R. L., Jenkins, P., & Gullotta, T. P. (Eds.). (1996). *Preventing violence in America.* Thousand Oaks, CA: Sage.

Handal, P., & Moore, C. (1987). The influence of physical, psychosocial, and sociocultural supplies on mental health and life satisfaction: A test of Caplan's Supply Model. *Journal of Primary Prevention, 7*(3), 132-142.

Hansen, W. B., & Graham, J. W. (1991). Preventing alcohol, marijuana, and cigarette use among adolescents: Peer pressure resistance training versus establishing conservative norms. *Preventive Medicine, 20,* 414-430.

Hansen, W. B., Johnson, C. A., Flay, B. R., Graham, J. W., & Sobel, J. (1988). Affective and social influences approaches to the prevention of multiple substance abuse among seventh grade students: Results from Project SMART. *Preventive Medicine, 17,* 135-154.

Harvey, P., Forehand, R., Brown, C., & Holmes, R. (1988). The prevention of sexual abuse: Examination of the effectiveness of a program with kindergarten-age children. *Behavior Therapy, 19,* 429-435.

Harwood, R. L., & Weissberg, R. P. (1992). A conceptual framework for context-sensitive prevention programming: A symbolic interactionist perspective. *Journal of Primary Prevention, 13*(2), 85-114.

Haskell, W. L. (1985). Exercise programs for health promotion. In J. C. Rosen & L. J. Solomon (Eds.), *Prevention in health psychology.* Hanover, NH: University Press of New England.

Hatcher, R. A. (1990). Sexual etiquette 101. *SIECUS, 18*(5), 9.

Hathaway, W. L., & Pargament, K. I. (1991). The religious dimensions of coping: Implications for prevention and promotion. *Prevention in Human Services, 9*(2), 65-92.

Hauser, S., Vieyra, M., Jacobson, A., & Wertlieb, D. (1985). Vulnerability and resilience in adolescence: Views from the family. *Journal of Early Adolescence, 5*(1), 81-100.

Haven, G. G., & Stolz, J. W. (1989). Students teaching AIDS to students: Addressing AIDS in the adolescent population. *Public Health Reports, 104*(1), 75-79.

Hawkins, J. D., Catalano, R. F., & Kent, L. A. (1991). Combining broadcast media and parent education to prevent teenage drug abuse. In L. Donohew, H. E. Sypher, & W. J. Bukoski (Eds.), *Persuasive communication and drug abuse prevention*. Hillsdale, NJ: Lawrence Erlbaum.

Hawkins, J. D., Catalano, R. F., Morrison, D. M., O'Donnell, J., Abbott, R. D., & Day, L. E. (1989). The Seattle Social Development Project: Effects of the first four years on protective factors and problem behaviors. In J. McCord & R. Tremblay (Eds.), *The prevention of antisocial behavior in children*. New York: Guilford.

Hawkins, J. D., Doueck, H. J., & Lishner, D. M. (1988). Changing teaching practices in mainstream classrooms to improve bonding and behavior in low achievers. *American Educational Research Journal, 25*(1), 31-50.

Hawkins, J. D., & Lam, T. (1987). Teacher practices, social development, and delinquency. In J. Burchard & S. Burchard (Eds.), *Prevention of delinquent behavior*. Newbury Park, CA: Sage.

Hawkins, J. D., Von Cleve, E., & Catalano, R. F. (1991). Reducing early childhood aggression: Results of a primary prevention program. *Journal of the American Academy of Child and Adolescent Psychiatry, 30*(2), 208-217.

Hawkins, J. D., & Weis, J. G. (1985). The social development model: An integrative approach to delinquency prevention. *Journal of Primary Prevention, 6*(2), 73-97.

Hay, D. F. (1994). Prosocial development. *Journal of Child Psychiatry and Psychology, 35*(1), 29-71.

Heller, K., Price, R., Reinherz, S., Riger, S., Wandersman, A., & D'Aunno, T. A. (Eds.). (1984). *Psychology and community change: Challenges of the future*. Homewood, IL: Dorsey.

Heller, K., & Swindle, R. W. (1983). Social networks, perceived social support, and coping with stress. In R. Felner, L. A. Jason, J. N. Moritsugu, & S. S. Farber (Eds.), *Preventive psychology*. New York: Pergamon.

Herrenkohl, E. C., Herrenkohl, R. C., & Egolf, B. (1994). Resilient early school-age children from maltreating homes: Outcomes in late adolescence. *American Journal of Orthopsychiatry, 64*(2), 301-309.

Hersey, J. C., Klibanoff, L. S., Clyburn, S., & Probst, J. C. (1981). *Evaluation of the "Friends Can Be Good Medicine" pilot project*. Arlington, VA: Kappa Systems.

Hess, R. (1983). Early intervention with the unemployed: Employment transition program of the University of Michigan. *Journal of Primary Prevention, 4*(2), 129-131.

Higgins, A. (1991). The just community approach to moral education: Evaluation of an idea and recent findings. In W. Kurtines & J. Gewirtz (Eds.), *Handbook of moral behavior and development*. Hillsdale, NJ: Lawrence Erlbaum.

Hinkle, L. E., Jr., & Loring, W. C. (1977). *The effects of the man-made environment on health and behavior*. Washington, DC: Government Printing Office.

Hjorther, A., Nielsen, F. M., & Segest, E. (1990). Prevention of AIDS: Free condoms to drug abusers in the municipality of Copenhagen. *International Journal of the Addictions, 25*(7), 745-753.

Holahan, C. J., & Spearly, J. L. (1980). Coping and ecology: An integrative model for community psychology. *American Journal of Community Psychology, 8*, 671-685.

Hollister, W. (1967). The concept of strens in education: A challenge to curriculum development. In E. Bower & W. Hollister (Eds.), *Behavioral science frontiers in education*. New York: John Wiley.

Holmes, T. H., & Rahe, R. H. (1967). The social readjustment rating scale. *Journal of Psychosomatic Research, 11,* 213-218.

Hong, L. (1992). *Safer sex menu* [Mimeo]. New Haven, CT: Yale School of Medicine, Department of Epidemiology and Public Health, reproduced by the University of Connecticut Health Education Office.

Hooked on tobacco: The teen epidemic. (1995, March). *Consumer Reports, 60,* 142-147.

Howard, E. (1902/1965). *Garden cities of tomorrow*. Cambridge: MIT Press.

Howell, J. C. (1995). *Guide for implementing the comprehensive strategy for serious, violent, and chronic juvenile offenders*. Washington, DC: Office of Juvenile Justice and Delinquency Prevention.

Hraba, J. (1979). *American ethnicity*. Itasca, IL: F. E. Peacock.

Huey, W., & Rank, R. (1984). Effects of counselor and peer led assertiveness training groups for black adolescents who are aggressive. *Journal of Counseling Psychology, 31,* 193-203.

Hulley, S. B., & Hearst, N. (1989). The worldwide epidemiology and prevention of AIDS. In V. Mays, G. Albee, & S. Schneider (Eds.), *Primary prevention of AIDS* (Vol. 12). Newbury Park, CA: Sage.

Hunter, D. J., & Chen, L. C. (1992). The impact of AIDS, and AIDS education, in the context of health problems of the developing world. In J. Sepulveda, H. Fineberg, & J. Mann (Eds.), *AIDS prevention through education: A world view*. New York: Oxford University Press.

Hutchins, S. S., Gindler, J., Atkinson, W., Mihalek, E., Ewert, D., LeBarron, C., Swint, E., & Hadler, S. (1993). Preschool children at high risk for measles: Opportunities to vaccinate. *American Journal of Public Health, 83*(6), 862-867.

Huxley, P., & Warner, R. (1993). Primary prevention of parenting dysfunction in high-risk cases. *American Journal of Orthopsychiatry, 63*(4), 582-588.

Insel, P. M. (1980). *Environmental variables and the prevention of mental illness*. Lexington, MA: Lexington Books.

Institute of Medicine. (1991). *Improving American's diet and health: From recommendations to action* (P. R. Thomas, Ed.). Washington, DC: Committee on Dietary Guidelines.

Is there lead in your water? (1993, February). *Consumer Reports, 58,* 73-78.

Iscoe, I., Bloom, B., & Spielberger, C. (Eds.). (1977). *Community psychology in transition*. New York: John Wiley.

Israel, B. A., & Schurman, S. J. (1990). Social support, control, and the stress process. In K. Glanz, F. M. Lewis, & B. K. Rimer (Eds.), *Health behavior and health education*. San Francisco: Jossey-Bass.

Ito, J. R., Donovan, D. M., & Hall, J. J. (1988). Relapse prevention in alcohol aftercare: Effects on drinking outcome, change process, and aftercare attendance. *British Journal of Addiction, 83,* 171-181.

Ittelson, W. H., Proshansky, H. M., Rivlin, G. G., Winkel, G. H., & Dempsey, D. (1974). *An introduction to environmental psychology*. New York: Holt, Rinehart & Winston.

Ivey, A. E., & Authier, J. (1978). *Microcounseling: Innovations in interviewing, counseling, psychotherapy, and psychoeducation* (2nd ed.). Springfield, IL: Charles C Thomas.

Jaccard, J., Turrisi, R., & Wan, C. (1990). Implications of behavioral decision theory and social marketing for designing social action programs. In J. Edwards, R. S. Tindale, L. Heath, & E. J. Posavac (Eds.), *Social influence processes and prevention*. New York: Plenum.

Jacobson, E. (1934). *You must relax: A practical method of reducing the strain of modern living.* New York: McGraw-Hill.

Janis, I. L. (1983). Stress inoculation in health care. In D. Meichenbaum & M. Jaremko (Eds.), *Stress reduction and prevention.* New York: Plenum.

Jansson, B., & Haglund, B. (1991). Intervention strategies directed at exposure to organic solvents at work sites: A case study. *Journal of Primary Prevention, 11*(4), 295-317.

Janz, N. K., & Becker, M. H. (1984). The health belief model: A decade later. *Health Education Quarterly, 11,* 1-47.

Jason, L. A. (1992). Eco-transactional behavioral research. *Journal of Primary Prevention, 13*(1), 37-72.

Jason, L. A., Crawford, I., & Gruder, C. L. (1989). Using a community model in media-based health promotion intervention. *Journal of Primary Prevention, 9*(4), 233-236.

Jason, L. A., Durlak, J. A., & Holton-Walter, E. (1984). Prevention of child problems in the schools. In M. Roberts & L. Peterson (Eds.), *Prevention of problems in childhood.* New York: John Wiley.

Jason, L. A., Johnson, J., Danner, K., Taylor, S., & Kurasaki, K. (1993). A comprehensive, preventive, parent-based intervention for high-risk transfer students. *Prevention in Human Services, 10*(2), 27-38.

Jason, L. A., Kurasaki, K. S., Neuson, L., & Garcia, C. (1993). Training parents in a preventive intervention for transfer children. *Journal of Primary Prevention, 13*(3), 213-227.

Jason, L. A., LaPointe, P., & Billinghom, S. (1986). The media and self-help: A preventive community intervention. *Journal of Primary Prevention, 6*(3), 156-167.

Jason, L. A., Lesowitz, T., Michaels, M., Blitz, C., Victars, L., Lean, L., & Yeager, E. (1989). A worksite smoking cessation intervention involving the media and incentives. *American Journal of Community Psychology, 17*(6), 785-799.

Jason, L. A., & Rhodes, J. E. (1989). Children helping children: Implications for prevention. *Journal of Primary Prevention, 9*(4), 203-212.

Jeffery, R. W., Forster, J., French, S., Kelder, S., Lando, H., McGovern, P., Jacobs, Jr., D., & Baxter, J. (1993). The healthy worker project: A work-site intervention for weight control and smoking cessation. *American Journal of Public Health, 83,* 395-401.

Jeger, A. M., & Slotnick, R. S. (Eds.). (1982). *Community mental health and behavioral-ecology: A handbook of theory, research, and practice.* New York: Plenum.

Jemmott, J. B., & Jemmott, J. S. (1994). Interventions with adolescents in community settings. In R. J. DiClemente & J. L. Peterson (Eds.), *Preventing AIDS: Theories and methods of behavioral interventions.* New York: Plenum.

Joffe, J. M. (1982). Approaches to prevention of adverse developmental consequences of genetic and prenatal factors. In L. A. Bond & J. M. Joffe (Eds.), *Facilitating infant and early childhood development.* Hanover, NH: University Press of New England.

Joffe, J. M., & Albee, G. W. (Eds.). (1981a). *Prevention through political action and social change* (Vol. 5). Hanover, NH: University Press of New England.

Joffe, J. M., & Albee, G. W. (1981b). Powerlessness and psychopathology. In J. Joffe & G. Albee (Eds.), *Prevention through political action and social change.* Hanover, NH: University Press of New England.

Johnson, D. L. (1988). Primary prevention of behavior problems in young children: The Houston Parent-Child Development Center. In R. Price, E. L. Cowen, R. P. Lorion, & J. Ramos-McKay (Eds.), *14 ounces of prevention.* Washington, DC: American Psychological Association.

Johnson, D. W., Johnson, R., Tiffany, M., & Zaidman, B. (1984). Cross-ethnic relationships: The impact of intergroup cooperation and intergroup competition. *Journal of Educational Research, 78*(2), 75-79.

Johnson, D. W., Maruyama, G., Johnson, R., Nelson, D., & Skon, L. (1981). Effects of cooperative, competitive and individualistic goal structures on achievement: A meta-analysis. *Psychological Bulletin, 89*(1), 47-62.

Johnson, J., Williams, M., & Kotarba, J. (1990). Proactive and reactive strategies for delivering community-based HIV prevention services: An ethnographic analysis. *AIDS Education and Prevention, 2*(3), 191-200.

Jung, C. G. (1957). *Collected works.* New York: Pantheon.

Kadushin, A. (1977). *Consultation in social work.* New York: Columbia University Press.

Kahn, N. (1984). *More learning in less time: A guide to effective study* (2nd ed.). Upper Montclair, NJ: Boynton/Cook.

Kalafat, J., Elias, M., & Gara, M. A. (1993). The relationship of bystander intervention variables to adolescents' responses to suicidal peers. *Journal of Primary Prevention, 13*(4), 231-244.

Kanfer, F. H., & Phillips, S. (1970). *Learning foundations of behavior therapy.* New York: John Wiley.

Kapila, M., & Pye, M. J. (1992). The European response to AIDS. In J. Sepulveda, H. Fineberg, & J. Mann (Eds.), *AIDS: Prevention through education: A world view.* New York: Oxford University Press.

Kaplan, R. M. (1993). *The Hippocratic predicament: Affordability, access, and accountability in American medicine.* New York: Academic Press.

Karsk, R., & Klein, D. C. (1978). Teenagers in Columbia. In D. C. Klein (Ed.), *Psychology of the planned community: The new town experience.* New York: Plenum.

Katcher, M. L. (1987). Prevention of tap water scald burns: Evaluation of a multi-media injury control program. *American Journal of Public Health, 77*(9), 1195-1197.

Katlin, C. S., & Goldband, S. (1980). Biofeedback. In F. Kanfer & A. Goldstein (Eds.), *People helping people change* (2nd ed.). New York: Pergamon.

Katz, A. H. (1993). *Self-help in America: A social movement perspective.* New York: Twayne.

Katz, D. (1960). The functional approach to the study of attitudes. *Public Opinion Quarterly, 24*(2), 163-204.

Kauffman, C., Grunebaum, H., Cohler, B., & Garner, E. (1979). Superkids: Competent children of psychotic mothers. *American Journal of Psychiatry, 36,* 1389-1402.

Kazdin, A. E. (1990). Prevention of conduct disorder. In NIMH, *The prevention of mental disorders: Progress, problems, and prospects [Preliminary report of the National Conference on Prevention Research].*

Keeler, K., & Swift, C. (1982). The community baby shower: Detroit packages prevention messages to teenage parents. *Journal of Primary Prevention, 3*(1), 48-51.

Kellam, S. G. (1975). *Mental health and going to school: The Woodlawn Program of Assessment, Early Intervention, and Evaluation.* Chicago: University of Chicago Press.

Kellam, S. G. (1990). Developmental epidemiological framework for family research on depression and aggression. In G. R. Patterson (Ed.), *Depression and aggression in family interaction.* Englewood Cliffs, NJ: Lawrence Erlbaum.

Kellam, S. G., & Werthamer-Larsson, L. (1986). Developmental epistemiology: A basis for prevention. In M. Kessler & S. Goldston (Eds.), *A decade of progress in primary prevention.* Hanover, NH: University Press of New England.

Keller, E. F. (1985). *Reflections on gender and science.* New Haven, CT: Yale University Press.

Kelly, J. A., St. Lawrence, J. S., Brasfield, T. L., & Hood, H. V. (1989). Group intervention to reduce AIDS risk behavior in gay men: Applications of behavioral principles. In

V. Mays, G. Albee, & S. Schneider (Eds.), *Primary prevention of AIDS*. Newbury Park, CA: Sage.

Kelly, J. G. (1988). *A guide to conducting prevention research in the community: First steps*. New York: Haworth.

Kelly, J. G., & Hess, R. E. (1987). *The ecology of prevention: Illustrating mental health consultation*. New York: Haworth.

Kelly, L. D. (1982). Between the dream and the reality: A look at programs nominated for the Lela Rowland Prevention Award of the National Mental Health Association. *Journal of Primary Prevention, 2*(4), 217-229.

Kenkel, M. B. (1986). Stress-coping support in rural communities: A model for primary prevention. *American Journal of Community Psychology, 14L5*, 457-478.

Kennell, J. H., Jerauld, R., Wolfe, H., Chesler, D., Kreger, N., McAlpine, W., Steffa, M., & Klaus, M. H. (1974). Maternal behavior one year after early and extended post-partum contact. *Developmental Medicine and Child Neurology, 16*, 172-179.

Kenney, K. C. (1986). Research in mental health consultation: Emerging trends, issues, and problems. In F. V. Mannino, E. J. Trickett, M. F. Shore, M. G. Kidder, & G. Levin (Eds.), *Handbook of mental health consultation*. Washington, DC: U.S. Department of Health and Human Services.

Kennie, D. C. (1993). *Preventive care for elderly people*. Cambridge, UK: Cambridge University Press.

Kent, M. W., & Rolf, J. E. (Eds.). (1979). *Social competence in children* (Vol. 3). Hanover, NH: University Press of New England.

Kessler, M., & Goldston, S. E. (Eds.). (1986). *A decade of progress in primary prevention* (Vol. 9). Hanover, NH: University Press of New England.

Kessler, M., Goldston, S. E., & Joffe, J. M. (Eds.). (1992). *The present and future of prevention: In honor of George W. Albee* (Vol. 15). Newbury Park, CA: Sage.

Kessler, S. (Ed.). (1979). *Genetic counseling: Psychological dimensions*. New York: Academic Press.

Ketterer, R. E., Bader, B., & Levy, M. (1980). *Strategies and skills for promoting mental health*. Beverly Hills, CA: Sage.

Kidder, M. G., Tinker, M. B., Mannino, F. V., & Trickett, E. J. (Compilers). (1986). An annotated reference guide to the consultation literature, 1978-1984. In F. V. Mannino, E. J. Trickett, M. F. Shore, M. G. Kidder, & G. Levin (Eds.), *Handbook of mental health consultation*. Washington, DC: U.S. Department of Health and Human Services.

Killen, J. D., Fortmann, S. P., Newman, B., & Varady, A. (1990). Evaluation of a treatment approach combining nicotine gum with self-guided behavioral treatments for smoking relapse prevention. *Journal of Consulting and Clinical Psychology, 58*(1), 85-92.

Killen, J. D., Telch, M. J., Robinson, T. N., Maccoby, N., Taylor, C. B., & Farquhar, J. W. (1988). Cardiovascular disease risk reduction for tenth graders: A multiple-factor school-based approach. *Journal of the American Medical Association, 260*(12), 1728-1733.

Kim, S. (1983). The short-term effect of a national prevention model on student drug abuse. *Journal of Primary Prevention, 4*(2), 118-128.

King, E. S., Rimer, B., Seay, J., Balshem, A., & Engstrom, P. (1994). Promoting mammography use through progressive interventions: Is it effective? *American Journal of Public Health, 84*, 104-106.

King, G. D. (1977). An evaluation of the effectiveness of a telephone counseling center. *American Journal of Community Psychology, 5*, 75-83.

Kirby, D., & DiClemente, R. J. (1994). School-based interventions to preventing unprotected sex and HIV among adolescents. In R. J. DiClemente & J. L. Peterson (Eds.), *Preventing AIDS: Theories and methods of behavioral interventions*. New York: Plenum.

Kirkham, M. A., & Schilling, R. (1990). Life skills training with mothers of handicapped children. *Advances in Group Work,* 67-87.

Kirscht, J. P., & Joseph, J. G. (1989). The health belief model: Some implications for behavior change, with reference to homosexual males. In V. Mays, G. Albee, & S. Schneider (Eds.), *Primary prevention of AIDS.* Newbury Park, CA: Sage.

Klaus, M. H., Jerauld, R., Kreger, N. C., McAlpine, W., Steffa, M., & Kennell, J. H. (1972). Maternal attachment: Importance of the first postpartum days. *New England Journal of Medicine, 286,* 460.

Klaus, M. H., & Kennell, J. H. (1976). *Maternal-infant bonding.* St. Louis: C. V. Mosby.

Klein, D. (Ed.). (1978). *Psychology of the planned community: The new town experience.* New York: Human Sciences Press.

Klein, D. C., & Goldston, S. E. (1977). Primary prevention: An idea whose time has come. *Proceedings of the Pilot Conference on Primary Prevention, April 24, 1976* (DHEW Publication No. ADM 77-447). Washington, DC: Government Printing Office.

Kline, M. L., & Snow, D. L. (1994). Effects of a worksite coping skills intervention on the stress, social support, and health outcomes of working mothers. *Journal of Primary Prevention, 15*(2), 105-122.

Klitzner, M., Bamberger, E., & Gruenewald, P. J. (1990). The assessment of parent-led prevention programs: A national descriptive study. *Journal of Drug Education, 20*(2), 111-125.

Knollmueller, R. N. (Ed.). (1993). *Prevention across the life span: Healthy people for the twenty-first century.* Washington, DC: American Nurses Publishing.

Kobasa, S. C., Maddi, S. R., & Kahn, S. (1982). Hardiness and health: A prospective study. *Journal of Personality and Social Psychology, 42,* 168-177.

Kohlberg, L. (1981). *Essays on moral development* (Vol. 1). New York: Harper & Row.

Kohlberg, L. (1983). *Moral stages: A current formulation and a response to critics.* New York: Karger.

Kohlberg, L. (1987). *Child psychology and childhood education.* New York: Longman.

Kolbert, E. (1994, December 14). Television gets closer look as a factor in real violence. *New York Times,* pp. A1, D20.

Kornberg, M. S., & Caplan, G. (1980). Risk factors and preventive intervention in child psychopathology: A review. *Journal of Primary Prevention, 1*(2), 71-133.

Kumpfer, K. L., Shur, G. H., Ross, J. G., Bunnelli, K. K., Librett, J. L., & Millward, A. R. (1993). *Measurements in prevention: A manual on selecting and using instruments to evaluate prevention programs.* CSAP Technical Report—8. Rockville, MD: U.S. Department of Health and Human Services.

Kunz, J. R. M., & Finkel, A. J. (Eds.). (1987). *The American medical association family medical guide* (rev. ed.). New York: Random House.

Kurtines, W. M., & Gewirtz, J. L. (1984). *Morality, moral behavior, and moral development.* New York: John Wiley-Interscience.

Kurtines, W. M., & Gewirtz, J. L. (Eds.). (1991). *Handbook of moral behavior and development* (Vols. 1-3). Hillsdale, NJ: Lawrence Erlbaum.

Last, J. M. (Ed.). (1980). *Maxey-Roxenau public health and preventive medicine* (11th ed.). New York: Appleton-Century-Crofts.

Laurendeau, M., Gagnon, G., Desjardins, N., Perreault, R., & Kishchuk, N. (1991). Evaluation of an early, mass media parental support intervention. *Journal of Primary Prevention, 11*(3), 207-226.

Lavigne, V. V., Reisinger, J. J., Bernard, I., & Stewart, C. (1983). Prevention and early intervention: An operational model. *Journal of Primary Prevention, 4*(2), 107-117.

Lawrence, L., & McLeroy, K. R. (1986). Self-efficacy and health education. *Journal of School Health, 56*(8), 317-321.

Lawton, M. P., Liebowit, B., & Charon, H. (1970). Physical structure and the behavior of senile patients following ward remodeling. *Aging and Human Development, 1*(3), 231-239.

Lazarus, R. S. (1984). The costs and benefits of denial. In S. Brenitz (Ed.), *Denial of stress.* New York: International Universities Press.

Lazarus, R. S. (1985). The trivialization of distress. In J. Rosen & L. Solomon (Eds.), *Prevention in health psychology.* Hanover, NH: University Press of New England.

Lazarus, R. S., & Folkman, S. (1984). *Stress, appraisal, and coping.* New York: Springer.

Leavell, H. R., & Clark, E. G. (Eds.). (1953). *Textbook of preventive medicine.* New York: McGraw-Hill.

Lee, P. R., & Moss, A. R. (1987). AIDS prevention: Is cost-benefit analysis appropriate? *Health Policy, 8,* 193-196.

Lemkau, P. V. (1969). The planning project for Columbia. In M. F. Shore & F. V. Mannino (Eds.), *Mental health and the community: Problems, programs, and strategies.* New York: Behavioral Publications.

Lent, R. W., & Hackett, G. (1987). Career self-efficacy: Empirical status and future directions. *Journal of Vocational Behavior, 30,* 347-382.

Levant, R. (1983). Client-centered skills training programs for the family: A review of the literature. *The Counseling Psychologist, II*(3), 29-46.

Levenstein, P. (1988). *Messages from home: The mother-child home program and the prevention of school disadvantage.* Columbus: Ohio State University Press.

Leventhal, H., Prohaska, T., & Hirschman, R. (1985). Preventive health behavior across the life span. In J. Rosen & L. Solomon (Eds.), *Prevention in health psychology.* Hanover, NH: University Press of New England.

Levin, J. S., & Vanderpool, H. Y. (1991). Religious factors in physical health and the prevention of illness. *Prevention in Human Services, 9*(2), 41-64.

Levine, E. M., & Kanin, E. J. (1987). Sexual violence among dates and acquaintances: Trends and their implications for marriage and family. *Journal of Family Violence, 2*(1), 55-65.

Levine, M., & Perkins, D. V. (1987). *Principles of community psychology: Perspectives and applications.* New York: Oxford University Press.

Levy, S. M. (1985). Emotional response to disease and its treatment. In J. Rosen & L. Solomon (Eds.), *Prevention in health psychology.* Hanover, NH: University Press of New England.

Lewin, K. (1951). *Field theory in social sciences* (D. Cartwright, Ed.). New York: Harper.

Libassi, M. F., & Maluccio, A. (1986). Competence-centered social work: Prevention in action. *Journal of Primary Prevention, 6*(3), 168-180.

Lieberman, M. A., & Videka-Sherman, L. (1986). The impact of self-help groups on the mental health of widows and widowers. *American Journal of Orthopsychiatry, 56*(3), 435-449.

Lindemann, E. (1944). Symptomatology and management of acute grief. *American Journal of Psychiatry, 101,* 141-148.

Lindsley, O. R. (1964). Geriatric behavioral prosthetics. In R. Kastenbaum (Ed.), *New thoughts on old age.* New York: Springer.

Lin-Fu, J. S. (1970). Childhood lead poisoning: An eradicable disease. *Children, 17*(1), 2-9.

Lin-Fu, J. S. (1979). Lead poisoning in children. *Children Today, 8*(1), 9-14.

Linkenbach, J. (1990). An Adlerian technique for substance abuse prevention and intervention. *Individual Psychology, 46,* 203-207.

Little, L. F., Gaffney, I. C., & Grissmer, J. (1991). A stress management, crisis prevention, and crisis intervention program for commercial airline pilots. In A. R. Roberts (Ed.),

Contemporary perspectives on crisis intervention and prevention. Englewood Cliffs, NJ: Prentice Hall.

Litwin, H. (1985). Ombudsman services. In A. Monk (Ed.), *Handbook of gerontological services.* New York: Van Nostrand Reinhold.

Lockwood, A. (1978). The effects of value clarification and moral development curricula on school-age subjects: A critical review of recent research. *Review of Educational Research, 48,* 325-364.

Loewenberg, F. M., & Dolgoff, R. (1992). *Ethical decisions for social work practice* (4th ed.). Itasca, IL: F. E. Peacock.

Lofquist, W. A. (1983). *Discovering the meaning of prevention: A practical approach to positive change.* Tucson, AZ: AYD.

Long, B. B. (1986). The view from the top: National prevention policy. In M. Kessler & S. Goldston (Eds.), *A decade of progress in primary prevention.* Hanover, NH: University Press of New England.

Long, B. B. (1992). Developing a constituency for prevention. In M. Kessler, S. Goldston, & J. Joffe (Eds.), *The present and future of prevention.* Newbury Park, CA: Sage.

Lorion, R. P., Hightower, A. D., Work, W. C., & Shockley, P. (1987). The basic academic skills enhancement program: Translating prevention theory into action research. *Journal of Community Psychology, 15,* 63-77.

Louria, D. B., Kidwell, A. P., Lavenhar, M. A., Thind, I. S., & Najem, R. G. (1976). Primary and secondary prevention among adults: An analysis with comments on screening and health education. *Preventive Medicine, 5*(4), 549-572.

Lowenthal, M. F., & Havens, C. (1968). Interaction and adaptation. *American Sociological Review, 33,* 20-30.

Lozoff, B., Brittenham, G. M., Trause, M. A., Kennell, J. H., & Klaus, M. H. (1977). The mother-newborn relationship: Limits of adaptability. *Journal of Pediatrics, 9*(1), 1-12.

Lum, D. (1986). *Social work practice and people of color: A process-stage approach.* Monterey, CA: Brooks/Cole.

Lustig, S. L. (1994). The AIDS prevention magic show: Avoiding the tragic with magic. *Public Health Reports, 109*(2), 162-167.

Luthar, S. S., & Zigler, E. (1991). Vulnerability and competence: A review of research on resilience in childhood. *American Journal of Orthopsychiatry, 61*(1), 6-22.

Lutzer, V. D. (1987). An educational and peer support group for mothers of preschoolers at-risk for behavior disorder. *Journal of Primary Prevention, 7*(3), 153-161.

Lutzker, J. R., Wesch, D., & Rice, J. M. (1984). A review of Project "12-Ways": An ecobehavioral approach to the treatment and prevention of child abuse and neglect. *Advanced Behavioral Research Therapy, 6,* 63-73.

Maccoby, N., & Altman, D. G. (1988). Disease prevention in communities: The Stanford Heart Disease Prevention Program. In R. Price, E. L. Cowen, R. P. Lorion, & J. Ramos-McKay (Eds.), *14 ounces of prevention.* Washington, DC: American Psychological Association.

Maccoby, N., Farquhar, J. W., Wood, P. D., & Alexander, J. (1977). Reducing the risk of cardiovascular disease: Effects of a community-based campaign on knowledge and behavior. *Journal of Community Health, 3*(2), 100-114.

MacKinnon, D. P., Pentz, M. A., & Stacy, A. W. (1993). The alcohol warning label and adolescents: The first year. *American Journal of Public Health, 83*(4), 585-587.

MacMahon, B., & Pugh, T. F. (1970). *Epidemiology: Principles and methods.* Boston: Little, Brown.

Madava, E. J. (1990). Maximizing the potential for community self-help through clearing house approaches. *Prevention in Human Service, 7*(2), 109-138.

Magen, R. H., & Rose, S. D. (1994). Parents in groups: Problem solving versus behavior skill training. *Research in Social Work Practice, 4*(2), 172-191.

Maguire, L. (1991). *Social support systems in practice: A generalist approach.* Silver Spring, MD: National Association of Social Workers.

Magrab, P. R., Sostek, A. M., & Powell, B. A. (1984). Prevention in the perinatal period. In M. Roberts & L. Peterson (Eds.), *Prevention of problems in childhhod.* New York: Wiley-Interscience.

Mahoney, M. J. (1974). *Cognition and behavior modification.* Cambridge, MA: Ballinger.

Malow, R. M., West, J., Corrigan, S., Pena, J., & Cunningham, S. (1994). Outcome of psychoeducation for HIV risk reduction. *AIDS Education and Prevention, 6*(2), 113-125.

Maluccio, A. N., Washitz, S., & Libassi, M. F. (1992). Ecologically oriented, competence-centered social work practice. In C. W. LeCroy (Ed.), *Case studies in social work practice.* Belmont, CA: Wadsworth.

Manger, T. H., Hawkins, J. D., Haggerty, K. P., & Catalano, R. F. (1992). Mobilizing communities to reduce risks for drug abuse: Lessons on using research to guide prevention practice. *Journal of Primary Prevention, 13*(1), 3-22.

Manning, M. M., & Wright, T. L. (1983). Self-efficacy expectations, outcome expectancies, and the persistence of pain control in childbirth. *Journal of Personality and Social Psychology, 45,* 421-431.

Mannino, F. V. (1981). Empirical perspective in mental health consultation. *Journal of Prevention, 1*(3), 147-155.

Mannino, F. V., Trickett, E. J., Shore, M. F., Kidder, M. G., & Levin, G. (1986). *Handbook of mental health consultation* (DHHS Publication No. ADM 86-1446). Washington, DC: Government Printing Office.

Mannino, F. V., & Shore, M. F. (1986). History and development of mental health consultation. In F. V. Mannino, E. J. Trickett, M. F. Shore, M. G. Kidder, & G. Levin (Eds.), *Handbook of mental health consultation.* Washington, DC: Department of Health and Human Services.

Manson, S. P. (Ed.). (1982). *New directions in prevention among American Indians and Alaska Native communities.* Portland: Oregon Health Sciences University.

Mantell, J. E., & Schinke, S. P. (1991). The crisis of AIDS for adolescents: The need for preventive intervention. In A. R. Roberts (Ed.), *Contemporary perspectives on crisis intervention and prevention.* Englewood Cliffs, NJ: Prentice Hall.

Manuso, J. S. J. (1981). Corporate mental health programs and policies. In L. K. Y. Ng & D. L. Davis (Eds.), *Strategies for public health.* New York: Van Nostrand Reinhold.

Markman, H. J., Floyd, F. J., Stanley, S. M., & Storaasli, R. D. (1988). Prevention of marital distress: A longitudinal investigation. *Journal of Consulting and Clinical Psychology, 56*(2), 210-217.

Marlatt, G. A., & George, W. H. (1984). Relapse prevention: Introduction and overview of the model. *British Journal of Addiction, 79,* 261-273.

Marlatt, G. A., & George, W. H. (1990). Relapse prevention and the maintenance of optimal health. In S. Shumaker et al. (Eds.), *The handbook of health behavior change.* New York: Springer.

Martin, S. L., Ramey, C. T., & Ramey, S. (1990). The prevention of intellectual impairment in children of impoverished families: Findings of a randomized trial of educational day care. *American Journal of Public Health, 80*(7), 844-847.

Marx, R. D., & Ivey, A. E. (1988). Communication skills programs that last: Face to face and relapse prevention. *International Journal for the Advancement of Counseling, 11,* 135-151.

Mason, J. O., & McGinnis, J. M. (1990). "Healthy People 2000": An overview of the national health promotion and disease prevention objectives. *Public Health Reports, 105*(5), 441-446.

Masterpasqua, F., & Swift, M. (1984). Prevention of problems in childhood on a community-wide basis. In M. Roberts & L. Peterson (Eds.), *Prevention of problems in childhood.* New York: John Wiley.

Mata, A., & Jorquez, J. S. (1989). Mexican-American intravenous drug users' needle-sharing practices: Implications for AIDS prevention. In V. Mays, G. Albee, & S. Schneider (Eds.), *Primary prevention of AIDS.* Newbury Park, CA: Sage.

Maton, K. I. (1989a). Community settings as buffers of life stress? Highly supportive churches, mutual help groups, and senior centers. *American Journal of Community Psychology, 17*(2), 203-232.

Maton, K. I. (1989b). Towards an ecological understanding of mutual-help groups: The social ecology of "fit." *American Journal of Community Psychology, 17*(6), 729-753.

Matsushima, J. (1990). Interviewing for alleged abuse in the residential treatment center. *Child Welfare, 69*(4), 321-331.

May, P. A., & Hymbaugh, K. J. (1989). A macro-level fetal alcohol syndrome prevention program for Native Americans and Alaska Natives: Description and evaluation. *Journal of Studies on Alcohol, 50*(6), 508-518.

Mayer, J. (1975). *A diet for living.* New York: David McKay.

Mayer, J. A., Dubbert, P. M., Scott, R. R., Dawson, B. L., Ekstrand, M. L., & Fondren, T. G. (1987). Breast self-examination: The effects of personalized prompts on practice frequency. *Behavior Therapy, 2,* 135-146.

Mays, V. M. (1989). AIDS prevention in black populations: Methods of a safer kind. In V. Mays, G. Albee, & S. Schneider (Eds.), *Primary prevention of AIDS.* Newbury Park, CA: Sage.

Mays, V. M., Albee, G. W., & Schneider, S. F. (Eds.). (1989). *Primary prevention of AIDS: Psychological approaches* (Vol. 13). Newbury Park, CA: Sage.

Mays, V. M., & Cochran, S. D. (1987). Acquired immunodeficiency syndrome and black Americans: Special psychosocial issues. *Public Health Reports, 102*(2), 224-231.

McAnarney, E. R., & Schreider, C. (1984). *Identifying social and psychological antecedents of adolescent pregnancy: The contribution of research to concepts of prevention.* New York: W. T. Grant Foundation.

McAuley, E., & Courneya, K. S. (1993). Adherence to exercise and physical activity as health-promoting behaviors: Attitudinal and self-efficacy influences. *Applied and Preventive Psychology, 2,* 65-77.

McCann, B. S., Retzlaff, B., Walden, C., & Knopp, R. (1990). Dietary intervention for coronary heart disease prevention. In S. A. Shumaker, E. Schron, & J. Ockene (Eds.), *The handbook of health behavior change.* New York: Springer.

McCord, J. (1978). A thirty-year follow-up of treatment effects. *American Psychologist, 33,* 284-289.

McCord, J., & Tremblay, R. E. (Eds.). (1992). *Preventing antisocial behavior: Interventions from birth through adolescence.* New York: Guilford.

McCormick, M. (Ed.). (1980). *Prevention of mental retardation and other developmental disabilities.* New York: Marcel Dekker.

McCrady, B. S. (1989). Extending relapse prevention models to couples. *Addictive Behavior, 14,* 69-74.

McElhaney, S. J., & Barton, H. A. (1995). Advocacy and services: The National Mental Health Association and prevention. *Journal of Primary Prevention, 15*(3), 313-322.

McGuffin, P., & Katz, R. (1986). Genetics and psychopathology: Prospects for prevention. In M. Kessler & S. Goldston (Eds.), *A decade of progress in primary prevention.* Hanover, NH: University Press of New England.

McGuire, W. J. (1968). The nature of attitudes and attitude change. In G. Lindzey & E. Aronson (Eds.), *The handbook of social psychology* (2nd ed., Vol. 3). Reading, MA: Addison-Wesley.

McGuire, W. J. (1984). Public communication as a strategy for inducing health-promoting behavior change. *Preventive Medicine, 13,* 299-319.

McKusick, L., Hoff, C. C., Stall, R., & Coates, T. J. (1991). Tailoring AIDS prevention differences in behavioral strategies among heterosexual and gay bar patrons in San Francisco. *AIDS Education and Prevention, 3*(11), 1-9.

McPhail, R., Ungood-Thomas, J., & Chapman, H. (1975). *Learning to care: Rationale and method of the lifeline curriculum.* Niles, IL: Argus.

Mead, G. H. (1934). *Mind, self, and society: From the standpoint of a social behaviorist.* Chicago: University of Chicago Press.

Meade, C. D., McKinney, W. P, & Barnas, G. P. (1994). Educating patients with limited literacy skills: The effectiveness of printed and videotaped materials about colon cancer. *American Journal of Public Health, 84*(1), 119-121.

Meador, B. D., & Rogers, C. R. (1984). Person-centered therapy. In R. Corsini (Ed.), *Current psychotherapies* (3rd ed.). Itasca, IL: F. E. Peacock.

Mecca, A. M., Smelser, N. J., & Vasconcellos, J. (Eds.). (1989). *The social importance of self-esteem.* Berkeley: University of California Press.

Mednick, S. A., Baert, A. E., & Backmann, B. P. (1981). *Prospective longitudinal research: An empirical basis for the primary prevention of psychosocial disorders.* New York: Oxford University Press.

Meichenbaum, D. (1977). *Cognitive-behavior modification: An integrated approach.* New York: Plenum.

Meichenbaum, D. (1985). *Stress inoculation training.* New York: Pergamon.

Meichenbaum, D., & Jaremko, M. E. (Eds.). (1983). *Stress reduction and prevention.* New York: Plenum.

Meichenbaum, D., & Turk, D. C. (1987). *Facilitating treatment adherence: A practitioner's handbook.* New York: Plenum.

Meissen, G. J., & Berchek, R. L. (1988). Intentions to use predictive testing by those at risk for Huntington's disease: Implications for prevention. *American Journal of Community Psychology, 16*(2), 261-277.

Merritt, A. L. (1987). The tort liability of hospital ethics committees. *Southern California Law Review, 60,* 12-41.

Michelson, L. (1987). Cognitive-behavioral strategies in the prevention and treatment of antisocial disorders in children and adolescents. In J. Burchard & S. Burchard (Eds.), *Prevention of delinquent behavior.* Newbury Park, CA: Sage.

Milgram, G. G., & Nathan, P. E. (1986). Efforts to prevent alcohol abuse. In B. A. Edelson & L. Michelson (Eds.), *Handbook of prevention.* New York: Plenum.

Miller, F. E. (1977). The program movement: ZIA-A model of capital formation. In G. Whittaker (Ed.), *Capital formation: Challenge for the third century.* Ann Arbor: University of Michigan Press.

Miller, H. L., Coombs, D., Leeper, J., & Barton, S. (1984). An analysis of the effects of suicide-prevention facilities on suicide rates in the United States. *American Journal of Public Health, 74*(4), 340-343.

Miller, S. D., O'Neal, G. S., & Scott, C. (Eds.). (1982). *Primary prevention approaches to the development of mental health services for ethnic minorities: A challenge to social work education and practice.* New York: Council on Social Work Education.

Mitchell, S. K., Magyary, D., Barnard, K., Sumner, G., & Booth, C. (1988). A comparison of home-based prevention programs for families of newborns. In L. Bond & B. Wagner (Eds.), *Families in transition.* Newbury Park, CA: Sage.

Monahan, J. T., & Vaux, A. (1980). Macroenvironment and community mental health. In P. M. Insel (Ed.), *Environmental variables and the prevention of mental illness.* Lexington, MA: Lexington Books.

Monat, A., & Lazarus, R. S. (Eds.). (1985). *Stress and coping: An anthology.* New York: Columbia University Press.

Moncher, M., & Schinke, S. P. (1994). Group intervention to prevent tobacco use among Native American youth. *Research on Social Work Practice, 4*(2), 160-171.

Monk, A., & Kaye, L. W. (1982). Assessing the efficacy of ombudsman services for the aged in long-term care institutions. *Evaluation and Program Planning, 5*(4), 363-370.

Moore, C. (1995, January-February). Green revolution in the making. *Sierra,* pp. 50-52, 126-130.

Moos, R. H. (1985). Creating healthy human contexts: Environmental and individual strategies. In J. Rosen & L. Solomon (Eds.), *Prevention in health psychology.* Hanover, NH: University Press of New England.

Moos, R. H. (1992). Understanding individuals' life contexts: Implications for stress reduction and prevention. In M. Kessler, S. Goldston, & J. Joffe (Eds.), *The present and future of prevention.* Newbury Park, CA: Sage.

Moos, R. H., & Brownstein, R. (1977). *Environment and utopia: A synthesis.* New York: Plenum.

Morris, M., & Frisman, L. K. (1987). The competent community revisited: A case study of networking in policy implementation. *Journal of Community Psychology, 15*(1), 29-34.

Morse, W. (1968). Training teachers in life space interviewing. In D. Hamacheck (Ed.), *Human dynamics in psychology and education.* Boston: Allyn & Bacon.

Morton, A. L. (1969). *The life and ideas of Robert Owen.* New York: International.

Mullooly, J. P., Schuman, K. L., Stevens, V. J., Glasgow, R. E., & Vogt, T. M. (1990). Smoking behavior and attitudes of employees of a large HMO before and after a work site ban on cigarette smoking. *Public Health Reports, 105*(6), 623-628.

Munoz, R. F. (1986). Opportunities for prevention among Hispanics. In R. L. Hough, P. Gongla, V. Brown, & S. Goldston (Eds.), *Psychiatric epidemiology and primary prevention: The possibilities.* Los Angeles: University of California, Neuropsychiatric Institute.

Munoz, R. F., Glish, M., Soo-Hoo, T., & Robertson, J. (1982). The San Francisco Mood Survey Project: Preliminary work toward the prevention of depression. *American Journal of Community Psychology, 10*(3), 317-329.

Munoz, R. F., Snowden, L. R., & Kelly, J. G. (Eds.). (1979). *Social and psychological research in community settings.* San Francisco: Jossey-Bass.

Murray, D. M., Pirie, P., Luepker, R. V., & Pallonen, U. (1989). Five- and six-year follow-up results from four seventh-grade smoking prevention strategies. *Journal of Behavioral Medicine, 12*(2), 207-218.

Nathan, P. E. (1985). Prevention of alcoholism: A history of failure. In J. Rosen & L. Solomon (Eds.), *Prevention in health psychology.* Hanover, NH: University Press of New England.

National Institute on Drug Abuse. (1981a). *Vol. 1: Prevention planning workbook* (DHHS Publication No. ADM 81-1061). Washington, DC: Government Printing Office.

National Institute on Drug Abuse. (1981b). *Vol. 2: A needs assessment workbook for prevention planning* (DHHS Publication No. ADM 81-1062). Washington, DC: Government Printing Office.

National Research Council. (1987). *Risking the future adolescent sexuality, pregnancy, and childbearing* (C. D. Haven, Ed.). Washington, DC: National Academy Press.

Neal-Cooper, R., & Scott, R. B. (1988). Genetic counseling in sickle cell anemia: Experiences with couples at risk. *Public Health Reports, 103*(2), 174-178.

Neighbors, B., Forehand, R., & McVicar, D. (1993). Resilient adolescents and interparental conflict. *American Journal of Orthopsychiatry, 63*(3), 462-471.

Neill, A. S. (1960). *Summerhill: A radical approach to child rearing.* New York: Hart.

Nelkin, D., & Tancredi, L. (1989). *Dangerous diagnostics: The social power of biological information.* New York: Basic Books.

Nelson, E. C., Keller, A., & Zubkoff, M. (1981). Incentives for health promotion: The government's role. In L. K. Y. Ng & D. L. Davis (Eds.), *Strategies for public health.* New York: Van Nostrand Reinhold.

Netting, F. E., & Hinds, H. N. (1984). Volunteer advocates in long-term care: Local implementation of a federal mandate. *The Gerontologist, 24*(1), 13-15.

Newman, O. (1972). *Defensible space.* New York: Macmillan.

Ng, L. K. Y., & Davis, D. L. (Eds.). (1981). *Strategies for public health: Promoting health and preventing disease.* New York: Van Nostrand Reinhold.

Nicol, S. E., & Erlenmeyer-Kimling, L. (1986). Genetic factors in psychopathology: Implications for prevention. In B. Edelstein & L. Michelson (Eds.), *Handbook of prevention.* New York: Plenum.

Nielsen, M., Blenkner, M., Bloom, M., Downs, T., & Beggs, H. (1972). Older persons after hospitalization: A controlled study of home aide services. *American Journal of Public Health, 62*(8), 1094-1101.

Nietzel, M. T., & Himelein, M. J. (1987). Crime prevention through social and physical environment change. *Behavior Analyst, 10*(1), 69-74.

Noble, K. D. (1987). The dilemma of gifted women. *Psychology of Women Quarterly, 11,* 367-378.

Noble, M. (Ed.). (1981). *Primary prevention in mental health and social work: A sourcebook of curriculum and teaching materials.* New York: Council on Social Work Education.

Norman, E., & Turner, S. (1993). Adolescents' substance abuse prevention programs: Theories, models, and research in the encouraging 80's. *Journal of Primary Prevention, 14*(1), 3-20.

Northeast Utilities Service Company. (1992). *Spectrum lighting catalog.* Greenwich, CT: Author.

Novaco, R. (1977). A stress inoculation approach to anger management in the training of law enforcement officers. *American Journal of Community Psychology, 5,* 327-346.

Nuehring, E. M., Abrams, H. A., Fike, D. F., & Ostrowsky, E. F. (1983). Evaluating the impact of prevention programs aimed at children. *Social Work Research and Abstracts, 19,* 11-18.

Nutrition Action Health Letter, 22 (1995). [Special Issue]. 8.

Ojemann, R. H. (1972). Education in human behavior in perspective. *People Watching, 1*(2), 1-14.

Okun, M. A., Sandler, I. N., & Baumann, D. J. (1988). Buffer and booster effects as event-support transactions. *American Journal of Community Psychology, 16*(3), 435-449.

Okwumabua, J. O., Okwumabua, T. M., Hayes, A., & Stovall, K. (1994). Cognitive level and health decision-making in children: A preliminary study. *Journal of Primary Prevention, 14*(4), 279-287.

Olds, D. L. (1988). The prenatal/early infancy project. In R. Price, E. L. Cowen, R. P. Lorion, & J. Ramos-McKay (Eds.), *14 ounces of prevention.* Washington: American Psychological Association.

O'Neill, P. (1989). Responsibility to whom? Responsible for what? Some ethical issues in community intervention. *American Journal of Community Psychology, 17*(3), 323-341.

Orlandi, M. A. (1986). Community-based substance abuse prevention: A multicultural perspective. *Journal of School Health, 56*(9), 394-401.

Osborn, J. E. (1991). Women and HIV/AIDS: The silent epidemic? *SIECUS Report, 19*(2), 14.

Osofsky, J. D. (1986). Perspectives on infant mental health. In M. Kessler & S. Goldston (Eds.), *A decade of progress in primary prevention.* Hanover, NH: University Press of New England.

Oster, R. A. (1983). Peer counseling: Drug and alcohol abuse prevention. *Journal of Primary Prevention, 3*(3), 188-199.

Oxford, J. (1990). *Community psychology: Theory and practice.* New York: John Wiley.

Oxford English Dictionary (compact edition). (1971). New York: Oxford University Press.

Ozawa, M. (1986). The nation's children: Key to a secure retirement. *New England Journal of Human Services, 6*(3), 12-19.

Padian, N. S., van de Wijgert, J. H. H. M., & O'Brien, T. R. (1994). Interventions for sexual partners of HIV-infected or high-risk individuals. In R. J. DiClemente & J. L. Peterson (Eds.), *Preventing AIDS: Theories and methods of behavioral interventions.* New York: Plenum.

Pagel, M. D., & Davidson, A. R. (1984). A comparison of three social-psychological models of attitude and behavior plan: Prediction of contraceptive behavior. *Journal of Personality and Social Psychology, 47,* 517-533.

Park, C. A. (1982). Combining prevention and remediation services in a church-related agency. *Child Welfare, 62*(5), 289-296.

Parker, G. R., Cowen, E. L., Work, W. C., & Wyman, P. A. (1990). Test correlates of stress resilience among urban school children. *Journal of Primary Prevention, 11*(1), 19-35.

Parkes, C. M., Stevenson-Hinde, J., & Marris, P. (Eds.). (1991). *Attachment across the life cycle.* London: Tavistock/Routledge.

Patrick, L. F., & Minish, P. A. (1985). Child-rearing strategies for the development of altruistic behavior in young children. *Journal of Primary Prevention, 5*(3), 154-168.

Patterson, G. R. (1982). *A social learning approach* (Vol. 3). Eugene, OR: Castalia.

Payne, I. R., Bergin, A. E., Bielema, K. A., & Jenkins, P. H. (1991). Review of religion and mental health: Prevention and the enhancement of psychosocial functioning. *Prevention in Human Services, 9*(2), 11-40.

Pearson, C. (1981). The role of the insurance industry in health education. In L. K. Y. Ng & D. L. Davis (Eds.), *Strategies for public health.* New York: Van Nostrand Reinhold.

Pearson, J. L., Cowan, P. A., Cowan, C. P., & Cohn, D. A. (1993). Adult attachment and adult child-older parent relationships. *American Journal of Orthopsychiatry, 63*(4), 606-613.

Pentz, M. A., Dwyer, J. H., MacKinnon, D. P., Flay, B. R., Hansen, W. B., Wang, E. Y., & Johnson, C. A. (1989). A multicommunity trial for primary prevention of adolescent drug abuse: Effects on drug use prevalence. *Journal of the American Medical Association, 261*(22), 3259-3266.

Peplau, L. A., & Goldston, S. E. (Eds.). (1984). *Preventing the harmful consequences of severe and persistent loneliness* (DHHS Publication No. ADM 84-1312). Washington, DC: Government Printing Office.

Perez-Escamilla, R., Pollitt, E., Lonnerdal, B., & Dewey, K. (1994). Infant feeding policies in maternity wards and their effect on breast-feeding success: An analytical overview. *American Journal of Public Health, 84*(1), 89-97.

Perlman, D., & Peplau, L. A. (1984). Loneliness research: A survey of empirical findings. In L. Peplau & S. Goldston (Eds.), *Preventing the harmful consequences of severe and persistent loneliness* (DHHS Publication No. ADM 84-1312). Washington, DC: Government Printing Office.

Perlmutter, A. H. (Prod.). (1992). *An ounce of prevention* (Videotape, part of a telecourse, "The World of Abnormal Psychology"). Washington, DC: T. Levine Communications, Inc., & the Annenberg/Corporation for Public Broadcasting.

Perlmutter, F. (Ed.). (1982a). *New directions for mental health services: Mental health promotion and primary prevention*. San Francisco: Jossey-Bass.

Perlmutter, F. (1982b). *Mental health promotion and primary prevention*. San Francisco: Jossey-Bass.

Peterman, P. J. (1981). Parenting and environmental considerations. *American Journal of Orthopsychiatry, 51*(2), 351-355.

Petersen, W. (1977). The ideological origins of Britain's new towns. In I. Allen (Ed.), *New towns and the suburban dream*. Port Washington, NY: Kennikat.

Peterson, C., & Bossio, L. M. (1991). *Health and optimism*. New York: Free Press.

Peterson, C., Seligman, M. E. P., & Vaillant, G. E. (1988). Pessimistic explanatory style as a risk factor for physical illness: A thirty-five year longitudinal study. *Journal of Personality and Social Psychology, 55,* 23-27.

Peterson, L. (1984). Teaching home safety and survival skills to latch-key children: A comparison of two manuals and methods. *Journal of Applied Behavior Analysis, 17*(3), 279-293.

Peterson, L., Farmer, J., & Mori, L. (1987). Process analysis of injury situations: A complement to epidemiological methods. *Journal of Social Issues, 43*(2), 33-44.

Peterson, L., & Mori, L. (1985). Prevention of child injury: An overview of targets, methods, and tactics for psychologists. *Journal of Consulting and Clinical Psychology, 53*(5), 586-595.

Peterson, L., & Mori, L. (1986). Training preschoolers in home safety skills to prevent inadvertent injury. *Journal of Clinical Child Psychology, 15*(2), 106-114.

Peterson, L., Mori, L., Selby, V., & Rosen, B. N. (1988). Community interventions in children's injury prevention: Differing costs and differing benefits. *Journal of Community Psychology, 16,* 188-204.

Phillips, D. P., & Carstenson, L. L. (1986). Clustering of teenage suicides after television news stories about suicide. *New England Journal of Medicine, 315,* 685-689.

Phinney, J. S. (1989). Stages of ethnic identity in minority group adolescence. *Journal of Early Adolescence, 9,* 34-49.

Phinney, J. S. (1990). Ethnic identity in adolescents and adults: Review of research. *Psychological Bulletin, 108,* 499-514.

Pierson, D. E. (1988). The Brookline Early Education Project. In R. Price, E. L. Cowen, R. P. Lorion, & J. Ramos-McKay (Eds.), *14 ounces of prevention*. Washington, DC: American Psychological Association.

Pilisuk, M., & Parks, S. H. (1986). *The healing web: Social networks and human survival*. Hanover, NH: University Press of New England.

Pilisuk, M., Parks, S. H., Kelly, J., & Turner, E. (1982). The helping network approach: Community promotion of mental health. *Journal of Primary Prevention, 3*(2), 116-132.

Pill, C. J. (1981). A family life education group for working with stepparents. *Social Casework, 62*(3), 159-166.

Pithers, W. D., Kashima, K. M., Cumming, G. F., Beal, L. S., & Buell, M. M. (1988). Relapse prevention of sexual aggression. *Annuals of the New York Academic of Science, 528,* 244-260.

Pless, I. B., & Arsenault, L. (1987). The role of health education in the prevention of injuries to children. *Journal of Social Issues, 43*(2), 87-103.

Plimpton, S., & Root, J. (1994). Materials and strategies that work in low literacy health communications. *Public Health Reports, 109*(1), 89-92.

Ponterotto, J. G., & Pedersen, P. B. (1993). *Prevention prejudice: A guide for counselors and educators.* Newbury Park, CA: Sage.

Pope, K. S. (1990). Identifying and implementing ethical standards for primary prevention. *Prevention in Human Services, 8*(2), 43-64.

Porter, R. A. (1983). Ecological strategies of prevention in rural community development. *Journal of Primary Prevention, 3*(4), 235-243.

Poser, E. G. (1970). Toward a theory of behavioral prophylaxis. *Journal of Behavior Therapy and Experimental Psychiatry, 1,* 39-45.

Powell, S., & Berg, R. C. (1987). When the elderly are abused: Characteristics and interventions. *Educational Gerontology, 13,* 71-83.

Powell, T. J., & Enright, S. J. (1990). *Anxiety and stress management.* London: Routledge.

Pransky, J. (1986, March-April). Can you legislate prevention? *New Designs for Youth Development,* pp. 15-20.

President's Commission on Mental Health. (1978). Report of Task Force on Prevention. In D. G. Forgays (Ed.), *Primary prevention of psychopathology* (Vol. 3). Hanover, NH: University Press of New England.

Prestby, J. E., Wandersman, A., Florin, P., Rich, R., & Chavis, D. (1990). Benefits, costs, incentive management and participation in voluntary organizations: A means to understanding and promoting empowerment. *American Journal of Community Psychology, 18*(1), 117-149.

Price, R. H., Cowen, E. L., Lorion, R. P., & Ramos-McKay, J. (Eds.). (1988). *14 ounces of prevention: A casebook for practitioners.* Washington, DC: American Psychological Association.

Price, R. H., Ketterer, R. F., Bader, B. C., & Monahan, J. (Eds.). (1980). *Prevention in mental health: Research, policy, and practice.* Beverly Hills, CA: Sage.

Price, R. H., & Smith, S. E. (1985). *A guide to evaluating prevention programs in mental health* (Publication No. ADM 85-1365). Washington, DC: Government Printing Office.

Protective role of bicycle safety helmet confirmed. (1994). *Public Citizen Health Research Group Health Letter, 10*(8), 4.

Puska, P., McAlister, A., Niemensivu, H., Piha, T., Wiil, J., & Koskela, K. (1987). A television format for national health promotion: Finland's "Keys to Health." *Public Health Reports, 102*(3), 263-270.

Rainwater, L. (1970). *Behind ghetto walls: Black families in a federal slum.* Chicago: Aldine.

Ramey, C., Bryant, D., Campbell, F., Sparling, J., & Wasik, B. (1988). Early intervention for high-risk children: The Carolina early intervention program. In R. Price, E. L. Cowen, R. P. Lorion, & J. Ramos-McKay (Eds.), *14 ounces of prevention.* Washington, DC: American Psychological Association.

Rappaport, J. (1981). In praise of paradox: A social policy of empowerment over prevention. *American Journal of Community Psychology, 9,* 1-25.

Rauch, J. B. (1988). Social work and the genetics revolution. *Social Work, 33*(5), 389-395.

Reid, W., & Epstein, L. (1972). *Task-centered casework.* New York: Columbia University Press.

Reinherz, H., & Griffin, C. L. (1977). Identifying children at risk: A first step to prevention. *Health Education, 8*(4), 14-16.

Reinherz, H., Frost, A. B., Stewart-Berghauer, G., Pakiz, B., Kennedy, K., & Schille, C. (1990). The many faces of correlates of depressive symptoms in adolescents. *Journal of Early Adolescence, 10*(4), 455-471.

Reisman, L. Z., & Matheny, A. P. (1969). *Genetics and counseling in medical practice.* St. Louis, MO: C. V. Mosby.

Reiss, Jr., A. J., & Roth, J. A. (1993). (Eds.). *Understanding and preventing violence.* New York: Academic Press.

Renzulli, J. S. (1973). Talent potential in minority group students. *Exceptional Children, 39,* 437-444.

Reppucci, J., Revenson, R., Aber, M., & Reppucci, N. D. (1991). Unrealistic optimism among adolescent smokers and nonsmokers. *Journal of Primary Prevention, 11*(3), 227-236.

Richardson, F., Reinhard, G., Rosenthal, A., Hayes, C., & Silver, R. (1987). *Review of the research literature on the effects of health warning labels: A report to the United States Congress.* Washington, DC: Macro Systems, Inc. for NIAAA/ADAMHA.

Rieman, D. W. (1992). *Strategies in social work consultation.* New York: Longman.

Riessman, F. (1965, April). The "helper" therapy principle. *Social Work,* 27-32.

Riessman, F. (1976, September-October). How does self-help work? *Social Policy,* 41-45.

Rigotti, N. A., Stoto, M. A., Bierer, M. F., Rosen, A., & Schelling, T. (1993). Retail stores' compliance with a city no-smoking law. *American Journal of Public Health, 83*(2), 227-232.

Rimer, B. K. (1990). Perspectives on interpersonal theories in health education and health behavior. In K. Glanz, F. M. Lewis, & B. K. Rimer (Eds.), *Health behavior and health education.* San Francisco: Jossey-Bass.

Rimm, D. C., & Masters, J. C. (1974). *Behavior therapy: Techniques and empirical findings.* New York: Academic Press.

Ringler, N., Kennell, J. H., Jarvella, R., Novojosky, B., & Klaus, M. H. (1975). Mother-to-child speech at 2 years: Effects of early postnatal contact. *Journal of Pediatrics, 86,* 141.

Ringler, N., Trause, M., Klaus, M., & Kennell, J. (1978). The effect of extra postpartum contact and maternal speech patterns on children's IQs, speech, and language comprehension at five. *Child Development, 49,* 862-865.

Ripple, L., Alexander, E., & Polemis, B. (1964). *Motivation, capacity, and opportunity: Studies in casework theory and practice.* Chicago: University of Chicago Press.

Ritter, D. R. (Ed.). (1982). *Consultation, education, and prevention in community mental health.* Springfield, IL: Charles C Thomas.

Rivlin, L. G., & Imbimbo, J. E. (1989). Self-help efforts in a squatter community: Implications for addressing contemporary homeless. *American Journal of Community Psychology, 17*(6), 705-728.

Roberts, A. R. (Ed.). (1991). *Contemporary perspectives on crisis intervention and prevention.* Englewood Cliffs, NJ: Prentice Hall.

Roberts, B., & Thorsheim, H. (1986). A partnership approach to consultation: The process and results of a major primary prevention field experiment. *Prevention in Human Services, 4*(3 & 4), 151-186.

Roberts, M., & Peterson, L. (Eds.). (1984). *Prevention of problems in childhood: Psychological research and applications.* New York: John Wiley.

Robertson, L. S. (1986). Injury. In B. Edelstein & L. Michelson (Eds.), *Handbook of prevention.* New York: Plenum.

Robin, A. (1981). A controlled evaluation of problem-solving communication training with parent-adolescent conflict. *Behavior Therapy, 12,* 593-609.

Robins, L. N., & Rutter, M. (Eds.). (1990). *Straight and devious pathways from childhood to adulthood.* New York: Cambridge University Press.

Robins, L. N., & Wish, E. (1977). Childhood deviance as a developmental process: A study of 223 urban black men from birth to 18. *Social Forces, 56*(2), 448-471.

Roesch, R. (1988). Community psychology and the law. *American Journal of Community Psychology, 16*(4), 451-463.

Rogers, A. B., Kessler, L., Portnoy, B., Potosky, L., Patterson, B., Tenney, J., Thompson, F., Krebs-Smith, S., Breen, N., Mathews, O., & Kahle, L. (1994). "Eat for Health": A supermarket intervention for nutrition and cancer risk reduction. *American Journal of Public Health, 84*(1), 72-76.

Rogers, E. M. (1973). *Communication strategies for family planning.* New York: Free Press.

Rogers, E. M. (1983). *Diffusion of innovations* (3rd ed.). New York: Free Press.

Rook, K. S. (1984). Interventions for loneliness: A review and analysis. In L. Peplau & S. Goldston (Eds.), *Preventing the harmful consequences of severe and persistent loneliness* (DHHS Publication No. ADM 84-1312). Washington, DC: Government Printing Office.

Rooney-Rebeck, P., & Jason, L. (1986). Prevention of prejudice in elementary school children. *Journal of Primary Prevention, 7*(2), 63-73.

Roosa, M. W., & Christopher, F. S. (1990). Evaluation of an abstinence-only adolescent pregnancy prevention program: A replication. *Family Life Education, 39,* 363-367.

Roper, W. L. (1991). Current approaches to prevention of HIV infections. *Public Health Reports, 106*(2), 111-115.

Roppel, C. E., & Jacobs, M. K. (1988). Multimedia strategies for mental health promotion. In L. A. Bond & B. M. Wagner (Eds.), *Families in transition.* Newbury Park, CA: Sage.

Rosen, G. (1958). *A history of public health.* New York: MD.

Rosen, J. C., & Solomon, L. J. (Eds.). (1985). *Prevention in health psychology* (Vol. 8). Hanover, NH: University Press of New England.

Rosenberg, M. L., Tolsma, D. D., Kolbe, L. J., Kroger, F., Cynamon, M. L., & Bowen, G. S. (1992). The role of behavioral sciences and health education in HIV prevention: Experience at the U.S. Centers for Disease Control. In J. Sepulveda, H. Fineberg, & J. Mann (Eds.), *AIDS: Prevention through education: A world view.* New York: Oxford University Press.

Rosenfield-Schlichter, M. D., Sarber, R. E., Bueno, G., Greene, B. F., & Lutzker, J. R. (1983). Maintaining accountability for an ecobehavioral treatment of one aspect of child neglect: Personal cleanliness. *Education and Treatment of Children, 6*(2), 153-164.

Rosenstock, I. M. (1990). The health belief model: Explaining health behaviors through expectancies. In K. Glanz, F. M. Lewis, & B. K. Rimer (Eds.), *Health behavior and health education.* San Francisco: Jossey-Bass.

Rosenstock, I. M., Strecher, V. J., & Becker, M. H. (1994). The health belief model and HIV risk behavior change. In R. DiClemente & J. Peterson (Eds.), *Preventing AIDS.* New York: Plenum.

Roskin, M. (1982). Coping with life changes: A preventive social work approach. *American Journal of Community Psychology, 10*(3), 331-340.

Ross, C. (1980). Mobilizing schools for suicide prevention. *Suicide and Life-Threatening Behavior, 107,* 239-244.

Ross, J. W. (1991). Oregon's response to the health care crisis. *Health and Social Work, 16*(3), 147-149.

Rothman, J. (1979). Three models of community organization practice. In F. M. Cox, J. L. Erlich, J. Rothman, & J. E. Tropman (Eds.), *Strategies of community organization* (3rd ed.). Itasca, IL: F. E. Peacock.

Rotter, J. B. (1982). *The development and application of social learning theory: Selected papers.* New York: Praeger.

Rouse, J. W. (1978). Building a sense of place. In D. C. Klein (Ed.), *Psychology of the planned community: The new town experience.* New York: Human Sciences Press.

Rubenstein, J. L., Heeren, T., Housman, D., Rubin, C., & Stechler, G. (1989). Suicidal behavior in "normal" adolescents: Risk and protective factors. *American Journal of Orthopsychiatry, 59*(1), 59-71.

Rudd, J., & Glanz, K. (1990). How individuals use information for health action: Consumer information processing. In K. Glanz, F. M. Lewis, & B. K. Rimer (Eds.), *Health behavior and health action.* San Francisco: Jossey-Bass.

Rundall, T. G., & Bruvold, W. H. (1988). A meta-analysis of school-based smoking and alcohol use prevention programs. *Health Education Quarterly, 15*(3), 317-334.

Russell, L. B. (1986). *Is prevention better than cure?* Washington, DC: Brookings Institution.

Russell, L. B. (1994). *Educated guesses: Making policy about medical screening tests.* Berkeley: University of California Press.

Rutter, M. (1979). Protective factors in children's responses to stress and disadvantage. In M. Kent & J. Rolf (Eds.), *Social competence in children.* Hanover, NH: University Press of New England.

Rutter, M. (1981). *Maternal deprivation reassessed* (2nd ed.). New York: Penguin.

Rutter, M. (1987). Psychosocial resilience and protective mechanisms. *American Journal of Orthopsychiatry, 57,* 316-331.

Sameroff, A. J., & Chandler, M. J. (1975). Reproductive risk and the continuum of caretaking casualty. In F. Horowitz & E. M. Hertherington (Eds.), *Review of child research development* (Vol. 4). Chicago: University of Chicago Press.

Samuels, S. E. (1993). Project LEAN—lessons learned from a national social marketing campaign. *Public Health Reports, 108*(1), 45-53.

Sandahl, C., & Rönnberg, S. (1990). Brief group psychotherapy in relapse prevention for alcohol dependent patients. *International Journal of Group Psychotherapy, 40*(4), 453-476.

Sarason, I., Johnson, J., Berberich, J., & Siegel, J. (1979). Helping police officers to cope with stress: A cognitive-behavioral approach. *American Journal of Community Psychology, 7,* 593-603.

Satir, V. (1972). *People making.* Palo Alto, CA: Science and Behavior Books.

Satir, V. (1983). *Conjoint family therapy: A guide to therapy and technique* (3rd ed.). Palo Alto, CA: Science and Behavior Books.

Sawhill, J. C. (1995, January-February). Wild life and ways of life: Seeking greener pastures. *Nature Conservancy, 45*(1), 5-9.

Scarr-Salapetek, S., & Williams, M. L. (1973). The effects of early stimulation on low-birth-weight infants. *Child Development, 44,* 94-101.

Schatz, B. (1989). *Protection against AIDS-related discrimination under state handicap laws: A fifty state analysis.* San Francisco: National Gay Rights Advocates.

Schauffler, H. H. (1993). Integrating smoking control policies into employee benefits: A survey of large California corporations. *American Journal of Public Health, 83*(9), 1226-1230.

Schechter, C., Vanchieri, C., & Crofton, C. (1990). Evaluating women's attitudes and perceptions in developing mammography promotion messages. *Public Health Reports, 105*(3), 253-256.

Scheier, M. F., Matthews, K., Owens, J., Magovern, G., Lefebvre, R., Allott, R., & Carver, C. (1989). Dispositional optimism and recovery from coronary artery bypass surgery: The beneficial effects on physical and psychological well-being. *Journal of Personality and Social Psychology, 57,* 1024-1040.

Schelkun, R. E. (1990). Twenty years of primary prevention: Consultation, education and prevention at the Washtenau County Community Mental Health Center. *Prevention in Human Services, 7*(2), 49-73.

Schiff, S. K., & Kellam, S. G. (1967). A community-wide mental health program of prevention and early treatment in first grade. In M. Greenblatt, P. E. Emery, & B. C. Glueck, Jr. (Eds.), *Poverty and mental health.* Psychiatric Research Report #21. Washington, DC: American Psychiatric Association.

Schild, S. (1977). Social work with genetic problems. *Health and Social Work, 2,* 58-77.

Schild, S., & Black, R. B. (1984). *Social work and genetics: A guide for practice.* New York: Haworth.

Schilling, R., El-Bassel, N., Serrano, Y., & Wallace, B. (1992). AIDS prevention strategies for ethnic-racial minority substance users. *Psychology of Addictive Behaviors, 6*(2), 81-90.

Schilling, R., Schinke, S., Nichols, S., Zayas, L., Miller, S., Orlandi, M., & Botvin, G. (1989). Developing strategies for AIDS prevention research with black and Hispanic drug users. *Public Health Reports, 104*(1), 2-10.

Schinke, S. P., Botvin, G., Orlandi, M., Schilling, R., & Gordon, A. (1990). African-American and Hispanic-American adolescents, HIV infection, and preventive intervention. *AIDS Education and Prevention, 2*(4), 305-312.

Schinke, S. P., & Gilchrist, L. D. (1984). *Life skills counseling with adolescents.* Baltimore: University Park Press.

Schinke, S. P., Gilchrist, L. D., & Small, R. W. (1979). Preventing unwanted adolescent pregnancy: A cognitive-behavioral approach. *American Journal of Orthopsychiatry, 49*(1), 81-88.

Schinke, S. P., Schilling, R. F., Barth, R. P., Gilchrist, L. D., & Maxwell, J. S. (1986). Stress-management intervention to prevent family violence. *Journal of Family Violence, 1*(1), 13-26.

Schmidt, S. E., & Tate, D. R. (1988). Employer-supported child care: An ecological model for supporting families. In L. Bond & B. Wagner (Eds.), *Families in transition.* Newbury Park, CA: Sage.

Schnelle, J., Gendrich, J., Beegle, G., Thomas, M., & McNees, M. (1980). Mass media techniques for prompting behavior change in the community. *Environment and Behavior, 12,* 157-166.

Schofield, M. J., Considine, R., Boyle, C., Sanson-Fisher, R. (1993). Smoking control in restaurants: The effectiveness of self-regulation in Australia. *American Journal of Public Health, 83*(9), 1284-1288.

Schorr, A. (1963). *Slums and social insecurity.* New York: Macmillan.

Schulberg, H. C., & Killilea, M. (Eds.). (1982). *The modern practice of community mental health.* San Francisco: Jossey-Bass.

Schwarz, D. F., Grisso, J., Miles, C., Holmes, J., & Sutton, R. (1993). An injury prevention program in an urban African-American community. *American Journal of Public Health, 83*(5), 675-680.

Schwebel, M. (1992). Making a dangerous world more tolerable for children: Implications of research on reactions to nuclear war, threat, war, and disaster. In G. Albee, L. A. Bond, & T. V. C. Monsey (Eds.), *Improving children's lives: Global perspectives on prevention.* Newbury Park, CA: Sage.

Schweinhart, L. J., & Weikart, D. B. (1988). The High/Scope Perry preschool program. In R. Price, E. L. Cowen, R. P. Lorion, & J. Ramos-McKay (Eds.), *14 ounces of prevention.* Washington, DC: American Psychological Association.

Searight, H. R., & Handal, P. J. (1986). Premature birth and its later effects: Towards preventive intervention. *Journal of Primary Prevention, 7*(1), 3-16.

Segal, J. (1986). Translating stress and coping research into public information and education. In M. Kessler & S. Goldston (Eds.), *A decade of progress in primary prevention.* Hanover, NH: University Press of New England.

Seiban, E. (Ed.). (1977). *New trends of psychiatry in the community.* Cambridge, MA: Ballinger.

Seligman, M. E. P. (1975). *Helplessness: On depression, development, and death.* San Francisco: Freeman.

Seligman, M. E. P. (1991). *Learned optimism.* New York: Knopf.

Selye, H. (1956). *The stress of life.* New York: McGraw-Hill.

Selye, H. (1976). *Stress in health and disease.* Reading, MA: Butterworth.

Sepulveda, J., Fineberg, H., & Mann, J. (Eds.). (1992). *AIDS: Prevention through education: A world view.* New York: Oxford.

Seuss, Dr. (1961). *The sneetches.* New York: Random Books for Young Readers.

Shaffer, D., Garland, A., Gould, M., Fisher, P., & Trautman, P. (1988). Preventing teenage suicide: A critical review. *Journal of the American Academy of Child and Adolescent Psychiatry, 27*(6), 675-687.

Shannon, M. T. (1989). Health promotion and illness prevention: A biopsychosocial perspective. *Health and Social Work, 14*(1), 32-40.

Shapiro, J. (1969). Dominant leaders among slum hotel residents. *American Journal of Orthopsychiatry, 39,* 644-650.

Shaw, L. G. (1987). Designing playgrounds for able and disabled children. In C. Weinstein & T. David (Eds.), *Spaces for children.* New York: Plenum.

Sheline, J. L., Skipper, B., & Broadhead, W. E. (1994). Risk factors for violent behavior in elementary school boys: Have you hugged your child today? *American Journal of Public Health, 84*(4), 661-663.

Sherif, M., Harvey, O., White, J., Hood, W., & Sherif, C. (1961). *Intergroup conflict and cooperation: The robbers' cave experiment.* Norman: University of Oklahoma, Institute of Intergroup Relations.

Sherman, E., & Reid, W. J. (1994). *Qualitative research in social work.* New York: Columbia University Press.

Shi, L. (1993). A cost-benefit analysis of a California county's back injury prevention program. *Public Health Reports, 108*(2), 204-211.

Shiloh, S., Waisbren, S. E., & Levy, H. L. (1989). A psychosocial model of a medical problem: Maternal phenylketonuria. *Journal of Primary Prevention, 10*(1), 51-62.

Shoffeitt, L., & Shoffeitt, P. (1978). A new mental health delivery model in a new city. In D. C. Klein (Ed.), *Psychology of the planned community: The new town experience.* New York: Human Sciences Press.

Shor, I. (1987). *Freire for the classroom: A sourcebook for liberatory teaching.* Portsmouth, NH: Boynton/Cook.

Shulman, L., & Gitterman, A. (1994). The life model, mutual aid, oppression, and the mediating function. In A. Gitterman & L. Shulman (Eds.), *Mutual aid groups, vulnerable populations, and the life cycle* (2nd ed.). New York: Columbia University Press.

Shumaker, S. A., Schron, E. B., & Ockene, J. K. (Eds.). (1990). *The handbook of health behavior change.* New York: Springer.

Shure, M. B. (1988). How to think, not what to think: A cognitive approach to prevention. In L. Bond & B. Wagner (Eds.), *Families in transition.* Newbury Park, CA: Sage.

Shure, M. B., & Spivak, G. (1978). *Problem-solving techniques in childrearing.* San Francisco: Jossey-Bass.

Shure, M. B., & Spivak, G. (1988). Interpersonal cognitive problem-solving. In R. Price, E. L. Cowen, R. P. Lorion, & J. Ramos-McKay (Eds.), *14 ounces of prevention.* Washington, DC: American Psychological Association.

Siegel, B. (1986). *Love, medicine, and miracles.* New York: Harper & Row.

Silverman, M. M. (1989). Children of psychiatrically ill parents: A prevention perspective. *Hospital and Community Psychiatry, 40*(12), 1257-1265.

Silverman, P. R. (1970). The widow as caregiver. *Mental Hygiene, 54,* 540-547.

Silverman, P. R. (1978). *Mutual help groups: A guide for mental health workers* (DHEW Publication No. ADM 78-646). Washington, DC: Government Printing Office.

Silverman, P. R. (1988). Widow-to-widow: A mutual help program for the widowed. In R. Price, E. L. Cowen, R. P. Lorion, & J. Ramos-McKay (Eds.), *14 ounces of prevention.* Washington, DC: American Psychological Association.

Simmel, G. (1950). *The sociology of Georg Simmel* (K. H. Wolf, Trans.). New York: Free Press.

Simon, B. L. (1988). The feminization of poverty: A call for primary prevention. *Journal of Primary Prevention, 9*(1 & 2), 6-17.

Simon, B. L. (1994). *The empowerment tradition in American social work: A history.* New York: Columbia University Press.

Simpson, H. M. (1987). Community-based approaches to highway safety: Health promotion and drinking-driving. *Drug and Alcohol Dependence, 20,* 27-37.

Skinner, B. F. (1953). *Science and human behavior.* New York: Macmillan.

Slavin, S. (1981). Synthesis of research on cooperative learning. *Educational Leadership, 38*(8), 655-660.

Smith, A. (1990). Social influence and antiprejudice training programs. In J. Edwards, R. S. Tindale, L. Heath, & E. J. Posavac (Eds.), *Social influence processes and prevention.* New York: Plenum.

Smith, E. L. (1988). The role of exercise in the prevention of bone involution. In R. Chernoff & D. Lipschitz (Eds.), *Health promotion and disease prevention in the elderly.* New York: Raven.

Snyder, L. B., & Rouse, R. A. (1992). Targeting the audience for AIDS messages by actual and perceived risk. *AIDS Education and Prevention, 4*(2), 143-159.

Sobel, H., & Worden, J. (1981). *Helping cancer patients cope: A problem-solving intervention for health care professionals.* New York: BMA and Guilford.

Solomon, B. (1976). *Black empowerment.* New York: Columbia University Press.

Solomon, L., Frederiksen, L., Arnold, S., & Brehony, K. (1984). Stress management delivered over public television: Steps toward promoting community mental health. *Journal of Primary Prevention, 4*(3), 139-149.

Sorenson, J. R., Swazey, J., & Scotch, N. (1981). Reproductive pasts and reproductive futures: Genetic counseling and its effectiveness. *Birth Defects Original Article Series, 17*(4).

Sorokin, P. A. (Ed.). (1954). *Forms and techniques of altruistic and spiritual growth.* Boston: Beacon.

Sosa, R., Kennell, J., Klaus, M., Robertson, S., & Urrutia, J. (1980). The effect of a supportive companion on perinatal problems, length of labor, and mother-infant interactions. *New England Journal of Medicine, 303,* 597-600.

Sperling, M. B., & Berman, W. H. (Eds.). (1994). *Attachment in adults: Clinical and developmental perspectives.* New York: Guilford.

Spivak, G., & Cianci, N. (1987). High-risk early behavior pattern and later delinquency. In J. Burchard & S. Burchard (Eds.), *Prevention of delinquent behavior.* Newbury Park, CA: Sage.

Spivak, G., & Levine, M. (1963). *Self-regulation in acting-out and normal adolescents.* Report M4531. Washington, DC: National Institute of Health.

Spivak, G., Platt, J. J., & Shure, M. B. (1976). *The problem solving approach to adjustment: A guide to research and intervention.* San Francisco: Jossey-Bass.

Spivak, G., & Shure, M. B. (1974). *Social adjustment of young children: A cognitive approach to solving real-life problems.* San Francisco: Jossey-Bass.

Spivak, M. (1978, October). The design log: A new informational tool. *AIAJ,* pp. 76-78.

Sprafkin, J., Swift, C., & Hess, R. (Eds.). (1983). *Rx television: Enhancing the preventive impact of TV.* New York: Haworth.

Srebnik, D. S., & Elias, M. J. (1993). An ecological, interpersonal skills approach to drop-out prevention. *American Journal of Orthopsychiatry, 63*(4), 526-535.

Stark, M. J., Campbell, B. K., & Brinkerhoff, C. V. (1990). "Hello, may we help you?" A study of attrition prevention at the time of the first phone contact with substance-abusing clients. *American Journal of Drug and Alcohol Abuse, 16*(1 & 2), 67-76.

Stark, W. (1992). Empowerment and social change: Health promotion within the Healthy Cities Project of WHO—Steps toward a participative prevention program. In G. Albee, L. Bond, & T. V. C. Monsey (Eds), *Improving children's lives.* Newbury Park, CA: Sage.

Stehr-Green, P. A., Dini, E., Lindegren, M. L., & Patriarca, P. (1993). Evaluation of telephoned computer-generated reminders to improve immunization coverage at inner-city clinics. *Public Health Reports, 108*(4), 426-430.

Stiffman, A. R. (1992). Physical and sexual abuse of children: What, who, and where? In M. Bloom (Ed.), *Changing lives.* Columbia: University of South Carolina Press.

Stilwell, E., & Manley, B. (1990). A family focus approach to child abuse prevention. *Journal of Primary Prevention, 10*(4), 333-342.

Stolberg, A. L. (1988). Prevention programs for divorcing families. In L. Bond & B. Wagner (Eds.), *Families in transition.* Newbury Park, CA: Sage.

Stolberg, A. L., & Bloom, M. (1992). Child development and functioning: Bases of preventive helpings. In M. Bloom (Ed.), *Changing lives.* Columbia: University of South Carolina Press.

Stolberg, A. L., & Garrison, K. M. (1985). Evaluating a primary prevention program for children of divorce. *American Journal of Community Psychology, 13*(2), 111-124.

Stolberg, A., Kiluk, D., & Garrison, K. (1986). A temporal model of divorce adjustment with implications for primary prevention. In S. Auerback & A. Stolberg (Eds.), *Crisis intervention with children and families.* Washington, DC: Hemisphere.

Striegel-Moore, R., & Rodin, J. (1985). Prevention of obesity. In J. Rosen & L. Solomon (Eds.), *Prevention in health psychology.* Hanover, NH: University Press of New England.

Stunkard, A. J. (1981). The practice of health promotion: The case of obesity. In L. Ng & D. Davis (Eds.), *Strategies for public health.* New York: Van Nostrand Reinhold.

Stunkard, A. J., Felix, M., & Yopp Cohen, R. (1985). Mobilizing a community to promote health: The Pennsylvania County Health Improvement Program (CHIP). In J. Rosen & L. Solomon (Eds.), *Prevention in health psychology.* Hanover, NH: University Press of New England.

Sullivan, H. S. (1953). *The interpersonal theory of psychiatry.* New York: Norton.

Surgeon General of the United States. (1988). *Report on nutrition and health* (DHHS Publication No. 88-50210). Washington, DC: Government Printing Office.

Swift, C. F. (1988). Stopping the violence: Prevention strategies for families. In L. Bond & B. Wagner (Eds), *Families in transition.* Newbury Park, CA: Sage.

Swift, C. F. (1992) Empowerment: The greening of prevention. In M. Kessler, S. Goldston, & J. Joffe (Eds.), *The present and future of prevention.* Newbury Park, CA: Sage.

Swift, C. F., & Levin, G. (1987). Empowerment: An emerging mental health technology. *Journal of Primary Prevention, 8*(1 & 2), 71-94.

Swift, M. S., & Healey, K. N. (1986). Translating research into practice. In M. Kessler & S. Goldston (Eds.), *A decade of progress in primary prevention.* Hanover, NH: University Press of New England.

Swizer, E. B., Deal, T. E., & Bailey, J. (1977). The reduction of stealing in second graders using a group contingency. *Journal of Applied Behavior Analysis, 10,* 267-272.

Szasz, T. (1986). The case against suicide prevention. *American Psychologist, 41*(7), 806-812.

Tabakoff, B., & Hoffman, P. A. (1988). Genetics and biological markers of risk for alcoholism. *Public Health Reports, 103*(6), 690-698.

Tableman, B. (1986). Statewide prevention programs: The politics of the possible. In M. Kessler & S. Goldston (Eds.), *A decade of progress in primary prevention.* Hanover, NH: University Press of New England.

Tableman, B. (1989). Installing prevention programming in the public mental health system. *American Journal of Community Psychology, 17*(2), 171-183.

Tableman, B., & Hess, R. (1985). Prevention: The Michigan experience. *Prevention in Human Services, 3*(4), whole issue.

Tableman, B., Marciniak, D., Johnson, D., & Rodgers, R. (1982). Stress management training for women on public assistance. *American Journal of Community Psychology, 10*(3), 357-367.

Tadmor, C. S. (1988). The perceived personal control preventive intervention for a cesarean birth population. In R. E. L. Cowen, R. P. Lorion, & J. Ramos-McKay (Eds.), *14 ounces of prevention.* Washington, DC: American Psychological Association.

Tadmor, C. S., & Brandes, J. M. (1984). The perceived personal control crisis intervention model in the prevention of emotional dysfunction for a high risk population of cesarean birth. *Journal of Primary Prevention, 4*(4), 240-251.

Tafoya, T. (1989). Pulling the coyote's tale: Native American sexuality and AIDS. In V. Mays, G. Albee, & S. Schneider. (Eds.), *Primary prevention of AIDS.* Newbury Park, CA: Sage.

Tavris, C. (1992). *The mismeasure of woman.* New York: Simon & Schuster.

Taylor, S. E., & Brown, J. D. (1988). Illusion and well-being: A social psychological perspective on mental health. *Psychological Bulletin, 103,* 193-210.

Taylor, D. K., & Beauchamp, C. (1988). Hospital-based primary prevention strategy in child abuse: A multi-level needs assessment. *Child Abuse & Neglect, 12,* 343-354.

Taylor, R. L., Lam, D. J., Roppel, C. E., & Barter, J. T. (1984). Friends can be good medicine: An excursion into mental health promotion. *Community Mental Health Journal, 20*(4), 294-304.

Telch, M. J., Miller, L. M., Killen, J. D., Cooke, S., & Maccoby, N. (1990). Social influences approach to smoking prevention: The effects of videotape delivery with and without same-age peer leader participation. *Addictive Behavior, 15,* 21-28.

Tertinger, D. A., Greene, B. F., & Lutzker, J. R. (1984). Home safety: Development and validation of one component of an ecobehavioral treatment program for abused and neglected children. *Journal of Applied Behavior Analysis, 17,* 159-174.

Thyer, B. (1992). A behavioral perspective on human development. In M. Bloom (Ed.), *Changing lives.* Columbia: University of South Carolina Press.

Thyer, B., & Geller, E. S. (1987). The "buckle-up" dashboard sticker: An effective environmental intervention for safety belt promotion. *Environment and Behavior, 19,* 484-494.

Thyer, B., Geller, E. S., Williams, M., & Purcell, E. (1987). Community-based "flashing" to increase safety belt use. *Journal of Experimental Education, 55,* 155-159.

Tizard, B., & Hodges, J. (1978). The effect of early institutional rearing on the development of eight-year-old children. *Journal of Child Psychology and Psychiatry, 19,* 99-118.

Tobias, S. (1978). *Overcoming math anxiety.* New York: Norton.

Tobler, N. S. (1986). Meta-analysis of 143 adolescent drug prevention programs: Quantitative outcome results of a program participants compared to a control or comparison group. *Journal of Drug Issues, 16*(4), 537-567.

Tolan, P. H., & Lorion, R. P. (1988). Multivariate approaches to the identification of delinquency proneness in adolescent males. *American Journal of Community Psychology, 16*(4), 547-561.

Tolan, P. H., Perry, M. S., & Jones, T. (1987). Delinquency prevention: An example of consultation in rural community mental health. *Journal of Community Psychology, 15,* 43-50.

Tolman, R. M. & Molidor, C. (1994). A decade of social group work research: Trends in methodology, theory, and program development. *Research on Social Work Practice, 4*(2), 142-159.

Toomer, J. W. (1978). Black involvement in a new community. In D. C. Klein (Ed.), Psychology of the planned community: The new town experience. New York: Human Sciences Press.

Torre, E. (1988). Prevention strategies of a self-empowered group of professional women: Recharting familiar ground. *Journal of Primary Prevention, 9*(1 & 2), 66-76.

Trad, P. V. (1993). The therapeutic use of previewing to deter parental abuse. *Journal of Primary Prevention, 13*(4), 263-280.

Trinkoff, A. & Parks, P. L. (1993). Prevention strategies for infant walker-related injuries. *Public Health Reports, 108*(6), 764-788.

Turk, D., Meichenbaum, D., & Genest, M. (1983). *Pain and behavioral medicine.* New York: Guilford.

Tzeng, O. C. S., Jackson, J. W., & Karlson, H. C. (1991). *Theories of child abuse and neglect: Differential perspectives, summaries, and evaluations.* New York: Praeger.

Unger, D. G., & Wandersman, A. (1983). Neighboring and its role in block organizations: An exploratory report. *American Journal of Community Psychology, 11*(3), 291-311.

Unger, D. G., Wandersman, A., & Hallman, W. (1992). Living near a hazardous waste facility: Coping with individual and family distress. *American Journal of Orthopsychiatry, 62*(1), 55-70.

United Nations Environment Programme. (1989). *The state of the environment, 1989.* Nairobi, Kenya: United Nations.

Urbain, E. S., & Kendall, P. C. (1980). Review of social-cognitive problem-solving interventions with children. *Psychological Bulletin, 88*(1), 109-143.

Urton, M. M. (1991). A community home inspection approach to preventing falls among the elderly. *Public Health Reports, 106*(2), 192-195.

U.S. Bureau of the Census. *Statistical abstracts of the United States.* Washington, DC: Government Printing Office.

U.S. Department of Agriculture and U.S. Health and Human Services. (1990). *Nutrition and your health: Dietary guidelines for Americans* (3rd ed., Home and Garden Bulletin No. 232). Washington, DC: Government Printing Office.

U. S. Department of Health, Education, and Welfare. (1977). *Summary proceedings. Tripartite conference on prevention* (DHEW Publication No. ADM 77-484). Washington, DC: Government Printing Office.

Valentine, D. P., & Andreas, T. (1984). An expanded view of respite care: Supporting families. *Journal of Primary Prevention, 5*(1), 27-35.

Van Parijs, L. G. (1986). Public education in cancer prevention. *Bulletin of the World Health Organization, 64*(6), 917-927.

Venters, M. H. (1989). Family-oriented prevention of cardiovascular disease: A social epidemiological approach. *Social Science and Medicine, 28*(4), 309-314.

Vicary, J. R. (1994). Primary prevention and the workplace. *Journal of Primary Prevention, 15*(2), 99-104.

Vickery, D., & Fries, J. (1980). *Take care of yourself: A consumer's guide to medical care.* Reading, MA: Addison-Wesley.

Vinokur, A. D., & Caplan, R. (1987). Attitudes and social support: Determinants of job-seeking behavior and well-being among the unemployed. *Journal of Applied Social Psychology, 17,* 1007-1024.

Vinokur, A. D., Caplan, R., & Williams, C. (1987). Effects of recent and past stress on mental health: Coping with unemployment among Vietnam veterans and nonveterans. *Journal of Applied Social Psychology, 17,* 708-728.

Vinokur, A. D., Price, R., Caplan, R. (1990). *From field experiments to program implementation: Assessing the potential outcome of an experimental intervention program for unemployed persons.* Unpublished paper, Institute for Social Research, University of Michigan.

Vinokur, A. D., van Ryn, M., Gramlick, E., & Price, R. (1991). Long-term follow-up and benefit-cost analysis of the Jobs Program: A preventive intervention for the unemployed. *Journal of Applied Psychology, 76*(2), 213-219.

Violence Prevention Coalition of Greater Los Angeles. (n.d.). [A kit of materials—fact sheets, resource directory, brochures on actions citizens can take to prevent violence, meeting times for the year, and list of accomplishments.] 313 North Figueroa Street, Room 127, Los Angeles, CA 90012.

Volberg, R. A. (1994). The prevalence and demographics of pathological gamblers: Implications for public health. *American Journal of Public Health, 84*(2), 237-241.

Wagner, B. M., Compas, B. E. & Howell, D. C. (1988). Daily and major life events: A test of an integrative model of psychosocial stress. *American Journal of Community Psychology, 16*(2), 189-205.

Wall, J. S., Hawkins, J. D., Lishner, D., & Fraser, M. (1981). *Juvenile delinquency prevention: A compendium of thirty-six program models.* Washington, DC: Government Printing Office.

Wallace, B. C. (1989). Relapse prevention in psychoeducational groups for compulsive crack cocaine smokers. *Journal of Substance Abuse Treatment, 6,* 229-239.

Wallack, L. (1984). Practical issues, ethical concerns and future directions in the prevention of alcohol-related problems. *Journal of Primary Prevention, 4*(4), 199-224.

Waller, R. R., & Lisella, L. W. (1991). National AIDS hotline HIV and AIDS information service through a toll-free telephone system. *Public Health Reports, 106*(6), 628-634.

Wallston, K. A., McMinn, M., Katahn, M., & Pleas, J. (1983). The helper-therapy principle applied to weight management specialists. *Journal of Community Psychology, 11*(1), 58-66.

Walsh, D. (1988). Critical thinking to reduce prejudice. *Social Education, 52, 280-282.*

Walters, L. (1988). Ethical issues in the prevention and treatment of HIV infection and AIDS. *Science, 239,* 597-603.

Walther, D. J. (1986). Wife abuse prevention: Effects of information on attitudes of high school boys. *Journal of Primary Prevention, 7*(2), 84-89.

Wandersman, A. (1987). Environmental approaches to prevention. In J. A. Steinberg & M. M. Silverman (Eds.), *Preventing mental disorders: A research perspective.* Rockville, MD: National Institutes of Mental Health.

Wandersman, A., Andrews, A., Riddle, D., & Fancett, C. (1983). Environmental psychology and prevention. In R. Felner, L. A. Jason, J. N. Moritsugu, & S. S. Farber (Eds.), *Preventive psychology.* New York: Pergamon.

Wandersman, L. P. (1982). An analysis of the effectiveness of parent-infant support groups. *Journal of Primary Prevention, 3*(2), 99-115.

Wandersman, L. P. (1984). An introduction to environmental approaches and prevention. *Prevention in Human Services, 4*(1 & 2), 1-10.

Warheit, G. J., Auth, J. B., & Vega, W. A. (1985). Psychiatric epidemiological field surveys: A case for using them in planning assessment and prevention strategies. In P. Hough,

P. A. Gongla, V. B. Brown, & S. E. Goldston (Eds.), *Psychiatric epidemiology and prevention*. Los Angeles: University of California, Neuropsychiatric Institute.

Warner, K. E., & Murt, H. A. (1985). Economic incentives and health behavior. In J. Rosen & L. Solomon (Eds.), *Prevention in health psychology*. Hanover, NH: University Press of New England.

Warren, R. L. (1978). Some observations on the Columbia experience. In D. C. Klein (Ed.), *Psychology of the planned community: The new town experience*. New York: Human Sciences Press.

Wasik, B. (1984). *Teaching parents effective problem solving: A handbook for professionals*. Unpublished manuscript. University of North Carolina, Chapel Hill.

Wastie, P., & Klein, D. C. (1978). An approach to institutional development. In D. C. Klein (Ed.), *Psychology of the planned community: The new town experience*. New York: Human Sciences Press.

Weinberg, J. K., & Levine, D. I. (1990). A primer on tort liability of primary prevention programs. *Prevention in Human Services, 8*(2), 65-88.

Weiner, L., Morse, B. A., & Garrido, P. (1989). FAS/FAE: Focusing prevention on women at risk. *International Journal of the Addictions, 24*(5), 385-395.

Weinhouse, B. (1987). *The healthy traveler*. New York: Pocket Books.

Weinstein, C. S. & David, T. G. (Eds.) (1987). *Spaces for children: The built environment and child development*. New York: Plenum.

Weinstein, G., & Fantini, M. (1970). *Toward humanistic education: A curriculum of affect*. New York: Praeger.

Weinstein, N. D. (Ed.). (1987). *Taking care: Understanding and encouraging self-protective behavior*. New York: Cambridge University Press.

Weinstein, N. D. (1989). Perceptions of personal susceptibility to harm. In V. Mays, G. Albee, & S. Schneider. (Eds.), *Primary prevention of AIDS*. Newbury Park, CA: Sage.

Weissberg, R. P., & Allen, J. P. (1986). Promoting children's social skills and adaptive interpersonal behavior. In T. Michelson & B. Edelstein (Eds.), *Handbook of prevention*. New York: Plenum.

Weissberg, R. P., Caplan, M. Z., & Swo, P. J. (1989). A new conceptual framework for establishing school-based social competence promotion programs. In L. A. Bond & B. E. Compas (Eds.), *Primary prevention and promotion in the schools*. Newbury Park, CA: Sage.

Werner, E. E. (1987). Vulnerability and resiliency in children at risk for delinquency: A longitudinal study from birth to young adulthood. In J. Burchard & S. Burchard (Eds.), *Prevention of delinquent behavior*. Newbury Park, CA: Sage.

Werner, E. E. (1989a). High-risk children in young adulthood: A longitudinal study from birth to 32 years. *American Journal of Orthopsychiatry, 59*(1), 72-81.

Werner, E. E. (1989b, April). Children of the garden island. *Scientific American, 260*(4), 106-111.

Werner, E. E., & Smith, R. S. (1977). *Kauai's children come of age*. Honolulu: University of Hawaii Press.

Werner, E. E., & Smith, R. S. (1982). *Vulnerable but invincible: A longitudinal study of resilient children and youth*. New York: McGraw-Hill Book Company.

Werner, E. E., & Smith, R. S. (1992). *Overcoming the odds: High risk children from birth to adulthood*. Ithaca, NY: Cornell University Press.

West, D., Horan, J., & Games, P. (1984). Component analysis of occupational stress inoculation applied to registered nurses in an acute care hospital setting. *Journal of Counseling Psychology, 31*, 209-218.

Whiteman, M., Fanshal, D., & Grundy, J. F. (1987, November-December). Cognitive-be-havioral interventions aimed at anger of parents at risk of child abuse. *Social Work,* *32*(6), 469-474.

Whittaker, J. K., & Garbarino, J. (1983). *Social support networks: Informal helping in the human services.* New York: Aldine.

Whittaker, J. K., & Tracy, E. M. (1990). Social network intervention in intensive family-based preventive services. *Prevention in Human Services, 9*(1), 175-192.

Wilensky, H. L., & Lebeaux, C. N. (1965). *Industrial society and social welfare.* New York: Free Press.

Williams, C. (1986). Improving care in nursing homes using community advocacy. *Social Science and Medicine, 23,* 1297-1303.

Williams, C. L. (1989). Prevention programs for refugees: An interface for mental health and public health. *Journal of Primary Prevention, 10*(2), 167-186.

Williams, C. L., Solomon, S. D., & Bartone, P. (1988). Primary prevention in aircraft disasters. *American Psychologist, 43*(9), 730-739.

Wilner, D. N., Walkley, R., Pinkerton, T., & Tayback, M. (1962). *The housing environment and family life.* Baltimore: Johns Hopkins University Press.

Wilson, S. (1982). Peer review in California: Summary findings of 40 cases. *Professional Psychology, 13*(4), 517-521.

Windson, R. A., Warner, K. E., & Cutter, G. R. (1988). A cost-effectiveness analysis of self-help smoking cessation methods for pregnant women. *Public Health Reports, 103*(1), 83-88.

Windsor, R. A., Lowe, J., Perkins, L., Smith-Yoder, D., Artz, L., Crawford, M., Amburgy, K., & Boyd, N. (1993). Health education for pregnant smokers: Its behavioral impact and cost benefit. *American Journal of Public Health, 83*(2), 201-208.

Winer, J. I., Hilpert, P. H., Gesten, E. L., Cowen, E. L., & Schubin, W. E. (1982). The evaluation of a kindergarten social problem solving program. *Journal of Primary Prevention, 2*(4), 205-216.

Winett, R. A., Leckliter, I. N., Chinn, D. E., Stahl, B., & Love, S. (1985). Effects of television modeling on residential energy conservation. *Journal of Applied Behavior Analysis, 18*(1) 33-44.

Winett, R. A., Neale, M. S., & Williams, K. R. (1982). The effects of flexible work schedules on urban families with young children: Quasi-experimental ecological studies. *American Journal of Community Psychology, 10*(1), 49-64.

Winkler, G. E. (1992). Assessing and responding to suicidal jail inmates. *Community Mental Health Journal, 28*(4), 317-326.

Wittman, F. D. (1989). Planning and programming server intervention initiatives for fraternities and sororities: Experiences at a large university. *Journal of Primary Prevention, 9*(4), 247-269.

Wittman, R. D. (1980). Sociophysical settings and mental health: Opportunities for men-tal-health services planning. In P. Insel (Ed.), *Environmental variables and the prevention of mental illness.* Lexington, MA: Lexington Books.

Wodarski, J. S. (1978). The reduction of electrical energy consumption: The application of behavior analysis. *Behavior Therapy, 8,* 347-353.

Wolkon, G., & Moriwaki, S. (1973). The ombudsman programme: Primary prevention of psychological disorders. *International Journal of Social Psychiatry, 19*(3 & 4), 956/1-5.

Wollenberg, S. P. (1989). A comparison of body mechanic usage in employees participating in three back injury prevention programmes. *International Journal of Nursing Studies, 26*(1), 43-52.

Wolpe, J. (1958). *The practice of behavior therapy.* New York: Pergamon.

Woolf, A., Lewander, W., Filippone, G., & Lovejoy, F. (1987). Prevention of childhood poisoning: Efficacy of an educational program carried out in an emergency clinic. *Pediatrics, 80*(3), 359-363.

Work, W. C., Cowen, E. L., Parker, G. R., & Wyman, P. A. (1990). Stress resilient children in an urban setting. *Journal of Primary Prevention, 11*(1), 3-17.

World Health Organization. (1977). *Primary prevention of schizophrenia in high-risk groups: Report of a working group.* Copenhagen: Author.

World Health Organization. (1988). *Urbanization and its implications for child health: Potential for action.* Geneva: Author.

Wright, D. D. (1993). Something's missing from the video: An alternative instructional approach to "An ounce of prevention." *Journal of Primary Prevention, 14*(2). 149-166.

Wursten, A., & Sales, B. (1988). Community psychologists in state legislative decision making. *American Journal of Community Psychology, 16*(4), 487-502.

Wyman, P. A., Cowen, W. L., Work, W. C., & Parker, G. R. (1991). Developmental and family milieu correlates of resilience in urban children who have experienced major life stress. *American Journal of Community Psychology, 19*(3), 405-426.

Wynne, L. C., McDaniel, S. H., & Weber, T. T. (1986). *Systems consultation: A new perspective for family therapy.* New York: Guilford.

Yates, B. A., & Dowrick, P. W. (1991). Stop the drinking driver: A behavioral school-based prevention program. *Journal of Alcohol and Drug Education, 36*(2), 12-19.

Yoffe, E. (1992, December 13). Silence of the frogs. *New York Times Magazine,* pp. 36-39, 64, 66, 76.

Young, R. L., & Adams, G. R. (1984). The 4-H youth organization: Primary prevention through competence promotion. *Journal of Primary Prevention, 4*(4), 225-239.

Young, R. L., Elder, J. P., Green, M., de Moor, C., & Wildey, M. B. (1988). Tobacco use prevention and health facilitator effectiveness. *Journal of School Health, 58*(9), 370-373.

Zador, P. L., & Ciccone, M. A. (1993). Automobile driver fatalities in frontal impacts: Air bags compared with manual belts. *American Journal of Public Health, 83*(5), 661-666.

Zambelli, G. C., & DeRosa, A. P. (1992). Bereavement support groups for school-age children: Theory, intervention, and case example. *American Journal of Orthopsychiatry, 62*(4), 484-493.

Zarkin, G. A., Dean, N., Mauskopf, J. & Williams, R. (1993). Potential health benefits of nutrition label changes. *American Journal of Public Health, 83*(5), 717-724.

Ziegenfuss, J. T., Charette, J., & Guenin, M. (1984). The patients' rights representative project: Design of an ombudsman service for mental patients. *Psychiatric Quarterly, 56*(1), 3-12.

Zigler, E. (1985). Assessing Head Start at 20: An invited commentary. *American Journal of Orthopsychiatry, 55*(4), 603-609.

Zigler, E., & Styfco, S. J. (1993). *Head Start and beyond: A national plan for extending childhood intervention.* New Haven, CT: Yale University Press.

Zigler, E., & Valentine, J. (Eds.). (1979). *Project Head Start: A legacy of the war on poverty.* New York: Free Press.

Zimmerman, D. (1983). Moral education. In A. P. Goldstein (Ed.), *Prevention and control of aggression.* New York: Pergamon.

Zimmerman, M. A., & Rappaport, J. (1988). Citizen participation, perceived control, and psychological empowerment. *American Journal of Community Psychology, 16*(5), 725-750.

Zins, J. E. (1995). Has consultation achieved its primary prevention potential? *Journal of Primary Prevention, 15*(3), 285-301.

Zoucha-Jensen, J. M., & Coyne, A. (1993). The effects of resistance strategies on rape. *American Journal of Public Health, 83*(11), 1633-1634.

AUTHOR INDEX

SUBJECT INDEX

ABOUT THE AUTHOR

Martin Bloom obtained a PhD in social psychology from the University of Michigan in 1963 after receiving a diploma in social study from the University of Edinburgh (1958). He has been teaching in schools of social work for most of his career. Among his publications are *Primary Prevention: The Possible Science* (1981), *Configurations of Human Behavior* (1984), *Life Span Development: Bases for Preventive and Interventive Helping* (1985, 2nd ed.), *Introduction to the Drama of Helping* (1990), and *Evaluating Practice: Guidelines for the Accountable Professional* (1995, 2nd ed.). His current preoccupations include primary prevention, longitudinal research, and his first grandson—not necessarily in the order presented.